CONTINUOUS AMBULATORY PERITONEAL DIALYSIS IN THE USA

DEVELOPMENTS IN NEPHROLOGY

Volume 23

For a complete list of publications in this series see end of book

Continuous Ambulatory Peritoneal Dialysis in the USA

Final Report of
the National CAPD Registry 1981–1988

Edited by
ANNE S. LINDBLAD, MS and JOEL W. NOVAK, MS
Data Coordinating Center, The EMMES Corporation, Potomac, Maryland

and

KARL D. NOLPH, MD
University of Missouri, Columbia, Missouri

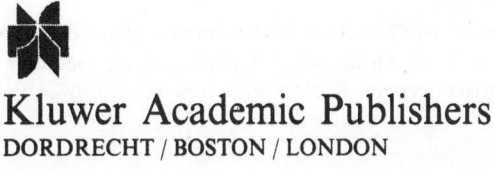

Kluwer Academic Publishers
DORDRECHT / BOSTON / LONDON

Library of Congress Cataloging in Publication Data

```
National CAPD Registry (U.S.)
   Continuous ambulatory peritoneal dialysis in the U.S.A. / final
report of the National CAPD Registry 1981-1988 ; edited by A.S.
Lindblad, J.W. Novak, and K.D. Nolph.
      p.   cm. -- (Developments in nephrology)
   Bibliography: p.
   1. Continuous ambulatory peritoneal dialysis--United States-
-Statistics.   I. Lindblad, A. S. (Ann S.)  II. Novak, J. W. (Joel
W.)  III. Nolph, Karl D.  IV. Title.  V. Series.
RC901.7.P48N38  1989
362.1'97461059--dc19                                          89-2686
```

ISBN-13: 978-94-010-6908-3   e-ISBN-13: 978-94-009-0931-1

DOI: 10.1007/978-94-009-0931-1

Published by Kluwer Academic Publishers,
P.O. Box 17, 3300 AA Dordrecht, The Netherlands.

Kluwer Academic Publishers incorporates
the publishing programmes of
D. Reidel, Martinus Nijhoff, Dr W. Junk and MTP Press.

Sold and distributed in the U.S.A. and Canada
by Kluwer Academic Publishers,
101 Philip Drive, Norwell, MA 02061, U.S.A.

In all other countries, sold and distributed
by Kluwer Academic Publishers Group,
P.O. Box 322, 3300 AH Dordrecht, The Netherlands

printed on acid free paper

National CAPD Registry

Principal Staff

CLINICAL COORDINATING CENTER
Division of Nephrology
University of Missouri
Columbia, Missouri

Karl D. Nolph, MD
Principal Investigator

Barbara Prowant, RN
Research Associate

DATA COORDINATING CENTER
The EMMES Corporation
11325 Seven Locks Road
Potomac, Maryland

Joel W. Novak, MS
Principal Investigator

Anne S. Lindblad, MS
Project Director

Sidney J. Cutler, ScD
Senior Epidemiologist

Donald M. Stablein, PhD
Statistician

Donald A. Vena, BS
Statistician

Marsha L. Denekas, AA, MLT
Operations Manager

Carol Smith, BS, MT
Data Manager

Acknowledgements

The authors wish to thank all participating centers for providing the data on which this report is based.

We gratefully acknowledge the assistance of the staff at The EMMES Corporation and the University of Missouri, without whom the report could not have been completed:

Cecily Fritz	Warren Pendleton
Jag Gill	Kelly Raygor
Jeanette Leroux	Phyllis Scholl
Maureen O'Connell	Tamara Voss

Contents

PREFACE   xiii

Section 1   INTRODUCTION   1

1.1 An Overview of Peritoneal Dialysis   3
1.2 The National CAPD Registry and the Registry Report   4
1.3 References   6

Section 2   REGISTRY PATIENT POPULATION   7

2.1 Classification of Patients   9
2.2 Registration by Class   10
2.3 Registration by Class and Year   10
2.4 Patient Follow-up and Data Currency   12
2.5 Registry Coverage   14
2.6 Census and Flow of CAPD Patients   14

Section 3   PATIENT CHARACTERISTICS   17

3.1 Sex and Age Distributions   21
3.2 Race and Age Distribution   22
3.3 Primary Renal Disease—CAPD   23
3.4 References   24

Section 4   COMPLICATIONS OF TREATMENT   27

4.1   Peritonitis—CAPD   30
4.2   Exit Site/Tunnel Infections—CAPD   33
4.3   Catheter Replacements—CAPD   35
4.4   Any Complications—CAPD   37
4.5   CCPD Complications   37
4.6   Hospitalizations—CAPD/CCPD   38
4.7   References   39

**Section 5   TERMINATION OF CONTINUOUS PERITONEAL
              DIALYSIS**   41

5.1   Probability of Transferring to an Alternate Dialysis
      Modality—CAPD   44
5.2   Probability of Transplantation—CAPD   45
5.3   Probability of Death While on CAPD   47
5.4   Probability of Discontinuing CAPD for any Reason   47
5.5   Probability of Discontinuing CCPD   47
5.6   Outcomes by Patient Type—CAPD/CCPD   49
5.7   Follow-up of Transfers to Hemodialysis—CAPD/CCPD   56
5.8   Follow-up of Kidney Transplants—CAPD/CCPD   58
5.9   Follow-up of Patient Deaths—CAPD/CCPD   58
5.10 References   60

Section 6   SPECIAL REPORTS—1988   61

A.   A Survey of Diabetics in the CAPD/CCPD Population   63
B.   Hematocrit Values in the CAPD/CCPD Population   75
C.   Timing and Characteristics of Multiple Peritonitis Epi-
     sodes   83
D.   Geographical Distribution of Registry Coverage   93
E.   Characteristics and Treatment Course of Long-term
     CAPD/CCPD Patients   101

Section 7   SPECIAL REPORTS—1987   109

A.   Update on Children Who Use CAPD/CCPD   111

B. First Exchange Device and Peritonitis among CAPD
   Patients   117
C. Follow-up of Transfer from CAPD/CCPD   125
D. Pediatric Population Evaluation   139
E. Complications of Peritoneal Catheters   157
F. The Effects of CAPD on Hypertension Control   167

Section 8 SPECIAL REPORTS—1986   177

Introduction   179
A. Factors Associated with First Hospitalization for CAPD-
   Related Complications   181
B. Factors Associated with Transfer off CAPD   189
C. Factors Associated with Death While on CAPD   199
D. Trends in the Occurrence of Complications and of Treat-
   ment Outcomes   209
E. Variation in Treatment Outcome According to Center
   Size   217
F. Variation in Treatment Outcome According to Treatment
   and Patient Characteristics   223
G. Some Additional Factors Associated with Transfer off
   CAPD   229
H. Characteristics of Patients Who Received a Kidney Trans-
   plant, Whose Kidney Function Returned, or Who Discon-
   tinued CAPD without Return of Kidney Function   233
I. Comparison of Outcomes for Patients with and without
   prior ESRD Therapy   237

Section 9 SPECIAL REPORT—1985   241

A. Prognostic Factors Associated with the First Episode of
   Peritonitis   243

Section 10 SPECIAL REPORT—1984   253

A. Considerations in Analysis of Complications   255

APPENDICES 275

  I. Executive Advisory Committee of the National CAPD
Registry of the National Institutes of Health 277
  II. Participating Centers of the National CAPD Registry of
the National Institutes of Health 279
  III. Bibliography of the National CAPD Registry of the
National Institutes of Health 291

TABLE OF EXHIBITS

Section 2 REGISTRY PATIENT POPULATION

Exhibit 2–1 Number of Patients Registered by Class and Type
of Dialysis 10
  2–2 Number of Patients Registered by Class and Year
of Registration 11
  2–3 Number of Patients with Follow-up by Class and
Type of Dialysis 11
  2–4 Last Contact and Status According to Activity
Classification of Center for Patients Last Reported
to be on CAPD/CCPD 12
  2–5 Currency of The National CAPD Registry Database by Class of Patient 13
  2–6 Number of Patients Receiving CAPD at Year
End 14
  2–7 Census and Flow of The National CAPD Registry
by Year 15

Section 3 PATIENT CHARACTERISTICS

Exhibit 3–1 Percent of Patients with Selected Characteristics by
Type of Therapy 20
  3–2 CAPD—Age Distribution by Sex 21
  3–3 CCPD—Age Distribution by Sex 22
  3–4 CAPD—Age Distribution by Race 23
  3–5 CCPD—Age Distribution by Race 24
  3–6 CAPD—Distribution of Patients by Primary
Renal Disease Type According to Year of Registration 25

Section 4   COMPLICATIONS

Exhibit   4–1   CAPD—Occurrence of Selected Complications by
Class of Patients   30

4–2   CAPD—Cumulative Probability of Experiencing
First Episode of Peritonitis (Class 1 Patients
Only)   31

4–3   CAPD—Complication Rates by Year of Registra-
tion   32

4–4   CAPD—Cumulative Probabilities and 95% Con-
fidence Intervals (C.I.) of Experiencing Selected
Events for the First Time by Year Registered
(Class 1 Patients Only)   33

4–5   CAPD—Cumulative Probability of Experiencing
First Exit Site/Tunnel Infection (Class 1 Patients
Only)   34

4–6   CAPD—Cumulative Probability of First Catheter
Replacement (Class 1 Patients Only)   35

4–7   CAPD—Cumulative Probability of First Compli-
cation (Class 1 Patients Only)   36

4–8   CCPD—Occurrence of Selected Complications by
Class of Patient   37

4–9   CCPD—Cumulative Probabilities and 95% Confidence Intervals (C.I.) of Experiencing Selected
Events for the First Time by Number of Months
on CCPD (Class 1 Patients Only)   38

Section 5   TERMINATION OF CONTINUOUS PERITONEAL DIALYSIS

Exhibit   5–1   CAPD—Cumulative Probability of Transfer
(Class 1 Patients Only)   44

5–2   CAPD—Cumulative Probability of Receiving a
Kidney Transplant (Class 1 Patients Only)   45

5–3   CAPD—Cumulative Probability of Death (Class 1
Patients Only)   46

5–4   CAPD—Cumulative Probability of Discontinuing
CAPD Therapy for any Reason (Class 1 Patients
Only)   48

5–5   CCPD—Cumulative Probability of Transfer
(Class 1 Patients Only)   49

5–6   CCPD—Cumulative Probability of Receiving a
      Kidney Transplant (Class 1 Patients Only)   50
5–7   CAPD—Cumulative Probability of Death (Class 1
      Patients Only)   51
5–8   CCPD—Cumulative Probability of Discontinuing
      CCPD Therapy for Any Reason (Class 1 Patients
      Only)   52
5–9   CAPD or CCPD—Cumulative Probability of
      Transplantation: Pediatrics vs. 'Standard' vs.
      'Other'   53
5–10 CAPD or CCPD—Cumulative Probability of
      Death: Pediatrics vs. 'Standard' vs. 'Other'   54
5–11 CAPD or CCPD—Cumulative Probability of
      'Technique Failure': Pediatrics vs. 'Standard' vs.
      'Other'   55
5–12 Follow–up of Transfers to Hemodialysis Sum-
      mary   56
5–13 Primary Reason for Leaving CAPD in Patients
      who Transferred from CAPD to Hemodialysis and
      Subsequently Returned to CAPD   57
5–14 Follow-up of Kidney Transplant Summary   58
5–15 Death Summary   59

Preface

The Final Report of the USA CAPD Registry summarizes eight years of observation and analysis that reflects the experiences of 485 clinical centers and over 25,000 CAPD patients. As such, it offers a wealth of information, available here for the first time to interested parties around the world.

Because the National Institutes of Health was quick to see the potential of CAPD as a promising therapy for patients with end stage renal disease, the Registry project was begun soon after its introduction into clinical practice in the USA. Accordingly, the Registry offered the nephrology community in the United States a special opportunity to study this emerging new therapy in some detail, an opportunity not previously available for any other form of dialysis. As will be seen in this report, the result of this early and intensive research effort has been the development of a vast amount of clinically important information regarding the utilization, safety, and efficacy of this important dialytic therapy.

Having documented the introduction of CAPD into medical practice in the USA, the Registry completed its objectives and the project came to an end in 1988. Given the unusual scientific productivity of the Registry project, this final report deserves the distinction and wide distribution that only a book provides. As the final report of the Registry, this volume presents the most recent analyses of the database, as well as summaries of all of the special studies undertaken by the project throughout its life (1981–1988). Because, the project was so unique in its scope and accomplishment, we expect that this report will serve as a standard reference for many years to come.

At the time of this writing (December, 1988), the number of patients in the USA using CAPD continues to increase with each passing year. While peritonitis remains one of the major factors contributing to patients' transfer off CAPD in favor of an alternative dialysis modality, we anticipate that situation will be modified with the introduction of new techniques, materials, and devices, e.g. the Y-set exchange device. Clearly, CAPD will continue to evolve and to mature. It is our hope that the innovations that are to come will be carefully evaluated in well controlled studies; and, we would like to think that this report will serve as a guide to the development of such studies, as well as a reference index for the progress that is anticipated.

It is important to note that participation of physicians and patients in this Registry was entirely voluntary, and that its success was due to the enthusiasm, dedication, meticulous effort, and intense interest of the nephrology community. The editors and staffs of the Coordinating Centers that prepared these materials take great pride and satisfaction in having been part of and witness to the phenomenon that was the USA NIH CAPD Registry.

Anne Lindblad
Joel Novak
Karl Nolph

SECTION ONE

Introduction

1. Introduction

Prior to the decade of the 1930's, the loss of renal function meant certain death—usually within days. In the thirty years that have followed, scientific, clinical and technological advances made possible the development of hemodialysis, thereby offering a new lease on life to those patients who could afford that replacement therapy. More recent medical and engineering developments have led to peritoneal dialysis becoming an alternative to hemodialysis as a replacement therapy for patients suffering from chronic renal failure.

Scientific, clinical and technological progress have continued. With advances in surgical technique, renal transplantation became a reasonable option for many patients with end-stage renal disease (ESRD), and it has become even more attractive with the recent introduction of cyclosporine and other anti-rejection therapies. Dialysis, however, continues to be an important therapeutic option for patients, who by choice or medical considerations are not transplant candidates.

1.1 An Overview of Peritoneal Dialysis

Peritoneal dialysis involves infusing a dialyzing fluid into the peritoneal cavity where the blood is cleansed of wastes across a living membrane, the peritoneum. Several forms of peritoneal dialysis are currently practiced including: continuous ambulatory peritoneal dialysis (CAPD), continuous cyclic peritoneal dialysis (CCPD), and intermittent peritoneal dialysis (IPD). Combination therapy with two or more of those modalities may also be practiced.

CAPD was first described in 1976 [1] but was not widely used until 1978, when the technique was improved by the introduction of plastic dialysis solution bags. CAPD utilizes a closed system composed primarily of the peritoneal cavity, a chronic in-dwelling catheter, connecting tubing, and a plastic dialysis solution container. Dialyzing fluid is gravity-infused into the patient's peritoneal cavity where it remains for four or more hours—after which the patient drains the peritoneal cavity by placing the dialysate bag lower than the abdomen, allowing the bag to be refilled by gravity. The filled bag is discarded, a fresh bag of solution is connected to the system and the cycle is repeated. Most patients perform four exchanges per day.

Continuous cyclic peritoneal dialysis (CCPD) is a variation of CAPD in which an automatic cycler machine delivers multiple overnight exchanges and an additional exchange in the morning. The dialysate then remains in the abdomen during the day for one long cycle.

Both CAPD and CCPD require the abdomen to be full on a continuous basis. An alternative to these methods is intermittent peritoneal dialysis (IPD)—a technique which allows for 'dry periods' when the abdomen is empty. Traditionally, IPD has been accomplished through a series of short dwell exchanges (1 hour) performed at least 3 times each week for a total of 40 hours of dialysis. One variation of IPD is nightly peritoneal dialysis, where the abdomen is empty during the day.

Intermittent and continuous forms of therapy provide much different weekly clearance spectrums. Clearances of very high molecular weight substances are usually reduced proportional to the cutbacks in time. Clearances of smaller solutes are also reduced, but this may be proportionally less if flow rates are increased during the dialysis treatment. As a result of these differences, the National CAPD Registry registers and follows only patients using CAPD or CCPD.

1.2 The National CAPD Registry and the Registry Report

The National CAPD Registry, sponsored by the National Institute of Diabetes and Digestive and Kidney Diseases (NIDDK), is responsible for developing information regarding the number of patients receiving CAPD and/or CCPD therapy, their characteristics, the extent of some of the more important treatment-related complications and selected outcomes to the therapy.

Registry operations are conducted through a Clinical Coordinating Center (CCC) at the University of Missouri, under the direction of Karl D. Nolph, M.D., and a Data Coordinating Center (DCC) located at The EMMES Corporation in Potomac, Maryland. Joel W. Novak, M.S. serves as principal director of the DCC; Anne S. Lindblad, M.S. serves as project director and Sidney Cutler, Sc.D. is the project's senior epidemiologist. The Clinical Coordinating Center acts as liaison between the Registry and the medical community, and specifically assists in information dissemination. The primary responsibility of the Data Coordinating Center is to operate the data collection and processing system, provide epidemiological and biostatistical support, and produce technical reports such as this, in collaboration with Dr. Nolph and his staff at the University of Missouri. Staff of the Kidney-Urology Branch (DKUHD), NIDDK, are collaborators in the project as are members of the Executive Advisory Committee (See Appendix I).

The Registry began operations on a pilot basis in January, 1981 with the participation of 15 centers; and, it became fully operational in October, 1981, with a roster of 184 participating centers. The National CAPD Registry is to be discontinued in July of 1988, but will be replaced by a total ESRD Registry which will monitor experiences with all types of therapies in ESRD patients. At the writing of this final report, 498 clinical centers in the United States have participated in the National CAPD Registry program.

This report summarizes data received by the Data Coordinating Center on 26,554 patients from the 498 participating centers. Information on the status of patients last reported as continuing CAPD/CCPD was requested through October 31, 1987 and the Data Coordinating Center received reports on over 90% of these patients prior to the closing of the data file. New registrations were accepted through January 31, 1988. Section 2 describes the size of the Registry and documents its growth. Further, it defines the patient cohorts that are available for analysis. In Sections 3, 4, and 5 we describe the characteristics of the patients who have been registered, the complications of treatment that they have experienced and outcomes of their treatment, e.g., death, transfer to another modality and transplantation.

Section 6 reports on the results of the special analyses undertaken in the last year. This section includes reports on the two special studies:
1. A Survey of Diabetics in the CAPD/CCPD Population (A).
2. Hematocrit Values in the CAPD/CCPD Population (B).

Both studies were prospective evaluations and were executed according to protocol specifications. Forms were pilot tested at selected institutions and modified as indicated. Samples of 771 and 812 patients were selected from among eligible Registry patients per protocol specifications for inclusion in the Diabetic and Hematocrit Special Studies, respectively. Data collection on these studies was initiated in July 1987 and terminated November 30, 1987, with both studies experiencing a return rate of over 90%.

The remainder of Section 6 presents analyses of registry data which deal with topics not routinely covered in our reports. Report C provides an in depth look at the timing and characteristics of peritonitis episodes subsequent to the first episode, Report D provides a graphical representation of the distribution of CAPD Registry Centers and patients in the United States, and the final Report describes the characteristics and treatment course of patients who have remained on CAPD/CCPD for 3 or more years. An additional 17 special studies, previously reported, are presented once again in this final report of the project. Those reports, which will be found in Sections 7–10, are grouped according to the year in which they appeared and are presented in descending order. A bibliography of all manuscripts published by the Registry follows those reports.

Clearly, CAPD as a replacement therapy has become firmly established as an alternate renal replacement therapy during the past eight years [2]. The authors hope that the clinical studies that we have been able to complete under this project have contributed to elucidating its advantages and disadvantages, with the result that physicians, nurses, and other health care professionals may now be able to use the technique more appropriately and with greater confidence.

A.L.
J.N.
K.N.

References

1. Popovich RP, Moncrief JW et al. The definition of a novel portable/wearable equilibrium peritoneal dialysis technique. Abstr Am Soc Artif Intern Organs 1976; 5:64.
2. Nolph KD, Lindblad AS, Novak JW. Current concepts: continuous ambulatory peritoneal dialysis. N Engl J Med 1988; 318:1595–1600.

SECTION TWO

Registry Patient Population

2. Registry Patient Population

As of January 31, 1988 when the Registry's files were closed for the current analysis, 26,554 patients had been registered with the National CAPD Registry. The majority of the patients, 92% (24,480), initially received CAPD; 1,833 (7%) initially received CCPD. An additional 241 patients were reported to have initially received combination therapy with both CAPD and CCPD. Follow-up information pertains to all events occurring on or before October 31, 1987, while new registrations are reported through January 31, 1988.

2.1 Classification of Patients

As might be expected, patients participating in the Registry vary widely. Two characteristics of unusual significance when analyzing patient responses to treatment are: experience on CAPD or CCPD prior to being registered and experience with an alternate ESRD therapy, prior to registration. Patients who received CAPD or CCPD prior to registration must be regarded as the survivors of a larger group of patients, who should not be grouped with newly treated patients when analyzing outcomes of CAPD or CCPD therapy. Similarly, patients who are known to have received (and may have failed) an alternate form of replacement therapy prior to commencing CAPD/CCPD should also be considered separately from previously untreated patients in analyses of outcomes since they may have very different prognoses.

To facilitate a discussion of the patient subgroups represented in the Registry, patients are classified with respect to prior CAPD, CCPD or other ESRD therapy. The classification scheme identifies four subgroups of particular interest:

1A — No replacement therapy for ESRD prior to registration.
1B — No CAPD/CCPD prior to registration but prior experience with alternative forms of replacement therapy.

10

2A — Experience with CAPD/CCPD prior to registration.
2B — Experience with both CAPD/CCPD and an alternative form of replacement therapy prior to registration.

Reference is made in all of our reports to these categories when describing the group(s) that are analyzed and the experiences reported.

2.2 Registration by Class

Of the 26,554 patients ever registered, 19,373 (73%) were registered at the time that CAPD or CCPD therapy was initiated (viz. Classes 1A (9,233) and 1B (10,140) as defined above). The remaining 7,181 patients (Class 2A and 2B) had been diagnosed earlier and treated with some other form of ESRD therapy (see Exhibit 2–1).

EXHIBIT 2-1

NUMBER OF PATIENTS REGISTERED BY CLASS*
AND TYPE OF DIALYSIS

| Type of Dialysis | Class* of Patient | | | | |
	1A	1B	2A	2B	Total
CAPD	8,445	9,430	2,612	3,993	24,480
CCPD	691	620	257	265	1,833
CAPD and CCPD	97	90	28	26	241
Total	9,233	10,140	2,897	4,284	26,554

* Class

1A - No replacement therapy for ESRD prior to registration.
1B - No CAPD/CCPD prior to registration but prior experience
     with alternative forms of replacement therapy.
2A - Experience with CAPD/CCPD prior to registration.
2B - Experience with both CAPD/CCPD and an alternative form
     of replacement therapy prior to registration.

2.3 Registration by Class and Year

Exhibit 2–2 details the yearly accrual of patients receiving CAPD and CCPD from the time of the Registry's activation. As of January 31, 1988, a total of 24,480 patients had been registered on CAPD. Note that from 1982 to 1986 the number of yearly registrants increased by more than 2,000 patients. These yearly increases of approximately 20–30% are thought to be the result of increases in the number of participating centers, the total number of ESRD patients and the fraction of ESRD patients being offered CAPD therapy. CCPD registrations have also been rising; more CCPD patients were registered in 1987 than in any previous year.

EXHIBIT 2-2

NUMBER OF PATIENTS REGISTERED AND YEAR*
OF REGISTRATION BY CLASS

Class	1981-1982	1983	1984	1985	1986	1987*	Total
			CAPD				
1A	921	891	1,355	1,637	1,826	1,815	8,445
1B	1,997	1,352	1,375	1,510	1,618	1,578	9,430
2A	658	153	242	448	595	516	2,612
2B	1,930	304	399	399	568	393	3,993
Total	5,506	2,700	3,371	3,994	4,607	4,302	24,480
			CCPD				
1A	33	42	84	95	176	261	691
1B	70	72	96	75	146	161	620
2A	13	23	15	17	101	88	257
2B	54	30	30	28	72	51	265
Total	170	167	225	215	495	561	1,833

*Includes information received through January 31, 1988.

Note: Table excludes the 241 patients treated by a combination of CAPD and CCPD.

EXHIBIT 2-3

NUMBER OF PATIENTS WITH FOLLOW-UP BY CLASS
AND TYPE OF DIALYSIS

| Type of Dialysis | Class of Patient | | | | |
	1A	1B	2A	2B	Total
CAPD	7,587	8,616	2,239	3,365	21,807
CCPD	603	557	233	236	1,629
CAPD and CCPD	79	72	24	23	198
Total	8,269	9,245	2,496	3,624	23,634

2.4 Patient Follow-up and Data Currency

Eighty-nine percent of the 26,554 registered patients (23,634) have follow-up information available and consequently are available for analysis in this report. Of those with follow-up, 16,203 received CAPD therapy (7,587 Class 1A and 8,616 Class 1B) and 1,160 received CCPD therapy (603 Class 1A and 557 Class 1B) as the initial treatment for end stage renal disease (see Exhibit 2–3).

EXHIBIT 2-4

LAST CONTACT AND STATUS ACCORDING TO ACTIVITY CLASSIFICATION
OF CENTER FOR PATIENTS LAST REPORTED TO BE ON CAPD/CCPD

ACTIVE CENTERS (412)

Date of last reported contact	Status at Last Contact		
	On CAPD/CCPD with follow-up data	Transferred to another center	Registered only
1981 - 1983	2	205	123
1984	0	147	9
1985 (Jan - April)	0	43	21
1985 (May - Aug)	0	61	9
1985 (Sept - Dec)	5	61	4
1986 (Jan - April)	11	63	5
1986 (May - Aug)	0	70	3
1986 (Sept - Dec)	12	110	18
1987 (Jan - April)	248	38	65
1987 (May - Aug)	414	94	167
1987 (Sept - Jan, 88)	7,220	45	812
Total	7,912	937	1,236

PROVISIONALLY INACTIVE CENTERS (86)

Date of last reported contact	Status at Last Contact		
	On CAPD/CCPD with follow-up data	Transferred to another center	Registered only
1981 - 1983	261	19	224
1984	95	20	18
1985 (Jan - April)	23	7	2
1985 (May - Aug)	78	13	29
1985 (Sept - Dec)	55	6	18
1986 (Jan - April)	95	4	57
1986 (May - Aug)	67	1	32
1986 (Sept - Dec)	29	0	19
1987 (Jan - April)	1	0	0
1987 (May - Aug)	0	0	0
1987 (Sept - Jan, 88)	0	0	0
Total	704	70	399

Exhibit 2–4 summarizes the status of patients reported to be on CAPD/ CCPD at the time of last reported contact. As of October 31, 1987, 83% of participating centers (412/498) had submitted follow-up reports regarding patient contacts during 1987; those centers are considered to be fully active. Eighty-six centers had not submitted follow-up reports in 1987 for any of their patients and are considered to be 'provisionally inactive'. Among the 412 actively participating centers, 90% of patients (9,103/10,085) last reported to be on CAPD/CCPD have data reflecting their status at some time during the preceding 13 month period (January 1, 1987–January 31, 1988). Over three-quarters of the patients (760/982) with last contact prior to January 1, 1987 were patients who transferred to another center. Note that if the patient's new center is not a Registry participant, further follow-up is considered unlikely. An additional 1,173 patients last reported as continuing on CAPD/CCPD are no longer being followed as the participating center is no longer an active Registry participant.

Exhibit 2–5 graphically illustrates the number of patients registered versus the number of patients with current follow-up by class of patient as defined earlier. The latter group includes patients continuing CAPD/CCPD and for whom information was received in the last 12 months, as well as patients who discontinued CAPD/CCPD as of the

EXHIBIT 2-5

CURRENCY OF THE NATIONAL CAPD REGISTRY DATABASE BY CLASS OF PATIENT

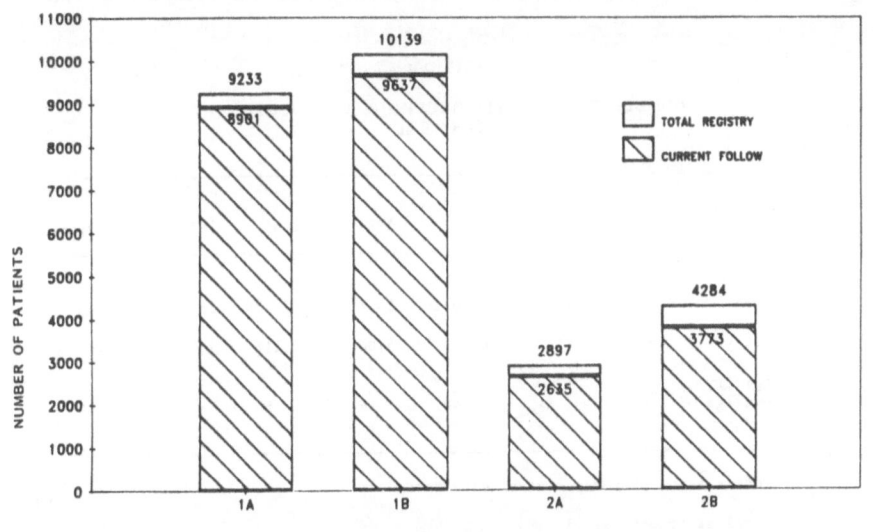

last report. For Class 1A and 1B patients data currency is in excess of 95%; for all classes of patients data currency exceeds 88%.

2.5 Registry Coverage

While the true number of patients receiving CAPD in the United States is not known, reports of the Health Care Financing Administration (HCFA) are available which indicate the number of patients reimbursed for CAPD as of December 31st of each year. Assuming HCFA's reports provide a reasonable estimate of the true size of the CAPD/CCPD population, we have estimated the Registry's coverage by comparing such data to the number of currently active patients reported by the Registry. Note that information provided by the HCFA does not report on CCPD patients prior to 1984. Exhibit 2–6 presents data on the number of patients receiving CAPD and CCPD; as of December 31st of each year, as reported by HCFA and estimated by the National CAPD Registry. Note that the data suggest that the National CAPD Registry has enrolled and followed approximately half of the CAPD population in the United States, through 1986.

2.6 Census and Flow of CAPD Patients

The National CAPD Registry has undergone constant change and growth since its inauguration in 1981. Every year an increasing number

EXHIBIT 2-6

NUMBER OF PATIENTS RECEIVING CAPD/CCPD
AT YEAR* END

				Year			
	1981	1982	1983	1984	1985	1986	1987**
CAPD/CCPD							
HCFA***	4,347	6,523	8,532	10,854	12,189	13,220	N.A.
Registry	1,949	3,553	4,073	5,004	6,118	7,170	8,181
% Registry Coverage	45	54	48	46	50	54	N.A.

* Totals as of December 31st of each year.

** Total as of October 31, 1987.

*** Includes patients reported to be on CCPD in 1984, 1985, and 1986.

EXHIBIT 2-7

CENSUS AND FLOW OF THE NATIONAL CAPD REGISTRY BY YEAR*
1981-1987**

	1981	1982	1983	1984	1985	1986	1987**
Newly Registered Patients	2,276	3,411	2,874	3,622	4,259	5,181	4,932
Transplants	31	164	265	361	476	699	623
Transfers	152	628	738	767	971	1,135	1,024
Deaths	106	428	630	841	1,028	1,360	1,259
On CAPD/CCPD as of December 31st of each year	1,949	3,553	4,073	5,004	6,118	7,170	8,181

* Totals as of December 31st of each year.

** Reflects the last reported status of all Registry patients received by the Data Coordinating Center as of October 31, 1987.

of patients receiving CAPD are registered. Notwithstanding the fact that patients routinely leave the Registry when they receive a kidney transplant, transfer to an alternate replacement therapy or die, the number of patients under follow-up at the end of each year has increased such that there has been an estimated four-fold increase since 1981. Exhibit 2–7 illustrates the yearly census and flow of CAPD Registry patients. For the purposes of Exhibit 2–7, patients who leave the Registry but return to CAPD/CCPD within 8 months are counted as continuing on CAPD/CCPD. Note that for later analysis regarding transfers off of CAPD/CCPD, patients who have discontinued CAPD/CCPD for more than 30 days are considered to have permanently transferred.

When the Registry began in 1981, a bolus of patients was entered as newly recruited centers registered patients already receiving CAPD. In 1983, a decrease in absolute numbers of new registrants was observed, as the influx of new centers stabilized. However, since 1983 a steady increase in registrations has been observed, as new centers continued to join the Registry, with the result that in 1986 newly registered patients increased markedly to 5,181. Note that new registrations exceed patient losses in every year.

SECTION THREE

Patient Characteristics

3. Patient Characteristics

This section details the characteristics of the 23,634 patients for whom outcome information is available, and who form the basis of the analyses that follow. At the time of registration 21,807 of those patients were receiving CAPD; 1,629 were receiving CCPD. As not all demographic data are available for all patients, patient totals on which percentages are based may vary slightly from characteristic to characteristic. Patients who reported using a combination of CAPD and CCPD are not reflected in this summary or in the outcome evaluations that follow.

Sex, age, race and primary renal disease type are summarized in Exhibit 3–1 for all CAPD and CCPD patients, irrespective of therapy received prior to registration. Overall, male patients outnumber female patients in the Registry; and, white patients outnumber blacks and those of 'other' races. The median age of Registry patients at CAPD/CCPD initiation is 53 years, and diabetic glomerulosclerosis, reported in 26% of patients, is the most frequently cited type of primary renal disease.

Exhibit 3–1 compares the distribution of patient characteristics in the National CAPD Registry with the distribution of characteristics of all persons with end-stage renal disease (ESRD) as reported by the Health Care Financing Administration [1]. The age distribution presented for Registry patients represents the age at CAPD or CCPD initiation of all patients ever registered. The age distribution for the total ESRD population considers the age, as of December 31, 1986, of all ESRD patients reporting chronic dialysis services in the calendar year 1986. Sixty-seven percent of Registry patients were under 60 years of age at registration. Considering only patients currently receiving CAPD/CCPD, sixty-one percent of Registry patients are under 60 years of age at last contact compared with 52% of all ESRD patients. Thus after adjustment for reporting differences, the Registry population appears to be younger than the total ESRD population. Several other

EXHIBIT 3-1

PERCENT OF PATIENTS WITH SELECTED CHARACTERISTICS
BY TYPE OF THERAPY

| Selected Characteristic | Therapy Type | | Total | Total ESRD[1] |
	CAPD (n=21,807)	CCPD (n=1,629)	(n=23,436)	(n=99,101)
SEX				
Male	55	51	55	53
Female	45	49	45	47
RACE				
White	76	74	76	63
Black	18	20	18	32
Other	6	6	6	5
PRIMARY RENAL DISEASE TYPE				
Diabetic Glomerulosclerosis	26	27	26	20
Chronic Glomerulonephritis	17	16	17	23
Hypertensive Renal Disease	15	11	15	23
Interstitial Nephritis/Chronic Pyelonephritis	8	8	8	*
Polycystic Kidney Disease	6	5	6	*
All Other Types	28	33	28	*
AGE (years)**				
< 5	1	4	1	<1
5-9	1	4	1	<1
10-19	3	9	4	1
20-39	24	24	24	18
40-59	37	29	37	32
≥ 60	33	30	33	48
MEDIAN AGE	53	47	53	*

1 End-Stage Renal Disease Patient Profile Tables - 1986. ESRD Information
Analysis Branch, Division of Information Analysis. U.S. Department of
Health and Human Services. Health Care Financing Administration, Bureau
of Data Management and Safety. Includes the characteristics of all patients
for whom a report of chronic dialysis services was provided in the calendar
year-1986.

* Not provided.
** Age for Registry patients calculated as of CAPD or CCPD initiation.
Age for total ESRD population calculated as of December 31, 1986.

differences in these populations are noteworthy. Whereas diabetic
glomerulosclerosis is the most frequently cited primary renal disease type
in the CAPD Registry, accounting for 26% of Registry patients, only
20% of the total ESRD population are so diagnosed. Chronic glomerulonephritis and hypertensive renal disease are more commonly reported
in the ESRD population, occurring in 23% and 23% of this cohort,
respectively. These two disease types account for only 17% and 15% of
Registry patients respectively. Approximately three-quarters (76%) of
Registry patients are white, whereas only 63% of all ESRD patients are

EXHIBIT 3-2

CAPD

AGE* DISTRIBUTION BY SEX

| Age Group in Years | Total Patients | | Sex | |
	N	%	Male %	Female %
<1	72	.3	.3	.4
1-4	114	.5	.6	.5
5-9	176	.8	.9	.8
10-14	269	1.2	1.2	1.3
15-19	353	1.6	1.4	1.9
20-29	1,966	9.0	7.9	10.4
30-39	3,337	15.3	15.7	15.0
40-49	3,417	15.7	15.9	15.4
50-59	4,743	21.8	21.0	22.8
60-69	4,845	22.3	23.0	21.4
70-79	2,140	9.8	10.5	9.0
80-89	311	1.4	1.6	1.3
≥ 90	8	< .1	< .01	< .01
Total Patients	21,751		11,984	9,767
Percent Patients	(100)		(55)	(45)

* Age at time of registration.

white. The distribution of sex appears to be similar between the Registry and the ESRD cohorts, with males accounting for more than half of both populations.

3.1 Sex and Age Distributions

Distributions of age by sex are provided separately for patients whose initial therapy was CAPD and CCPD (see Exhibits 3–2 and 3–3). Males and females are evenly distributed on CCPD therapy while a higher proportion of males (55%) are reported for CAPD. CCPD patients tend to be younger than CAPD patients, with 17% of CCPD patients being under the age of 20 years. In contrast only 5% of the CAPD population

EXHIBIT 3-3

CCPD

AGE* DISTRIBUTION BY SEX

Age Group in Years	Total Patients		Male	Female
	N	%	%	%
<1	21	1.3	1.7	.9
1-4	45	2.8	3.5	2.0
5-9	59	3.6	3.2	4.1
10-14	80	4.9	5.3	4.5
15-19	66	4.1	4.1	4.0
20-29	150	9.2	7.0	11.5
30-39	242	14.9	16.0	13.8
40-49	207	12.7	13.8	11.6
50-59	269	16.5	15.9	17.3
60-69	322	19.8	20.2	19.4
70-79	135	8.3	8.1	8.5
80-89	28	1.7	1.2	2.3
≥ 90	2	.1	0	.3
Total Patients	1,626		826	800
Percent Patients	(100)		(51)	(49)

* Age at time of registration.

is under the age of 20 years. From data presented in Exhibit 3–2, it is evident that males and females on CAPD are similarly distributed among age groups. Age distribution on CCPD is also similar for males and females with only minor differences observed in the 20–29 year-olds. Eleven percent of the females receiving CCPD are between age 20–29, while 7% of males are in their 20's. The median age for males and females on CCPD is 47 years and 48 years, respectively.

3.2 Race and Age Distribution

Distributions of race by age are also provided separately for CAPD (Exhibit 3–4) and CCPD (Exhibit 3–5) patients. Race categories are similarly distributed among patients using CAPD and CCPD, with

EXHIBIT 3-4

CAPD

AGE* DISTRIBUTION BY RACE

Age Group in Years	Total Patients		White	Black	Other
	N	%	%	%	%
<1	72	.3	.3	.3	.3
1-4	114	.5	.5	.4	1.0
5-9	176	.8	.8	.6	1.4
10-14	269	1.2	1.2	.9	2.7
15-19	354	1.6	1.5	1.8	2.4
20-29	1,963	9.0	8.9	9.1	10.7
30-39	3,336	15.4	14.8	17.7	15.1
40-49	3,408	15.7	14.2	20.7	19.4
50-59	4,743	21.8	21.0	24.8	23.1
60-69	4,845	22.3	23.7	18.3	17.0
70-79	2,136	9.8	11.3	4.8	6.2
80-89	311	1.4	1.7	.6	.9
≥ 90	8	< .1	< .1	< .1	0
Total Patients	21,735		16,550	3,823	1,362
Percent of Patients	(100)		(76)	(18)	(6)

* Age at time of registration.

three-quarters of patients reported as white. As noted in earlier Registry reports, white patients tend to be older with 37% being 60 years of age or older, while 24% of blacks and 'other' races fall into this age group. Patients classified in the 'other' race category tend to be younger; 19% of patients were under 30 years of age compared to 13% of white and blacks.

3.3 Primary Renal Disease—CAPD

The Registry collects frequency information on 16 primary renal disease diagnoses. Patients, whose primary renal disease diagnoses do not fall into one of these categories, are classified as 'other'. As indicated in Exhibit 3–6, five categories of renal disease account for 72% of all

EXHIBIT 3-5

CCPD

AGE* DISTRIBUTION BY RACE

Age Group in Years	Total Patients		White	Black	Other
	N	%	%	%	%
<1	21	1.3	1.1	1.5	3.0
1-4	45	2.8	2.6	2.1	7.0
5-9	59	3.6	3.3	3.0	10.0
10-14	80	4.9	5.2	3.9	5.0
15-19	67	4.1	3.7	4.6	8.0
20-29	150	9.2	9.5	8.8	8.0
30-39	242	14.9	14.8	17.3	8.0
40-49	206	12.7	11.8	15.8	13.0
50-59	269	16.5	16.6	17.0	14.0
60-69	322	19.8	20.2	17.9	21.0
70-79	135	8.3	9.5	5.8	3.0
80-89	28	1.7	1.8	2.1	0
≥ 90	2	.1	.1	.3	0
Total Patients	1,626		1,196	330	100
Percent of Patients	(100)		(74)	(20)	(6)

* Age at time of registration.

patients on CAPD: diabetic glomerulosclerosis (26%), chronic glomeru-lonephritis (17%), hypertensive renal disease (15%), interstitial nephritis/chronic pyelonephritis (8%), and polycystic kidney disease (6%). The remaining 28% of patients are distributed among 11 diagnostic categories, no one of which accounts for more than 3% of all patients.* Note that 11% of patients could not be classified into any one of the 16 disease types used; and, 6% of patients are coded as disease type unknown.

The distributions by primary renal disease of patients with follow-up information who were registered in 1981–82, 1983, 1984, 1985 and 1986 are given in Exhibit 3–6. Note that only 77% (3,310/4,302) of

* The reader should note that the diagnoses reported are the clinical impressions given by the attending physician and do not conform to uniform definitions.

EXHIBIT 3-6

CAPD

DISTRIBUTION OF PATIENTS BY PRIMARY RENAL DISEASE
TYPE ACCORDING TO YEAR* OF REGISTRATION

Renal Disease Type	Total Patients N (%)	1981-1983 %	1984 %	1985 %	1986 %	1987* %
Diabetic glomerulosclerosis	5,573 (26.4)	21.4	25.6	28.0	29.7	31.5
Chronic glomerulonephritis	3,558 (16.8)	21.3	17.0	14.4	14.3	12.8
Hypertensive renal disease	3,252 (15.4)	16.0	14.2	14.5	15.7	15.7
Polycystic kidney disease	1,330 (6.3)	7.5	6.3	5.6	5.5	5.4
Interstitial nephritis/ Chronic Pyelonephritis	1,630 (7.7)	6.6	8.7	8.7	8.3	7.7
Systemic immunological disease with renal involvement	604 (2.9)	3.1	3.1	3.1	2.5	2.4
Rapidly progressive glomerulonephritis	476 (2.3)	2.3	2.2	2.2	2.3	2.2
Obstructive uropathy	423 (2.0)	2.4	1.6	1.9	1.9	1.9
Familial nephritis	195 (.9)	1.3	.8	.6	.7	.7
Amyloidosis with renal involvement	114 (.5)	.6	.4	.6	.5	.5
Renal infarct, 2nd to vascular occlusion	120 (.6)	.5	.6	.6	.5	.7
Aplastic-hypoplastic kidney disease	98 (.5)	.6	.4	.5	.2	.4
Stone-forming renal disease	89 (.4)	.6	.4	.4	.4	.2
Nephrectomy, 2nd to cancer	83 (.4)	.4	.4	.4	.4	.3
Gouty nephropathy	40 (.2)	.2	.3	.1	.2	.1
Bilateral cortical necrosis	25 (.1)	.1	.1	.2	.2	.1
Other	2,217 (10.5)	8.9	11.6	12.0	10.4	11.4
Unknown	1,310 (6.2)	6.3	6.3	6.2	6.3	5.8
Number of Patients	21,139	7,105	2,823	3,662	4,239	3,310
Percent of Patients	100	34	13	17	20	16

* Follow-up information received as of October 31, 1987.

CAPD patients registered in 1987 are reported, as follow-up information has not been received for many newly registered patients. As can be seen, there continues to be an increase in the proportion of patients with diabetic glomerulosclerosis who enter the Registry each year. In 1981–83, 21.4% of the patients entered were diagnosed with diabetic glome-rulosclerosis increasing to 31.5% in 1987. Corresponding decreases are observed in patients with chronic glomerulonephritis and polycystic kidney disease. A noticeable increase in the percentage of patients entering the Registry after 1984 with interstitial nephritis/chronic pyelonephritis is also observed. These results are essentially identical for all registered patients irrespective of follow-up information status.

3.4 References

1. End-Stage Renal Disease Patient Profile Tables 1986. ESRD Information Analysis Branch, Division of Information Analysis. U.S. Department of Health and Human Services. Health Care Financing Administration, Bureau of Data Management and Safety.

SECTION FOUR

Complications of Treatment

4. Complications of Treatment

The National CAPD Registry routinely collects information on major complications associated with continuous peritoneal dialysis: peritonitis, exit site/tunnel infections and catheter replacements. Complications occurring in Class 1 and Class 2 patients are considered separately as the Registry has no knowledge of the problems experienced by Class 2 patients prior to registration. Note that the available data may overstate the number of episodes experienced by some patients as there are no clear criteria for differentiating between a new, distinct episode and the persistence of a previously reported complication.

Exhibits 4–1 through 4–9 detail complication rates and probability distributions for the time to first episode of selected complications. Rates are based on patient years of observation [1]. Class 1 patient years are calculated from the day CAPD/CCPD therapy was initiated to the last reported contact date or date of CAPD/CCPD termination. Observation times for Class 2 patients are calculated from the date of entry on the Registry to the date of last contact or CAPD/CCPD termination.

Rates per patient year are calculated as follows:

Rate per patient year =

$$\frac{\text{Total \# of Episodes Reported by the Cohort}}{\text{Total Years Cohort Under Observation}}.$$

Complication rates per patient year have been calculated separately by year of registration to assess possible time trends. Note that those rates are not strictly comparable as earlier cohorts have had more time for the development of repetitive complications. In addition, Registry forms utilized in 1981 through 1983, and in the last half of 1986 through 1987, required less rigorous documentation of complication episodes than those used in 1984 through the first 6 months of 1986. These changes in forms may have had an effect on the reporting practices of the centers.

The probability distributions which reflect the time of first episode of an event were estimated using the methods of Kaplan-Meier [2]. Distributions of first complications were calculated for Class 1 patients only, as Class 2 patients may have had a first event prior to being followed by the Registry.

Probability distributions have also been calculated separately by year of registration. As dates of complications were not reported prior to 1984 and are no longer reported as of October 31, 1986, times to first episode were estimated using the median of the interval in which the event was reported as the date of event.

4.1 Peritonitis—CAPD

The National CAPD Registry defines peritonitis as turbid dialysate with white blood count greater than 100 cells per cubic millimeter.

EXHIBIT 4-1

CAPD

OCCURRENCE* OF SELECTED COMPLICATIONS
BY CLASS** OF PATIENTS

Complication	TOTAL	1A	Class of Patients 1B	2A	2B
			RATES*		
Peritonitis	1.4	1.3	1.4	1.6	1.6
Exit Site/Tunnel Infections	.6	.6	.6	.6	.6
Catheter Replacement	.2	.2	.2	.3	.3
			BASED ON		
Patients	21,758	7,583	8,604	2,237	3,334
Patient Years	26,432	8,789	10,632	2,402	4,608

* Number of episodes per patient-year of observation.

** Class

    1A - No replacement therapy for ESRD prior to registration.
    1B - No CAPD/CCPD prior to registration but prior experience
        with alternative forms of replacement therapy.
    2A - Experience with CAPD/CCPD prior to registration.
    2B - Experience with both CAPD/CCPD and an alternative form
        of replacement therapy prior to registration.

Abdominal symptoms and/or positive culture are not required for diagnosis of peritonitis. Overall the peritonitis rate per patient year (ppy) for CAPD patients is 1.4 events. Class 1A patients experienced 1.3 peritonitis episodes ppy (Exhibit 4–1). The probability of Class 1 patients experiencing at least one episode of peritonitis is found to be 40% by the end of the sixth month of therapy; at the end of 24 months of therapy, the chances that a patient will have experienced at least one episode of peritonitis doubles to 80% (Exhibit 4–2). The median time to first peritonitis is estimated to be 8.4 months.

Despite the introduction of newer connection devices in recent years and single institutional reports of reduced rates of peritonitis, yearly

EXHIBIT 4-2

CAPD

CUMULATIVE PROBABILITY OF EXPERIENCING
FIRST EPISODE OF PERITONITIS
(CLASS 1 PATIENTS ONLY)

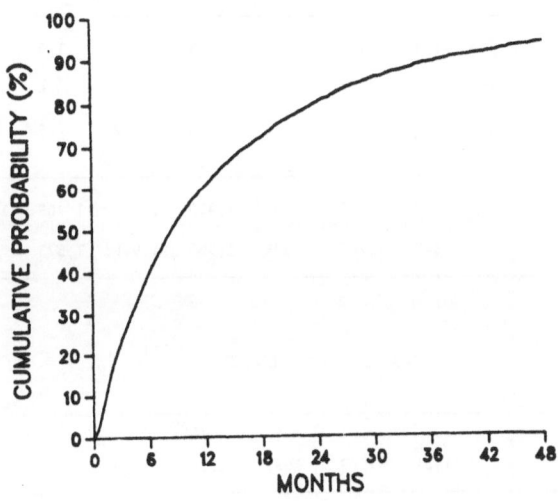

Cumulative Probabilities and 95% Confidence Intervals (C.I.) for Exhibit 4-2

	Months on CAPD					
	6	12	18	24	36	48
Cumulative Probability	40	60	72	80	89	93
95% C.I.	(39, 41)	(59, 61)	(71, 73)	(79, 81)	(87, 90)	(92, 94)

cohorts of Registry patients who are new to ESRD therapy at the time of registration (Class 1A) have experienced a constant rate of peritonitis. The peritonitis rate for Class 1A patients is 1.3 events per patient year for cohorts registered in 1983, 1984, 1985, 1986, and 1987, respectively (Exhibit 4–3). An increase in reported peritonitis episodes has been observed among Class 1B patients registered in 1986 and 1987. The estimated peritonitis rate per patient year in this cohort is 1.5 and 1.6 events respectively, compared with 1.3 episodes ppy for patients registered in 1983, 1984 and 1985.

The probability that a Class 1 CAPD patient who entered the Registry prior to 1984 experienced the first episode of peritonitis in the

EXHIBIT 4-3

CAPD

COMPLICATION RATES* BY YEAR OF REGISTRATION

CLASS 1A PATIENTS

| | YEAR | | | | | | |
	1981	1982	1983	1984	1985	1986	1987**
Peritonitis	1.3	1.4	1.3	1.3	1.3	1.3	1.3
Exit Site/Tunnel Inf.	.6	.7	.5	.5	.6	.6	.8
Catheter Replacement	.2	.3	.3	.3	.2	.2	.3
Patients	177	679	854	1,310	1,553	1,709	1,301
Patient Years	342	1,206	1,326	1,909	1,948	1,573	485

CLASS 1B PATIENTS

| | YEAR | | | | | | |
	1981	1982	1983	1984	1985	1986	1987**
Peritonitis	1.3	1.4	1.3	1.3	1.3	1.5	1.6
Exit Site/Tunnel Inf.	.6	.6	.6	.5	.5	.7	.8
Catheter Replacement	.2	.2	.2	.3	.2	.2	.3
Patients	424	1,403	1,313	1,329	1,425	1,519	1,191
Patient Years	872	2,277	2,152	1,876	1,701	1,320	432

* Number of episodes per patient year.

** Reflects information received through October 31, 1987.

EXHIBIT 4-4

CAPD

CUMULATIVE PROBABILITY AND 95% CONFIDENCE INTERVAL (C.I.)
OF EXPERIENCING SELECTED EVENTS FOR THE FIRST TIME
BY YEAR REGISTERED (CLASS 1 PATIENTS ONLY)

Events and Year of Registration	Months from Initiation of CAPD							
	6		12		18		24	
	Prob.	95% C.I.	Prob.	95% C.I.	Prob.	95% C.I.	Prob.	95% C.I.
Peritonitis								
1981-1983	43	(42,45)	63	(61,64)	72	(71,74)	80	(78,81)
1984-1987*	38	(37,39)	59	(57,61)	72	(70,73)	81	(79,82)
Exit Site/Tunnel Inf.								
1981-1983	26	(25,28)	37	(35,39)	45	(43,47)	51	(48,53)
1984-1987*	20	(19,21)	31	(30,33)	40	(38,42)	48	(46,51)
Catheter Replacement								
1981-1983	12	(11,13)	19	(18,21)	26	(24,28)	32	(30,35)
1984-1987*	9	(8,10)	17	(16,18)	25	(23,27)	33	(31,35)
Any of Above								
1981-1983	59	(57,60)	76	(74,77)	84	(83,85)	89	(88,90)
1984-1987*	51	(50,52)	72	(71,73)	82	(81,84)	89	(87,90)

* As of October 31, 1987

first 6 months on therapy is 43%; for the cohort registered after 1983 it is 38%. This observed decline in the probability of first peritonitis is maintained at 12 months, but disappears following 18 months (Exhibit 4-4). Median time to the first episode of peritonitis is 7.6 months for patients registered in 1981 through 1983 and 8.8 months for patients registered after 1983.

4.2 Exit Site/Tunnel Infections—CAPD

Differentiation between exit site and tunnel infections is difficult to determine in the usual clinical setting. Accordingly, the Registry classifies these events as one complication. The rate per patient year of observation for exit site/tunnel infections was 0.6 regardless of patient classification (Exhibit 4-1). Note that less than one quarter of the patients experience the first episode in the first 6 months of therapy and the probability that a patient has experienced at least one event by the

34

EXHIBIT 4-5

CAPD

CUMULATIVE PROBABILITY OF EXPERIENCING
FIRST EXIT SITE/TUNNEL INFECTION
(CLASS 1 PATIENTS ONLY)

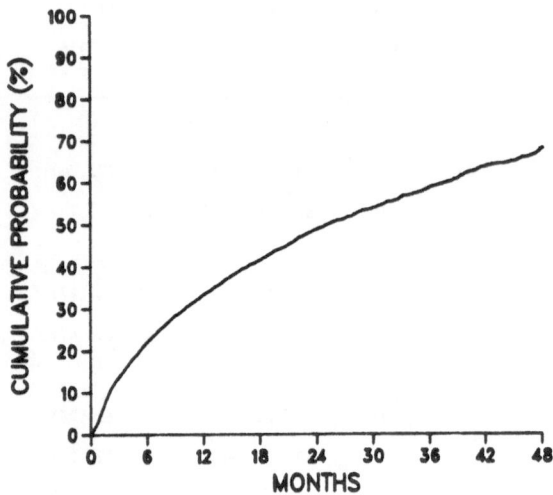

Cumulative Probabilities and 95% Confidence Intervals (C.I.) for Exhibit 4-5

	Months on CAPD					
	6	12	18	24	36	48
Cumulative Probability	22	33	41	49	59	68
95% C.I.	(21, 23)	(32, 34)	(40, 43)	(47, 50)	(56, 61)	(64, 71)

end of the second year is less than 50 % (Exhibit 4–5). The median time to first episode of exit site/tunnel infection is estimated to be 25.1 months.

An increase in the number of exit site tunnel infections reported per patient year has been observed for the 1987 cohort compared to previous yearly cohorts in both Class 1A and 1B patients (Exhibit 4–3). However, a decrease in the probability of experiencing a first episode of exit site/ tunnel infection continues to be noted for patients registered after 1983 compared to patients registered in 1981–1983. At one year, the probability of experiencing a first episode of exit site/tunnel infection is 37% for patients registered in 1981–1983; for patients registered after 1983, it is 31%. Note that confidence intervals are non-overlapping throughout the 18 month period.

4.3 Catheter Replacements—CAPD

Participating clinical centers are asked to report on the frequency of catheter replacements for those patients continuing with CAPD. Note that catheters that are removed due to failure and not replaced are not reported, nor is it likely that early catheter failures, i.e. prior to the first successful exchange are reported to the Registry. For these reasons, the catheter replacement rates reported by the Registry are considered to be underestimates of the true rate of catheter failure.

EXHIBIT 4-6

CAPD

CUMULATIVE PROBABILITY OF FIRST CATHETER REPLACEMENT
(CLASS 1 PATIENTS ONLY)

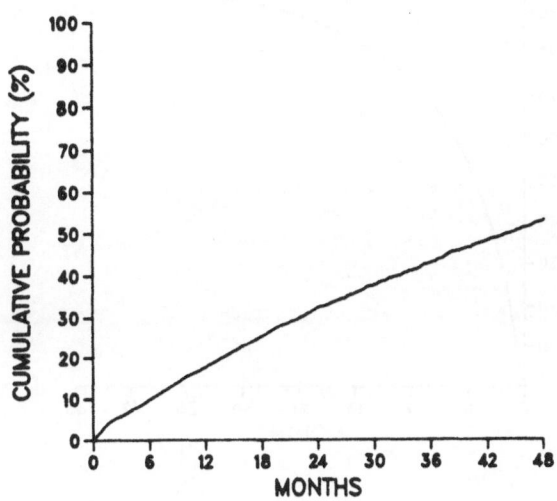

Cumulative Probabilities and 95% Confidence Intervals (C.I.) for Exhibit 4-6

	Months on CAPD					
	6	12	18	24	36	48
Cumulative Probability	10	18	25	32	43	53
95% C.I.	(9, 10)	(17, 19)	(24, 26)	(31, 34)	(40, 45)	(49, 56)

Overall catheter replacement rates for Class 1 patients were observed to be 0.2 events ppy; for Class 2 patients the observed rate is 0.3 events ppy (Exhibit 4–1). The probability of having at least one catheter replaced by end of two years of therapy was 32% (Exhibit 4–6). Catheter replacement rates and probabilities of the first replacement occurring do not appear to vary by year of registration (Exhibits 4–3 and 4–4). Probability estimates of a first catheter replacement for patients registered in 1981–1983 compared to patients registered in 1984–1986, remain within 3 percentage points throughout the observation period.

EXHIBIT 4-7

CAPD

CUMULATIVE PROBABILITY OF FIRST COMPLICATION*
(CLASS 1 PATIENTS ONLY)

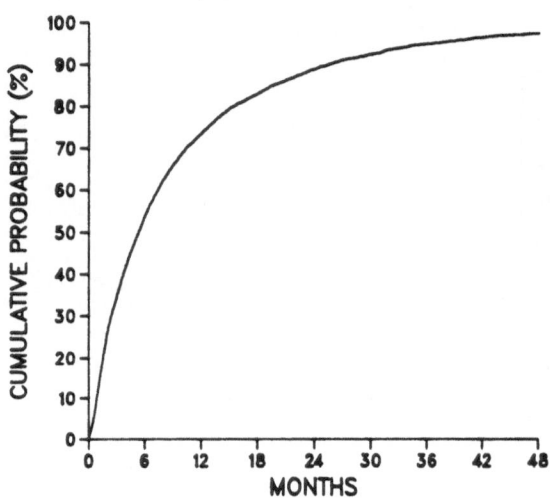

Cumulative Probabilities and 95% Confidence Intervals (C.I.) for Exhibit 4-7

	Months on CAPD					
	6	12	18	24	36	48
Cumulative Probability	53	73	83	89	95	97
95% C.I.	(53, 54)	(72, 74)	(82, 84)	(88, 90)	(94, 95)	(96, 98)

* Peritonitis, exit site/tunnel infection, catheter replacement.

4.4 Any Complications CAPD

Exhibit 4–7 illustrates the probability distribution estimate of the time to a first episode of peritonitis, exit site/tunnel infection or catheter replacement. Note that the chance that a CAPD patient will experience at least one of these three complications is 53% at 6 months. By the end of the second year of therapy, 89% of patients are expected to have experienced at least one of these three types of complications. The median time to experiencing a CAPD related complication of any type for the first time is 5.3 months.

4.5 CCPD Complications

Similar data summaries have been prepared for patients receiving CCPD. Complication rates and probability distribution estimates of the time to first complication are presented in Exhibits 4–8 and 4–9. As patients are not randomly allocated to treatment with CAPD or CCPD, comparisons of the two modalities are subject to selection biases; and hence, caution should be used when evaluating differences in complication rates and probability distributions for the two modalities.

As illustrated in Exhibit 4–8, complication rates per patient year across all categories were lower for Class 1 CCPD patients than for

EXHIBIT 4-8

CCPD

OCCURRENCE* OF SELECTED COMPLICATIONS
BY CLASS OF PATIENT

| Complication | Total | Class of Patient | | | |
		1A	1B	2A	2B
			RATES*		
Peritonitis	1.3	1.2	1.3	1.5	1.6
Exit Site/ Tunnel Inf.	0.6	0.6	0.6	0.7	0.6
Catheter Replacement	0.3	0.2	0.3	0.5	0.3
			BASED ON		
Patients	1,629	603	557	233	236
Patient Years	1,450	481	567	163	239

* Number of episodes per patient-year of observation.

38

EXHIBIT 4-9

CCPD

CUMULATIVE PROBABILITIES AND 95% CONFIDENCE INTERVALS (C.I.)
OF EXPERIENCING SELECTED EVENTS FOR THE FIRST TIME
BY NUMBER OF MONTHS ON CCPD (CLASS 1 PATIENTS ONLY)

Number of Months from Initiation of CCPD	EVENT TYPE							
	Peritonitis		Exit Site/ Tunnel Infection		Catheter Replacement		Any Complication	
	Prob.	95% C.I.	Prob.	95% C.I.	Prob.	95% C.I.	Prob.	95% C.I.
6	37	(33,40)	21	(18,24)	11	(9,14)	50	(47,54)
12	56	(52,61)	30	(26,35)	21	(17,26)	70	(66,74)
18	67	(61,72)	40	(34,47)	28	(22,34)	80	(75,85)
24	78	(71,84)	48	(40,57)	30	(23,39)	89	(83,92)
30	80	(73,86)	54	(46,63)	37	(28,47)	92	(87,95)
36	84	(76,90)	63	(50,73)	45	(33,57)	97	(92,99)

Class 2 CCPD patients. As in CAPD, peritonitis is the most frequently encountered complication among CCPD patients; and, over half (56%) of all Class 1 CCPD patients are expected to have experienced at least one episode of peritonitis by the end of their first year of therapy (Exhibit 4-9). First catheter replacements are expected to occur in 21% of CCPD patients by the end of one year of therapy; 30% of CCPD patients will have had a catheter replacement by the end of two years of therapy. Nearly half of all CCPD patients (48%) will have had a first exit site/tunnel infection by the end of two years. The median time to experience a first CCPD related complication of any type is 6 months.

4.6 Hospitalizations — CAPD/CCPD

Due to the restructuring of the data collection procedures of the National CAPD Registry, requests for detailed information on days hospitalized for CAPD/CCPD patients were terminated after October 31, 1986. Mean days hospitalized per patient year are based only on information received through October 31, 1986. CAPD and CCPD patients are reported to be hospitalized for 19.4 and 20.8 days ppy respectively for all causes, of which 7.7 and 8.3 days are directly attributed to CAPD and CCPD related complications such as peritonitis, exit site/tunnel infections, catheter replacements, etc. Patients with

CAPD or CCPD experience prior to entering the Registry (Class 2) are reported to have at least an additional day ppy of hospitalization for CAPD or CCPD related causes.

References

1. Kahn HA. *An Introduction to Epidemiologic Methods.* New York: Oxford University Press, 1983.
2. Kaplan E, Meier P. Nonparametric estimates from incomplete observations. J Am Stat Assoc 1958; 53:457–458.

Termination of Continuous Peritoneal Dialysis

5. Termination of Continuous Peritoneal Dialysis

For the most part, patients terminate CAPD or CCPD therapy for one of three reasons:
1. Transfer to another type of dialysis.
2. Transplantation.
3. Death.
On rare occasions CAPD/CCPD may be terminated because of a return of kidney function or because a patient refuses further therapy for end stage renal disease with no return of kidney function.

Patient transfers are considered to have occurred when a change to another dialysis modality is made with no intention to return to peritoneal dialysis or when a transfer of at least a four week duration is reported. Transfer to another replacement therapy often represents CAPD/CCPD failure—while the same cannot be said for transplants that are performed. Transplantation and transfer are routinely reported for patients followed by the Registry. Patient death is reported to the Registry only if it occurs while the patient is still receiving CAPD or CCPD—or if it occurs within two weeks of transfer to another therapy.

Probability distributions portraying the cumulative probability over time of transfer to another replacement therapy, transplantation, and death are estimated using the methods of Kaplan-Meier [1]. It is important to note that these probability distributions are not additive, in part due to the reporting of multiple events on a single patient. For example, patients who transfer to another modality and die within two weeks of that transfer will count as an event in both the transfer distribution and the death distribution. The results which follow reflect data submitted for Class 1 CAPD or CCPD patients only. Summaries for Class 2 patients are not provided as true time on peritoneal therapy cannot be estimated in previously treated patients.

5.1 Probability of Transferring to an Alternate Dialysis Modality— CAPD

Patients who have received CAPD for varying lengths of time may decide to discontinue CAPD in favor of hemodialysis, IPD or terminate all dialysis with no return of kidney function. Such patients are considered to be CAPD transfers for this analysis. Patients who die while on CAPD, transfer to another center and subsequently are lost to follow-up, receive a kidney transplant, discontinue dialysis due to a return in kidney function, or change to CCPD are not considered transfers. Such patients contribute information only for the time they are known to be receiving continuous peritoneal dialysis and are censored in the analyses that have been performed.

EXHIBIT 5-1

CAPD

CUMULATIVE PROBABILITY OF TRANSFER*
(CLASS 1 PATIENTS ONLY)

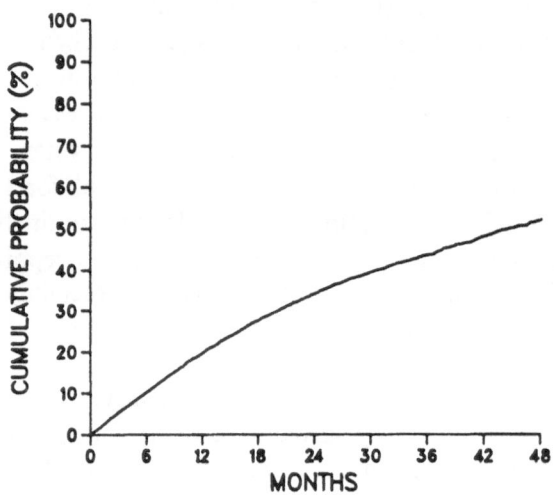

Cumulative Probabilities and 95% Confidence Intervals (C.I.) for Exhibit 5-1.

	Months on CAPD					
	6	12	18	24	36	48
Cumulative Prob.	10	20	28	34	44	52
95% C.I.	(10, 11)	(19, 20)	(26, 29)	(33, 35)	(42, 46)	(49, 54)

* Transfer to hemodialysis, IPD, or off dialysis with no return of kidney function

The estimated probability distribution for transferring off of CAPD is illustrated in Exhibit 5–1. Note that the probability of transferring to another modality doubles from 10% at 6 months to 20% at one year. After 18 months the probability of a transfer increases by approximately 6% every 6 months. By three years, 44% of patients have discontinued CAPD in favor of an alternate dialysis modality.

5.2 Probability of Transplantation—CAPD

An alternative to dialysis for the end stage renal disease patient is transplantation. The availability of a suitable kidney, patient preference

EXHIBIT 5-2

CAPD

CUMULATIVE PROBABILITY OF RECEIVING A KIDNEY TRANSPLANT
(CLASS 1 PATIENTS ONLY)

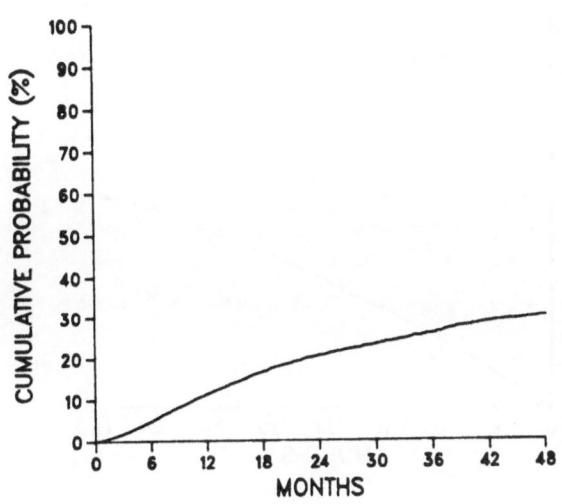

Cumulative Probabilities and 95% Confidence Intervals (C.I.) for Exhibit 5-2.

	Months on CAPD					
	6	12	18	24	36	48
Cumulative Prob.	5	11	17	20	26	30
95% C.I.	(4, 5)	(11, 12)	(16, 18)	(19, 22)	(24, 28)	(27, 33)

46

and medical considerations are all factors which influence the decision to transplant. For analysis purposes, patients receiving a transplant are counted as having experienced the event, all other patients, regardless of status (i.e., continuing CAPD, death, transfer, etc.) are censored as of the last day known to be on CAPD.

From Exhibit 5–2 it is evident that the majority of CAPD patients do not receive a transplant. Twenty percent of patients are reported to have received a transplant by the end of year two; and the cumulative probability of a transplant occurring increases to only 30% by the end of year four.

EXHIBIT 5-3

CAPD

CUMULATIVE PROBABILITY OF DEATH*
(CLASS 1 PATIENTS ONLY)

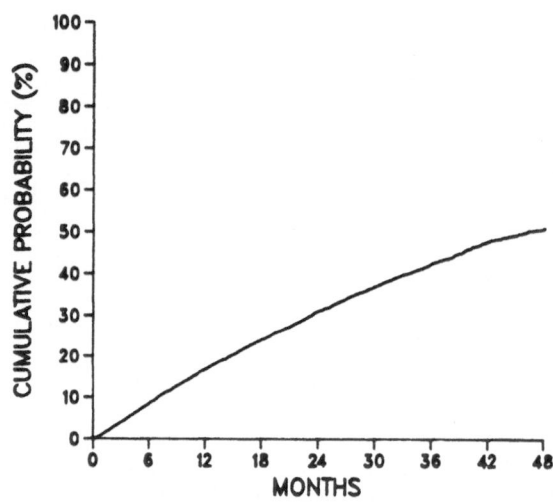

Cumulative Probabilities and 95% Confidence Intervals (C.I.) for Exhibit 5-3.

	Months on CAPD					
	6	12	18	24	36	48
Cumulative Prob.	8	17	24	31	42	51
95% C.I.	(8, 9)	(16, 17)	(23, 25)	(30, 32)	(40, 44)	(48, 54)

* While on CAPD or within two weeks of CAPD termination

5.3 Probability of Death While on CAPD

As previously indicated, deaths are reported to the Registry only if they occur while the patient is receiving CAPD or within two weeks of transfer to an alternative modality such as hemodialysis, IPD, or transplantation. Therefore, all patients not reported as dead provide information only for as long as they remain on CAPD. It should be understood, that those patients who subsequently die are not reflected in the Registry data base.

The probability distribution estimate of death while on CAPD, given in Exhibit 5–3, reveals a fairly constant increase in the cumulative probability of death with time. After six months on CAPD, deaths are observed to have occurred in 8% of patients, while the cumulative probability of death is 17% for patients who have been on treatment for twelve months. Increases of similar magnitude are observed at 18 months and 24 months. After four years on therapy, 51% of patients are reported as having died. The median time to death while receiving CAPD is 46.2 months.

5.4 Probability of Discontinuing CAPD for any Reason

As suggested earlier, patients who use CAPD as a replacement therapy for end stage renal disease can be expected to discontinue this treatment modality due to a variety of reasons: transfer to hemodialysis, IPD, discontinuation of all dialysis with or without return of kidney function, death or transplantation. Considering terminations for any reason as an event yields the probability distribution displayed in Exhibit 5–4. For patients coming to CAPD for the first time, over half (55%) may be expected to leave CAPD within 18 months; and after three years on therapy, three-quarters of the patients will have terminated CAPD. Of potential clinical significance are the patients who have remained on CAPD for 3 or more years. These patients may be considered 'long term' CAPD users, and are the subject of a special analyses appearing in Section 6 of this report.

5.5 Probability of Discontinuing CCPD

Probability distributions corresponding to patients beginning peritoneal-dialysis with CCPD were estimated in a similar manner to those for CAPD patients. Patients changing from CCPD to CAPD were not

48

EXHIBIT 5-4

CAPD

CUMULATIVE PROBABILITY OF DISCONTINUING
CAPD THERAPY FOR ANY REASON*
(CLASS 1 PATIENTS ONLY)

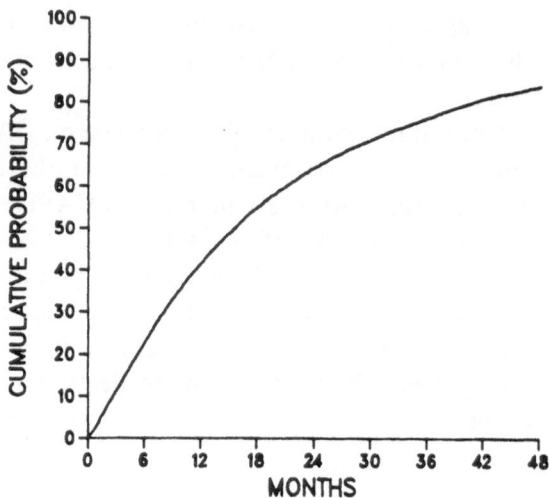

Cumulative Probabilities and 95% Confidence Intervals (C.I.) for Exhibit 5-4.

			Months on CAPD			
	6	12	18	24	36	48
Cumulative Prob.	22	41	55	64	76	84
95% C.I.	(22, 23)	(41, 42)	(54, 56)	(63, 65)	(75, 77)	(82, 85)

* Transfer to hemodialysis or IPD, transplantation, discontinuing dialysis with
  or without return of kidney function, death

considered transfers. Note that the estimates based on the CCPD patient population are subject to change as confidence bands at three years are rather sizeable. The probability of transferring from CCPD to hemodialysis or IPD, or discontinuing all dialysis with no return of kidney function, as shown in Exhibit 5–5, indicates that more than one-third of patients (36%) leave CCPD by two years in favor of an alternative dialysis modality. Transplants occur less frequently than transfers with approximately twenty-nine percent of the patients receiving a transplant within the first two years of therapy. However, a tripling of the probability of being transplanted was observed between the 0–6 month period (6%) and 6–12 month period (17%) (Exhibit 5–6). Similarly, the cumulative probability of death doubles the first six months (10%) to

EXHIBIT 5-5

CCPD

CUMULATIVE PROBABILITY OF TRANSFER*
(CLASS 1 PATIENTS ONLY)

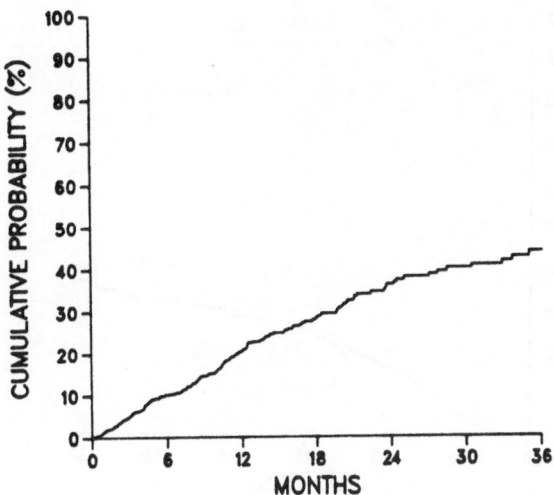

Cumulative Probabilities and 95% Confidence Intervals (C.I.) for Exhibit 5-5.

	Months on CCPD					
	6	12	18	24	30	36
Cumulative Prob.	10	20	28	36	40	44
95% C.I.	(8, 12)	(17, 24)	(23, 34)	(29, 44)	(32, 49)	(33, 55)

* Transfer to hemodialysis, IPD, or off dialysis with no return of kidney function

the second six months (22%); and, by 18 months approximately one-third of patients (31%) are reported as having died while on CCPD (Exhibit 5–7). The cumulative probability of discontinuing CCPD for any reason as illustrated in Exhibit 5–8 is estimated to be 50% at 1 year and 72% at 2 years.

5.6 Outcomes by Patient Type CAPD/CCPD

A symposium published in the ASAIO Journal in 1983 [2], defined a 'standard' population as nondiabetic patients, 20 to 59 years of age. A

EXHIBIT 5-6

CCPD

CUMULATIVE PROBABILITY OF RECEIVING A KIDNEY TRANSPLANT
(CLASS 1 PATIENTS ONLY)

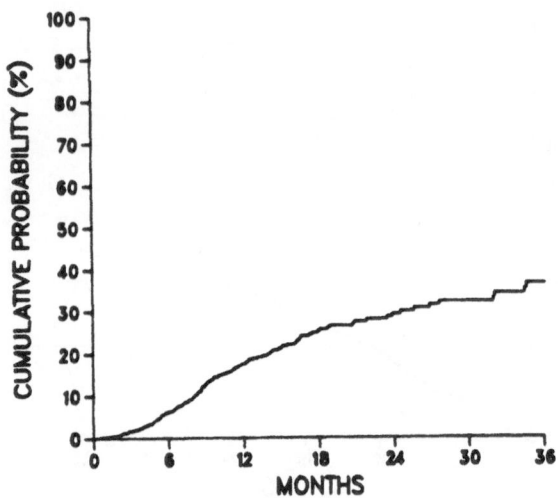

Cumulative Probabilities and 95% Confidence Intervals (C.I.) for Exhibit 5-6.

	Months on CCPD					
	6	12	18	24	30	36
Cumulative Prob.	6	17	25	29	32	37
95% C.I.	(5, 8)	(14, 21)	(20, 31)	(23, 37)	(24, 42)	(26, 48)

review of the Registry data base was made to assess the outcomes of such 'standard' patients and compare them with the outcomes of pediatric patients (< 20 years of age) and all other patients. 'Other' patients are defined as age > 59 years or adult patients diagnosed with Diabetic Glomerulosclerosis. All of the following analyses combine patients on CAPD with patients on CCPD.

5.6.1 Time to Transplant

As children are more likely to receive a transplant than adults, Exhibit 5–9 displays the probability separately for three groups of patients: age

EXHIBIT 5-7

CCPD

CUMULATIVE PROBABILITY OF DEATH*
(CLASS 1 PATIENTS ONLY)

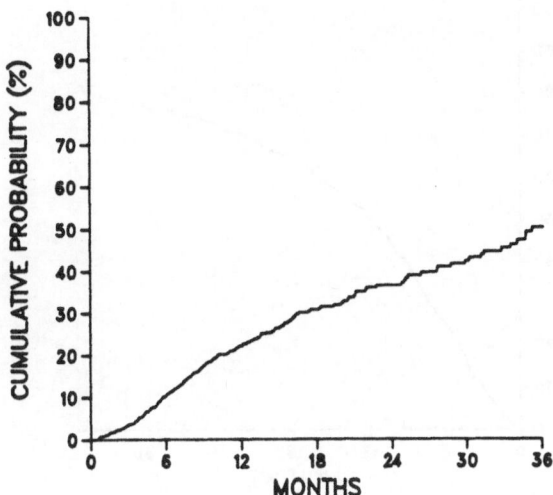

Cumulative Probabilities and 95% Confidence Intervals (C.I.) for Exhibit 5-7.

	Months on CCPD					
	6	12	18	24	30	36
Cumulative Prob.	10	22	31	37	42	50
95% C.I.	(8, 13)	(19, 26)	(26, 36)	(30, 44)	(35, 51)	(39, 61)

* While on CCPD or within two weeks of CCPD termination

< 20 years (pediatric), nondiabetics age 20–59 years ('standard'), diabetics and/or patients 60 years of age or older ('other'). For the purposes of this analysis all class 1 patients are considered regardless of therapy (i.e., CAPD or CCPD). The two year probability of a transplant is 26% for the 'standard' population, more than double the 12% transplant probability observed for diabetics or patients 60 years of age or greater. Children experience the greatest transplantation rate with 54% expected to receive a kidney transplant at two years; more than double the probability for the 'standard' group.

EXHIBIT 5-8

CCPD

CUMULATIVE PROBABILITY OF DISCONTINUING
CCPD FOR ANY REASON*
(CLASS 1 PATIENTS ONLY)

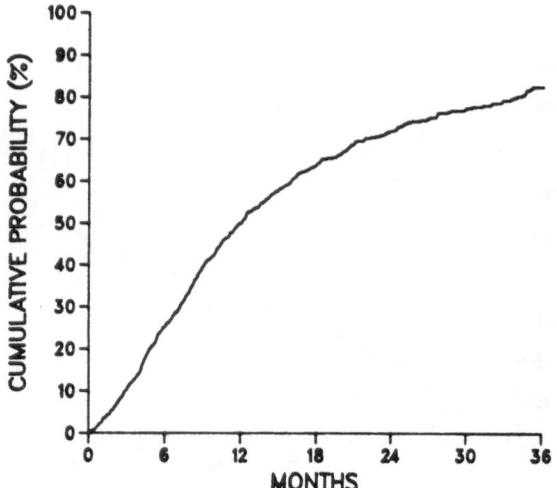

Cumulative Probabilities and 95% Confidence Intervals (C.I.) for Exhibit 5-8.

	Months on CCPD					
	6	12	18	24	30	36
Cumulative Prob.	25	50	64	72	77	82
95% C.I.	(22, 28)	(46, 54)	(60, 68)	(67, 76)	(72, 81)	(77, 87)

* Transfer to hemodialysis, IPD, transplantation, discontinuing dialysis with or without return of kidney function, death

5.6.2 Time to Death

Median time to death while on CAPD/CCPD for patients > 59 years of age or adult patients diagnosed with Diabetic Glomerulosclerosis is 29.5 months. The median has not been reached for pediatric or 'standard' patients. Two year probabilities of death are 11%, 17% and 43% for pediatric, 'standard', and 'other' patients respectively. Throughout the observation period, 'standard' patients and pediatric patients have an expected probability of dying while on continuous peritoneal dialysis of less than half that of 'other' patients (Exhibit 5–10).

EXHIBIT 5-9

CAPD/CCPD

CUMULATIVE PROBABILITY OF TRANSPLANTATION:
PEDIATRICS VS. "STANDARD" VS. "OTHER"

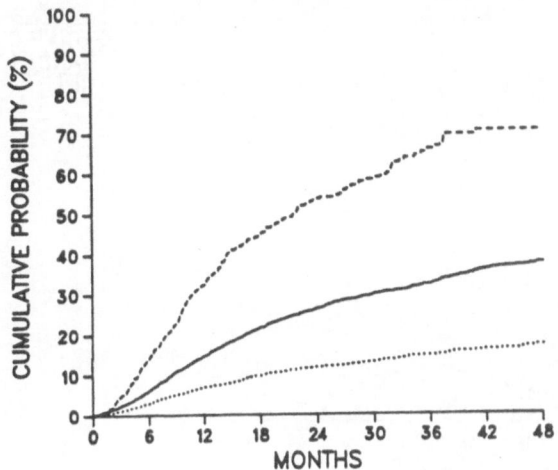

Cumulative Probabilities and 95% Confidence Intervals (C.I.) for Exhibit 5-9.

	Months on CAPD/CCPD					
	6	12	18	24	36	48
Pediatrics*						
Cumulative Prob.	14	32	45	54	66	70
95% C.I.	(12,17)	(28,36)	(40,50)	(48,59)	(58,73)	(58,80)
Standard**						
Cumulative Prob.	6	15	22	26	32	38
95% C.I.	(5,7)	(13,16)	(20,23)	(24,28)	(30,35)	(33,42)
Other***						
Cumulative Prob.	3	7	10	12	15	17
95% C.I.	(2,3)	(6,8)	(9,11)	(10,13)	(12,17)	(13,22)

*   Patients under 20 years of age
**   Patients between the ages of 20-59 years of age not diagnosed with Diabetic
      Glomerulosclerosis
*** Patients >59 years of age and/or adult patients diagnosed with Diabetic
      Glomerulosclerosis

5.6.3 Time to 'Technique Failure'

An assessment of the inability of peritoneal dialysis to adequately replace the functions of a failed kidney is complicated by the myriad of competing risks in the end stage renal disease population. Such risks include diabetes, cardiovascular complications, and age. Recognizing these limitations, an arbitrary definition of 'technique failure' can be

54

EXHIBIT 5-10

CAPD/CCPD

CUMULATIVE PROBABILITY OF DEATH:
PEDIATRICS VS. "STANDARD" VS. "OTHER"

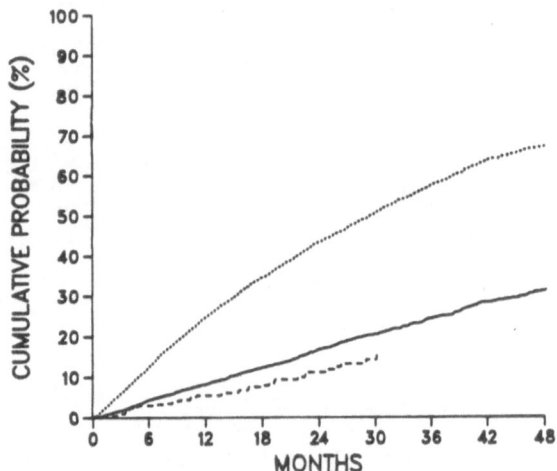

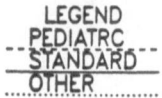

Cumulative Probabilities and 95% Confidence Intervals (C.I.) for Exhibit 5-10.

	Months on CAPD/CCPD					
	6	12	18	24	36	48
Pediatrics*						
Cumulative Prob.	3	5	7	11	-	-
95% C.I.	(2,5)	(3,8)	(5,12)	(7,17)	-	-
Standard**						
Cumulative Prob.	4	8	12	17	24	31
95% C.I.	(4,5)	(7,9)	(11,14)	(15,19)	(22,27)	(27,35)
Other***						
Cumulative Prob.	12	25	32	43	57	67
95% C.I.	(11,13)	(23,26)	(30,33)	(41,45)	(55,60)	(64,70)

*   Patients under 20 years of age
** Patients between the ages of 20-59 years of age not diagnosed with Diabetic
    Glomerulosclerosis
*** Patients >59 years of age and/or adult patients diagnosed with Diabetic
    Glomerulosclerosis
-   Rate unreliable; confidence interval width exceeds 95

made as follows: patients who transfer to an alternative dialysis
modality or die while on continuous peritoneal dialysis are considered
'technique failures'; patients who receive a kidney transplant, transfer
to another center and subsequently are lost to follow-up, or discontinue
dialysis due to a return in kidney function are not considered 'technique
failures'. These latter patients contribute information only for the time
they are known to be receiving continuous peritoneal dialysis and are
censored in the analysis.

EXHIBIT 5-11

CAPD/CCPD
CUMULATIVE PROBABILITY OF "TECHNIQUE FAILURE"[+]:
PEDIATRICS VS. "STANDARD" VS. "OTHER"

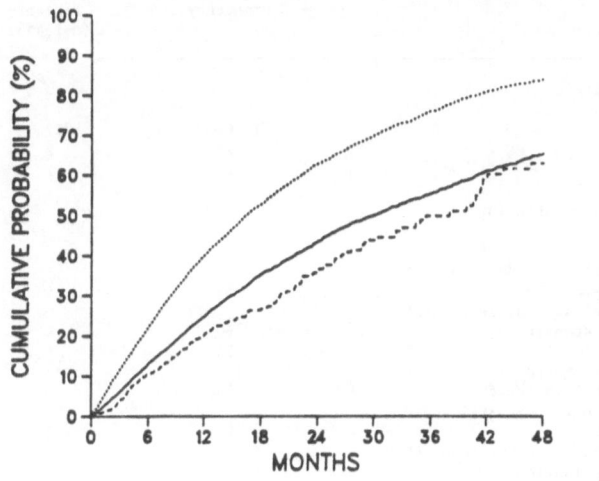

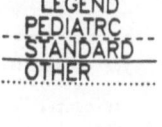

LEGEND
PEDIATRC
STANDARD
OTHER

Cumulative Probabilities and 95% Confidence Intervals (C.I.) for Exhibit 5-11.

		Months on CAPD/CCPD				
	6	12	18	24	36	48
Pediatrics*						
Cumulative Prob.	10	20	27	36	50	63
95% C.I.	(8,13)	(17,24)	(22,32)	(30,42)	(39,60)	(52,73)
Standard**						
Cumulative Prob.	13	25	35	43	55	65
95% C.I.	(12,14) ·	(23,26)	(34,37)	(41,45)	(53,58)	(62,68)
Other***						
Cumulative Prob.	22	40	53	63	76	84
95% C.I.	(21,23)	(39,41)	(51,54)	(61,64)	(74,77)	(82,86)

*   Patients under 20 years of age
** Patients between the ages of 20-59 years of age not diagnosed with Diabetic
     Glomerulosclerosis
*** Patients >59 years of age and/or adult patients diagnosed with Diabetic
     Glomerulosclerosis

\+   Transfer to hemodialysis or IPD, discontinuing dialysis without return of
     kidney function, death from any cause.

So defined, Exhibit 5–11 presents an estimate of the probability distribution for 'technique failure' for pediatric patients versus 'standard' patients versus all 'others'. Median time to technique failure is estimated to be 36 months for pediatric patients and 29.9 months for standard patients. Patients > 59 years of age and/or adult patients diagnosed with Diabetic Glomerulosclerosis have a median time to 'technique failure' of just 16.4 months. Two year probabilities of

56

EXHIBIT 5-12

FOLLOW-UP OF TRANSFERS TO HEMODIALYSIS SUMMARY

	Frequency	Percent (n=1,455)
Type of Hemodialysis:		
In-center	1,409	97
Home	25	2
Unknown	21	2
Primary Reason Discontinuing Peritoneal Dialysis:		
Peritoneal dialysis unable to meet fluid standard	59	4
Peritoneal dialysis unable to meet biochemical standard	60	4
Visual/manual impairment	15	1
Excessive peritonitis	384	27
Exit site/tunnel infection	133	9
Hospitalization for CAPD-related complications	25	2
Hospitalization for other than CAPD-related complications	17	1
Catheter leaks and malfunctions	55	4
Catheter failure	47	3
Hernia	28	2
Other medical reasons	226	16
Patient/family choice/inability to cope	217	15
Desire for change	34	2
Socioeconomic reasons	8	<1
Other	134	9
Unknown	13	<1

'technique failure' are 36%, 43% and 63% for the pediatric, 'standard', and 'other' cohorts respectively.

5.7 Follow-up of Transfers to Hemodialysis CAPD/CCPD

Although reasons for discontinuing CAPD/CCPD have previously been reported, a new follow-up form was instituted by the Registry in November, 1986 which provides more detailed information on this very important topic. Centers were requested to prospectively complete this form for all patients transferring to hemodialysis in the period July 1, 1986 to present. Information has been received on 1,455 patients and is summarized in Exhibit 5-12. Most patients transferring to hemodialysis receive in-center dialysis with only 2% of transferred patients utilizing home hemodialysis. Twenty-seven percent of the patients were reported to have discontinued CAPD/CCPD primarily due to excessive peritonitis, 15% due to patient or family choice or inability to cope, and 9% due to exit site/tunnel infections. In all, almost half of all patients'

(47%) primary reason for transferring to hemodialysis was due to a CAPD/CCPD related complication (peritonitis, exit site/tunnel infection, CAPD related hospitalization, catheter leak, malfunction or failure, or hernia). An additional 8% transferred because peritoneal dialysis could not meet the biochemical or fluid standard.

Eighty of the 1,455 patients (5%) who were reported to have transferred to hemodialysis since July 1, 1986, have subsequently returned to CAPD/CCPD as of January 31, 1988. Median time to return was 74 days with minimum and maximum time to return of 28 and 471 days respectively. Seventy-five percent of the patients who return due so within 4 months of leaving. The primary reasons these patients discontinued CAPD/CCPD are listed in Exhibit 5–13. Sixty-five percent (52/80) of patients had left CAPD/CCPD due to complications of peritoneal dialysis (peritonitis, exit site/tunnel infections, CAPD/CCPD related hospitalization, catheter leak, malfunction failure, or hernia). Of the 133 patients who discontinued CAPD/CCPD due to exit site/tunnel infections, 14% (19/133) have returned to CAPD/CCPD. Only 6% (24/384) of patients transferring to hemodialysis due to excessive peritonitis while on CAPD/CCPD have returned to CAPD/CCPD.

EXHIBIT 5-13

PRIMARY REASON FOR LEAVING CAPD IN PATIENTS
WHO TRANSFERRED FROM CAPD TO HEMODIALYSIS
AND SUBSEQUENTLY RETURNED TO CAPD

Primary Reason	Frequency	Percent (n=80)
Excessive Peritonitis	24	30
Exit Site/Tunnel Infection	19	24
Hospitalization for CAPD-related Complications	2	3
Catheter Leak/Malfunction	2	3
Catheter Failure	1	1
Hernia	4	5
Other Medical Reason	13	16
Patient/Family Choice/Inability to cope	3	4
Desire for Change	1	1
Other Reason	5	6
Not Stated	6	8

5.8 Follow-up of Kidney Transplants CAPD/CCPD

In the period beginning July 1, 1986 through October 31, 1987, 1070 reports have been received which summarize information concerning kidney transplants. From these reports, it is estimated that 20% of patients (209/1070) received a kidney from a living related donor (Exhibit 5–14). Four percent of patients received hemodialysis immediately prior to the transplant, and seventy percent of patients required no form of dialysis in the 2 week post-operative period. Of the 309 patients who required dialysis, the majority (73%) used peritoneal dialysis.

5.9 Follow-up of Patient Deaths CAPD/CCPD

Registry participants were requested to prospectively provide information with regard to events preceding a patient's death, as well as the probable cause of death for all deaths reported from July 1, 1986 to present. Forms summarizing these items have been received for 1,809

EXHIBIT 5-14

FOLLOW-UP OF KIDNEY TRANSPLANT SUMMARY

	Frequency	Percent (n=1070)
Transplanted Kidney - Living Related Donor		
No	855	80
Yes	209	20
Unknown	6	<1
Last Dialysis Prior to Transplant		
Peritoneal Dialysis	1,022	96
Hemodialysis	42	4
Unknown	6	<1
Dialysis Type in 2-week Post-op Period		
None	747	70
Peritoneal Dialysis	227	21
Hemodialysis	82	8
Unknown	14	1

EXHIBIT 5-15

DEATH SUMMARY

	Frequency	Percent (n=1,809)
Last Dialysis Type Prior to Death		
Peritoneal Dialysis	1,508	83
Hemodialysis	265	15
Unknown	39	2
Received Kidney Transplant Within 2 Weeks Prior to Death		
No	1,789	99
Yes	18	1
Unknown	1	<1
Complication of Peritoneal Dialysis Present at Death		
No	1,431	79
Yes, not contributing factor in patient's demise	173	10
Yes, minor contributing factor in patient's demise	101	6
Yes, major contributing factor in patient's demise	90	5
Unknown	14	1
Cause of Death		
Renal Disease only	221	12
Unrelated to Renal Disease or Peritoneal Dialysis	1,337	74
Both Renal Disease and Unrelated Causes	83	5
Unknown	168	9

patients, and the results are detailed in Exhibit 5–15. Eighty-three percent of the patients were reported to have used peritoneal dialysis up until the time of death. Only 15% reported to have received maintenance hemodialysis between the last peritoneal dialysis exchange and date of death. Only 18 patients (1%) received a transplanted kidney within two weeks of death. Eleven percent of patients were reported to have had a complication of peritoneal dialysis as a contributing factor in the patient's demise. An additional 10% had a complication present at the time of death, but it was not considered to have contributed to the patient's death. The majority of patients (74%) were claimed to have died from causes unrelated to renal disease or peritoneal dialysis. Twelve percent died as a consequence of renal disease and 5% succumbed due to both renal disease and causes unrelated to renal disease or peritoneal dialysis.

5.10 References

1. Kaplan E, Meier P. Nonparametric estimates from incomplete observations. J Am Stat Assoc 1958; 53:457–458.
2. Special Symposium on Morbidity and Mortality in Dialysis Treatment. ASAIO J 1983 Oct-Dec; 6(4).

Special Reports—1988

A. A Survey of Diabetics in the CAPD/CCPD Population*

Abstract

A survey of CAPD/CCPD patients with end-stage renal disease attributed to diabetes mellitus carried out by the USA NIH CAPD Registry, obtained results from 499 patients. These data suggest in diabetics with renal insufficiency, the time interval from age at diagnosis of diabetes to initiation of dialysis decreases as the age of diagnosis increases. Mean interval from the time of diabetes diagnosis to CAPD or CCPD initiation was 25 years for patients < 20 years of age at diagnosis and 17 years for patients ≥ 30 years of age. This trend is independent of the type of diabetes management and appeared to be independent of the type of diabetes. Patients were categorized on the basis of pre- and post-CAPD management of hyperglycemia. There were several associations noted between type of diabetes therapy and clinical findings. A higher proportion of legally blind patients had used insulin only (33%) compared to patients never using insulin (10%), and 78% of patients using insulin only were white compared with 49% among the never on insulin group. This latter result indicates that race influences the type of diabetes and/or progression of diabetes to renal insufficiency. Patients on insulin only reported parents and/or siblings with diabetes less often than patients using insulin and oral agents, some insulin, and never any insulin to manage their diabetes. We also noted that peritonitis rates are not increased in those patients who added insulin to dialysis solutions.

* The material contained in this report will be published as
  Lindblad AS, Nolph KD, Novak JW, Friedman EA. A survey of the NIH CAPD Registry with end-stage renal disease attributed to diabetic nephropathy. In press, *J Diabetic Complications*.

Introduction

Typically, the diabetic dependent on insulin throughout the course of the disease is highly suspect for deficient insulin production by the pancreas secondary to destruction of the islet cells where insulin is produced (so called type I diabetes). The nature of the destructive process may be variable but, in many instances, auto-immune mechanisms may be involved. In contrast, the diabetic that achieves acceptable control of serum glucose concentrations by dietary manipulation and/or oral hypoglycemic agents is more likely to have abnormal tissue responsivity to circulating insulin (so call type II diabetes); however, there may be an associated genetic susceptibility for inadequate reserves of islet cell activity and a resulting relative insulin deficiency [1]. Oral agents have been shown to increase endogenous insulin release at lower levels of glucose and to increase tissue responsivity to insulin in this second group [2].

Approximately 10 percent of all diabetic patients develop end-stage renal disease (ESRD). About 40 percent of type I patients develop ESRD between 10 and 20 years following the onset of diabetes [3]. A recently conducted survey of diabetic hemodialysis patients reported on a group of 232 patients under care in 14 dialysis centers in Brooklyn [4]. Unpublished results from this study suggest a constant interval from diagnosis of diabetes to initiation of therapy for end-stage renal disease which is independent of insulin dependency. Overall, patients from this study reported an average interval of 14.9 years from diabetes diagnosis to renal insufficiency. Additionally, blindness and family history were found to be equally prevalent in both the insulin-dependent and non-insulin dependent groups.

The purpose of the present registry survey of CAPD/CCPD patients whose end-stage renal disease is attributed to diabetes mellitus is to assess whether the results observed in diabetics on hemodialysis are applicable to diabetics treated by CAPD/CCPD. This study was designed to characterize, in CAPD/CCPD treated diabetics, the interval from diagnosis of diabetes mellitus to initiation of CAPD/CCPD, and to determine their family history of diabetes. We also ascertained the patient's degree of preserved vision as related to insulin dependency.

Material and Methods

To be eligible for study inclusion, patients must have been new to CAPD/CCPD at the time of entry in the registry, currently followed by the registry, and CAPD/CCPD must have been the patient's first treatment for end-stage renal disease. Only patients whose primary cause of renal disease was listed as diabetic glomerulosclerosis were eligible. All patients meeting the eligibility criteria were sampled with the restriction that no more than 10 patients were selected from any one center. For those centers with more than 10 eligible patients, a random sample of 10 was chosen. Telephone contact by the Data Coordinating Center to non-responding centers was used to maximize returns. Information pertaining to this study was prospectively collected by clinical center personnel (primarily nurses) for designated patients by telephone interview or at their next clinic visit.

Patients were asked by the interviewer to indicate 1) relatives with diabetes, 2) whether they were legally blind, 3) their age when first told they had diabetes, 4) their main successful therapy before and after starting CAPD/CCPD, and 5) the route of insulin administration, if any, on CAPD/CCPD. Main treatment categories to choose included 1) no treatment with diet, insulin, or oral agents, 2) diet modification only, 3) oral agent only (no insulin), 4) insulin only (no oral agent and never off insulin for more than 1 year since diagnosis, or 5) oral agents and insulin sequentially or combined.

McNemars test was used to identify differences in pre- and post-CAPD diabetes management plans, and the chi-square statistic was used to test for association between patient characteristics and pre- and post-CAPD diabetes management. Ninety-five percent confidence intervals were calculated for mean time intervals from diagnosis of diabetes to CAPD or CCPD initiation.

Results

Seven hundred seventy-one questionnaires were requested from the 239 participating centers with eligible patients. Ninety-six percent (739/771) were returned with a 4 percent (9/239) of centers unable to meet submission deadline. Of the 739 questionnaires received by the Data Coordinating Center, 33 percent (241/739) were coded as the patient was unwilling to participate or unavailable for an interview. The cause of this latter result was primarily due to transfer of the patient to a different center or modality 38 percent (91/241) or death of the patient 22 percent (52/241). In all, questionnaire information was received for 499 patients. This cohort forms the basis of the results which follow.

Characteristics of the patients who answered the questionnaire are detailed in Exhibit 1. The majority of patients are white (72%) and 54

EXHIBIT 1

SELECTED PATIENT CHARACTERISTICS

Characteristic	N (499)	% (100)
Race		
White	357	72
Black	82	16
Other	60	12
Sex		
Male	271	54
Female	228	46
Peritoneal Dialysis Type		
CAPD	457	92
CCPD or Both	42	8
Route of Insulin Administration		
No Insulin	63	13
Subcutaneous	157	31
Intraperitoneal	233	47
Both Sub Q and IP	46	9
Age at Diabetes Diagnosis		
Unknown	30	6
<20	156	31
20-29	78	16
30-49	80	16
50-59	140	28
≥60	15	3
Legally Blind	144	29
Family Members with Diabetes		
Parent(s)	213	43
Sibling(s)	165	33
Aunt(s) Uncle(s)	172	34
Children	43	9
At least one of the above	351	70
Parent(s) and sibling(s)	278	56

percent are male. Slightly less than a third of the patients (31%) were diagnosed with diabetes as a child (< 20 years of age). The median age of diabetes diagnosis of the entire cohort was 30 years of age. Twenty-nine percent of patients were considered legally blind, while a full 70 percent of patients reported at least one family member (i.e., parent, aunt, uncle, sibling, or child) with diagnosed diabetes. Fifty-six percent claimed to have a parent and/or a sibling with diabetes.

The majority of patients, 59 percent (295/499), had used insulin only to manage their diabetes both pre- and post-CAPD. These patients were not taking oral agents and had never been off insulin for more than one year since diabetes diagnosis (see Exhibit 2). Ninety-five patients were using no insulin prior to CAPD or CCPD initiation and 51 percent of these patients (48/95) changed to insulin only containing regimens.

EXHIBIT 2

NUMBER OF PATIENTS RECEIVING SPECIFIED DIABETES
MANAGEMENT THERAPY BY PRE- AND POST-CAPD STATUS

Pre-CAPD Initiation	Post-CAPD Initiation					
	No Therapy	Diet Only	Oral Only	Insulin and Oral	Insulin Only	Total
Unknown	0	0	1	0	8	9
No Therapy	1	0	1	0	3	5
Diet Only	1	13	2	0	6	22
Oral Only	3	10	13	3	39	68
Insulin and Oral	4	4	2	4	77	91
Insulin Only	3	5	0	1	295	304
Total	12	32	19	8	428	499

Similarly, of the 91 patients who were receiving a combination of insulin and oral agents prior to dialysis, 85 percent (77/91) changed to insulin only containing regimens. In contrast, only 3 percent (8/304) of patients on insulin only therapy prior to CAPD/CCPD initiation changed to regimens containing no insulin.

Lifetime diabetes management from diagnosis to the time of survey was divided into four categories based on insulin dependency. The first category includes patients whose main successful therapy has been to use insulin only with no oral agents throughout their diabetic history. Patients who have been using a combination of insulin and oral agents sequentially or in combination both pre- and post-CAPD/CCPD initiation, are classified as 'insulin and oral', and patients who have used insulin as part of their main successful therapy either pre- or post-CAPD initiation but not in both time periods are placed in the 'some insulin' category. Finally, patients who have never had insulin included as their main successful therapy at any time are grouped as 'never on insulin'. Characteristics of the patients in each of these groups are detailed in Exhibit 3. As was expected, patients in the insulin only group tend to have been younger at diabetes diagnosis (median age 19 years) compared to patients in the other categories where the median age at diagnosis was 37 years or greater. A greater proportion (p < .01) of patients in this insulin only group were white (78%) as compared with patients never on insulin (49%). Similarly, a higher proportion (p < .01) of legally blind patients (33%) are in the insulin only group compared

EXHIBIT 3

SELECTED PATIENT CHARACTERISTICS AND COMPLICATIONS
BY TYPE OF DIABETES MANAGEMENT

	Type of Diabetes Management				
	Insulin Only (n=279)	Insulin and Oral (n=76)	Some Insulin (n=72)	Never Any Insulin (n=42)	Total (469)*
Characteristics					
Median Age (years) at Diabetes Diagnosis	19	37	40	48	30
Median Age (years) at CAPD/CCPD Initiation	44	57	59	63	51
% White	78	70	67	49	73
% Legally Blind	33	28	25	10	29
% With at Least One Relative with Diabetes	67	78	78	69	71
% With Parent	38	51	53	42	42
% With Sibling	25	41	51	43	31
% With Parent and/or Sibling	48	66	74	60	56

*Age at diabetes diagnosis was unknown in 30 patients.

EXHIBIT 4

MEAN INTERVAL (YEARS) FROM DIAGNOSIS OF DIABETES
TO INITIATION OF CAPD OR CCPD (95% CONFIDENCE INTERVAL)
BY AGE AT DIABETES DIAGNOSIS AND
TYPE OF MAIN THERAPY FOR DIABETES

Diabetes Management	Age at Diabetes Diagnosis							
	<20 Years		20-29 Years		≥30 Years		Total	
	N	Mean	N	Mean	N	Mean	N	Mean
Insulin Only (95% C.I.)	141	25 (23, 26)	51	22 (20, 24)	87	17 (15, 18)	279	22 (21, 23)
Insulin and Oral (95% C.I.)	8	22 (19, 26)	15	23 (18, 28)	53	19 (17, 20)	76	20 (18, 21)
Some Insulin (95% C.I.)	7	32 (20, 44)	10	24 (18, 29)	55	16 (14, 18)	72	19 (16, 21)
Never on Insulin (95% C.I.)	0	* *	2	17 (9, 25)	40	14 (11, 16)	42	14 (11, 16)
Total (95% C.I.)	156	25 (24, 26)	78	22 (21, 24)	235	17 (16, 18)	469	20 (19, 21)

to the never on insulin group (10%). Patients on insulin only reported parents and/or siblings with diabetes less often than patients in the insulin and oral and some insulin groups (p < .01). Only 48 percent of insulin only diabetics reported having a parent and/or a sibling with diabetes compared with 60 percent, 66 percent, and 74 percent among the patients never on insulin, on insulin and oral agents, and some insulin, respectively.

The mean interval from diagnosis of diabetes to initiation of CAPD or CCPD and 95 percent confidence intervals were calculated for each diabetes management group by age of diabetes diagnosis (Exhibit 4). Overall, the interval between the diagnosis of diabetes and CAPD or

EXHIBIT 5

AGE AT DIABETES DIAGNOSIS VS.
LENGTH OF INTERVAL TO CAPD/CCPD INITIATION
BY TYPE OF DIABETES MANAGEMENT

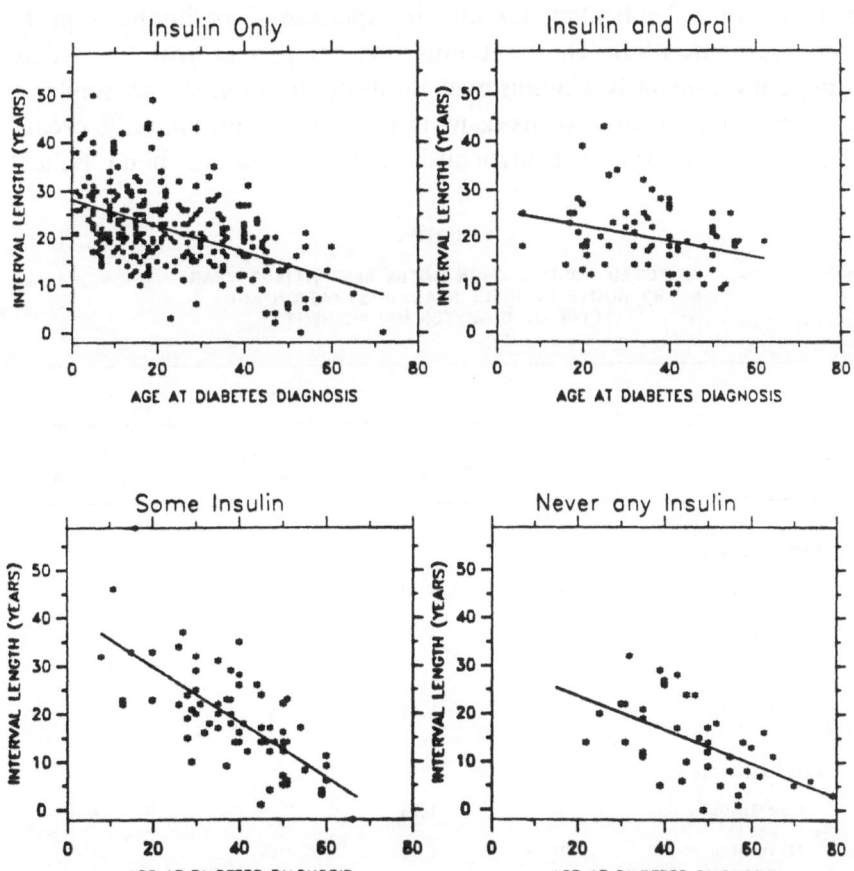

CCPD initiation was longer for those diagnosed before the age of 30 than for those diagnosed at 30 years or older (p < .05, adjusted comparison). Patients diagnosed with diabetes before the age of 20 years and patients 20 to 29 years of age at diagnosis reported mean intervals to first CAPD/CCPD exchange of 25 and 22 years, respectively. In contrast, patients whose diabetes diagnosis occurred at age 30 years or older, averaged only 17 years to CAPD/CCPD initiation. No patients under 20 (0/156) in this study began dialysis less than 10 years post-diabetes diagnosis compared with 16 percent (49/313) of patients over 20 years of age. Exhibit 5 demonstrates a decreasing interval to ESRD with increasing age of diabetes diagnosis regardless of type of diabetes management. Overall, the mean interval was 20 years with a 95 percent confidence interval of 19 years to 21 years. Complication rates per patient year by route of insulin administration and type of diabetes management were calculated and are presented in Exhibit 6. Although differences in rates were not large, diabetics never using insulin had the highest rate of peritonitis per patient year (1.31) while patients using a combination of subcutaneous and intraperitoneal peritonitis reported the lowest rate (.93). The peritonitis rate per patient year for patients using subcutaneously administered insulin (1.03 events) was similar to the rate reported for patients using intraperitoneal insulin (1.06 events). Blind patients using subcutaneously administered vs. blind patients

EXHIBIT 6

SELECTED COMPLICATION RATES PER PATIENT YEAR
BY ROUTE OF INSULIN ADMINISTRATION AND
TYPE OF DIABETES MANAGEMENT

		Complication		
	N	Peritonitis	Exit Site/Tunnel Infection	Catheter Replacement
Route of Insulin Administration				
Subcutaneous (SubQ)	156	1.03	.65	.20
Intraperitoneal (IP)	232	1.06	.60	.16
SubQ and IP	46	.93	.54	.23
No Insulin	62	1.31	.47	.17
Blind Patients				
Subq Insulin	44	1.05	.70	.18
IP Insulin	74	1.16	.64	.20

using intraperitoneal insulin post-CAPD initiation reported similar rates per patient year of peritonitis (1.05 vs. 1.16).

Discussion

The USA NIH CAPD Registry has previously analyzed diabetes mellitus as a risk factor for morbidity and mortality in patients maintained on CAPD [5]. The point prevalence survey herein reported was intended to characterize the type of diabetic enrolled in the CAPD Registry. We infer diabetes type from treatment history as neither C-peptide nor insulin measurements were practical for this survey. It is highly likely that diabetics whose age of diagnosis was less than 20 years and who were in the 'insulin only' category of treatment have type I diabetes. Those subjects who were never on insulin and had onset of diabetes (age of diagnosis) after 30 years, presumably have type II diabetes.

Overall, patients participating in this study reported a mean interval of 20 years from diabetes diagnosis to renal insufficiency. Although this average interval is longer than that reported in the Brooklyn study (14.9 years), the patients in the present study were younger with an average age at renal replacement therapy initiation of 51 years compared with 59.6 years for the Brooklyn population. The average interval to renal insufficiency among the 12 patients in the Brooklyn study who were considered clearly insulin dependent was similar to the estimate based on the 295 insulin-dependent patients in the present study (20.5 years and 25 years, respectively). This study demonstrated an inverse correlation between mean interval from diagnosis of diabetes to dialyzing and increasing age. The shorter the interval from diagnosis to dialysis at later ages of diagnosis does not necessarily imply that diabetes in older patients produces diabetic nephropathy at an accelerated rate. First, our study examines this interval only in patients who are already at end-stage nephropathy and does not prospectively follow the course of diabetic renal disease. Perhaps the progression of diabetic nephropathy in the entire diabetic population is quite different than in the select population whose kidneys are already destroyed. Second, it is possible that the diagnosis of diabetes is delayed in many older patients and that the duration of the disease is longer than what is realized or that older patients are more likely to have other more aggressive forms of renal disease mistakenly attributed to diabetes in the absence of a renal biopsy. Third, older diabetic patients have a higher expected mortality rate than younger patients. As patients must live long enough to have diabetic nephropathy observed, the distribution of time to nephropathy is likely biased low in the older cohort due to death. Finally, clinicians may be predisposed to earlier dialysis in older patients and more likely to delay dialysis as long as feasible in younger patients.

The higher percentages of legally blind patients in the 'insulin only' category (Exhibit 3) compared to the 'never any insulin' category may in part relate to the suggestion that the severest form of retinopathy occurs more frequently in the insulin-dependent diabetic [3]. In addition, many in the 'insulin only' group were diagnosed at younger ages and had a longer interval to dialysis. On the average, it would appear that the 'insulin only' group had their diabetes eight to eleven years longer at the time they started CAPD and came into the Registry.

Racial and genetic differences between diabetes types have been reported by others [3,6,7]. It has been suggested that non-insulin dependent diabetes has a stronger genetic basis than insulin dependent diabetes [6]. This observation is supported by the findings reported in this study as diabetics in patients and/or siblings was reported less frequently among patients managed by insulin only for the duration of their diabetes compared to other management plans. A much higher percentage of the 'never any insulin' patients were non-white (51%) compared to the 'insulin only' group (12%). Alternatively, while 78 percent of the 'insulin only' population were white, only 49 percent of the 'never any insulin' group were white. We cannot conclude from this data whether there are racial differences of distributions of type I and type II diabetes and/or selection biases of therapy based on racial, economic and social factors. However, other studies have shown that there is a higher incidence of non-insulin dependent diabetes mellitus among blacks than among whites [3] and higher incidence of insulin dependent diabetes among whites as compared to blacks [6].

Results from this survey indicate that following onset of ESRD there is an increase in the number of patients managed by insulin only as 304 of 499 patients were using insulin only pre-CAPD/CCPD compared with 428 patients post-CAPD/CCPD. Exposure to large amounts of glucose absorbed from the dialysate in peritoneal cavity probably explains this finding.

We have previously reported no increased risk of peritonitis in diabetics using intraperitoneal insulin than in those using subcutaneous insulin or no insulin at all [8]. In this point prevalence survey, we see this same trend. It is reassuring that sighted patients as well as blind patients adding insulin to their dialysis solutions can do so without an increase in contamination and subsequent peritonitis.

In summary, this survey provides some indications of the distributions of patient and treatment characteristics in a large group of diabetics with end-stage diabetic nephropathy who were receiving CAPD or CCPD. This study supports observations made by others with regards to racial and blindness prevalence imbalances among type I and type II diabetics. Further, it would appear that the time interval to the need for dialysis is longer in younger patients than intervals predicted from the general diabetic population, regardless of the type of therapy for diabetes. Fortunately, the time interval is still relatively long in all groups with an overall average near 20 years.

References

1. Davidson MB. Review: Pathogenesis of type II diabetes mellitus: an interpretation of current data. Am J Med 1986; 292:35–39.
2. Prosser PR, Kosola JW, Bowers CY. The 24–hour effects of glyburide and chlorpropamide after chronic treatment of type II diabetic patients. Am J Med 1985; 289:179–185.
3. Cutler RE, StJ-Hammond PG. Back to Basics: diabetic renal-eetinal syndrome, part 1 epidemiology and pathogenesis. Dial & Transplant 1987 Nov; 16(11):623–632.
4. Lowder GM, Perri NA, Thiruvengadam R, and Friedman EA. Employment, rehabilitation and diabetes type in diabetics on maintenance hemodialysis. Am Soc Neph 1986 Dec 7–10;19:81A. abstract.
5. Nolph KD, Cutler SJ, Steinberg SM, Novak JW, Hirschman GH. Factors associated with morbidity and mortality among patients on CAPD. Trans Am Soc Artif Intern Organs 1987 Apr-Jun; 23(2):57–65.
6. National Diabetes Data Group. Classification and diagnosis of diabetes mellitus and other categories of glucose intolerance. Diabetes 1987; 28:1044.
7. LaPorte RE, Tajima N, Dorman JS, et al. Differences between blacks and whites in epidemiology of insulin-dependent diabetes mellitus in Allegheny, Pennsylvania. Am J Epidemiol 1986; 123:592–603.
8. Nolph KD, Cutler SJ, Steinberg SM, Novak JW. Special studies from the NIH USA CAPD Registry. Peritoneal Dial Bull 1986 Jan-Mar; 6(1):28–35.

of patient mortality). Intervention in a large group of diabetes
subjects starting dialysis, reporting who were receiving CAPD or
CERA. The main cardiovascular outcomes under by this conservative,
multiply and illnesses in related with large sharing type I and type I
diabetes. Further, it would appear that the time allotted to the need for
dialysis. Sooner or later, transition from acute established after the
selected diabetes conditions, mortality in the cardiovascular for
diabetes. Furthermore, the CRA analysis, and some cases that all
group with an equal maintenance 10 years.

References

1. [reference text illegible]

2. [reference text illegible]

3. [reference text illegible]

4. [reference text illegible]

5. [reference text illegible]

6. [reference text illegible]

7. [reference text illegible]

8. [reference text illegible]

9. [reference text illegible]

B. Hematocrit Values in the CAPD/CCPD Population

Abstract

A survey of the National CAPD Registry population was conducted to assess the distribution of hematocrit in a large group of CAPD/CCPD patients to characterize the anemia of the population, and identify factors which relate to variation in hematocrit. A random sample of 812 patients was selected from the Registry population. Information was provided on 608 patients. Population characteristics were similar to the Registry population as a whole. Mean hematocrit was 29.4% and median hematocrit was 29%. Recent peritonitis, folate therapy, androgen therapy, and iron therapy had no obvious influences on hematocrit distributions. Significantly higher hematocrits were seen in males, whites, and patients with polycystic kidney disease. Significantly lower hematocrits were seen in surgically anephric patients and in patients who had received transfusions 60 days before the survey. Eighty-nine percent of patients had not received a transfusion 60 days prior to the survey. Some patients, especially those with hematocrits below the median, might benefit from recombinant erythropoietin therapy.

Introduction

Anemia in patients with chronic renal failure is related to multiple mechanisms including 1) a deficiency of erythropoietin, 2) the presence of inhibitors of erythropoiesis, and 3) shortened red cell survivals [1–2]. With the initiation of CAPD/CCPD, there is often a rise in hematocrit which has been attributed to a decrease in plasma volume with the removal of excessive body fluids and to an increase in red cell mass [3–5]. The increase in red cell mass may relate in part to increased red cell survival [6] and to removal of inhibitors of erythropoiesis [7]. Erythropoietin levels relative to hematocrit levels are inappropriately low in CAPD/CCPD patients and show no consistent change on the therapy [8–9]. Very low levels of erythropoietin have been associated with minimal or no increases in hematocrit following commencement of CAPD [8]. Thus, some minimal level of erythropoietin may play a permissive role for other beneficial mechanisms to be effective. With time on CAPD/CCPD, there may be return of hematocrit towards baseline levels subsequent to the rise seen in the early months of treatment [10]. Reasons for this late decline of the hematocrit are not known. Recently, in early clinical trials, recombinant erythropoietin has been administered intravenously to patients on chronic hemodialysis [11]. Increases in hematocrit over two or four weeks could be seen with administration of erythropoietin three times weekly. There is widespread interest in studies of the effects of intraperitoneal erythropoietin on the hematocrit of patients on CAPD/CCPD.

This survey of the National CAPD Registry population was conducted to provide information as to the distribution of hematocrit in a large group of CAPD/CCPD patients,to characterize the anemia of the CAPD/CCPD population in the Registry, identify factors which relate to the variation seen therein, and to evaluate the potential need for recombinant erythropoietin therapy in this population.

Materials and Methods

To be eligible for study inclusion, patients must have been new to CAPD/CCPD at the time of entry in the Registry, and currently followed by the Registry. Only patients who were 20 years of age or older at the time of CAPD/CCPD initiation were considered. A sample of 812 patients was randomly selected from the Registry population meeting the eligibility criteria. Institutions were required to prospectively complete a study specific form at the selected patient's next ambulatory visit. Telephone contact by the Data Coordinating Center to nonresponding centers was used to maximize returns.

The sample size of 812 patients was selected to provide for 150 completed records for patients on CAPD/CCPD for 2 or more years. The standard deviation for hematocrit levels is estimated to be approximately 5% and thus 5 unit changes in mean hematocrit levels for subgroups of size 30 can be reliably detected. Quantile estimation of hematocrit levels of the entire cohort as well as subgroups were calculated, and a regression analysis was used to identify factors which significantly affected hematocrit levels.

Results

Eight hundred-twelve requests for hematocrit values were made to 256 participating centers. Ninety-five percent (769/812) of the forms were returned to the Data Coordinating Center. One hundred-sixty-one patients were coded as having terminated CAPD/CCPD or transferred to a different center and hematocrit values were not provided. Information was provided on 608 patients, and these patients provide the basis for the analyses which follows.

Patient characteristics of the returned sample closely resemble the characteristics of the total Registry population from which the sample was selected (Exhibit 1). Fifty-three percent of the sampled patients are

EXHIBIT 1

PATIENT CHARACTERISTICS

Characteristic	N (608)	% (100)	Registry %
Therapy Type			
CAPD	569	93.6	92
CCPD	34	5.6	7
CAPD and CCPD	5	<1	1
Sex			
Male	321	52.8	55
Female	287	47.2	45
Race			
White	457	75.2	76
Black	112	18.4	17
Other	39	6.4	7
Prior ESRD Therapy			
No	321	52.8	45
Yes	287	47.2	55
Primary Renal Disease Type			
Diabetic glomerulosclerosis	144	23.7	25
Chronic glomerulonephritis	104	17.1	18
Hypertensive renal disease	95	15.6	15
Polycystic kidney disease	36	5.9	6
Other	229	37.7	36
Median Age	54 years		52 years
Duration on CAPD/CCPD			
0 - <3 months	45	7.4	*
3 - <6 months	59	9.7	*
6 - <9 months	71	11.7	*
9 - <12 months	67	11.0	*
1 - <2 years	201	33.1	*
2 - <3 years	80	13.2	*
3 or more years	85	14.0	*

* Not applicable

male, and three-quarters of the patients are white. Diabetic patients make up 24% of the sample, and the median age at CAPD or CCPD initiation is 54 years. More than half the sampled patients (53%) used CAPD as their first therapy for ESRD. Duration of CAPD/CCPD therapy at the time of hematocrit evaluation ranges from 1 month to more than 4 years. The majority of patients, 73% (443/608) have been on CAPD or CCPD for 2 years or less, and forty-five patients have been on therapy for 3 months or less at the time of hematocrit measurement.

Information on several factors which potentially relate to hematocrit levels was requested and the frequency of occurrence is provided in Exhibit 2. Eleven percent of the patients had undergone a transfusion within the preceding 60 days and an episode of peritonitis had occurred in 15% of patients within 30 days prior to hematocrit evaluation. The majority of patients, 73% (442/608) were taking a folate supplement of at least .5mg per day. Sixty-four percent of these patients (284/442) had folate included in a multivitamin supplement, and the remaining 158

EXHIBIT 2

PATIENT TRANSFUSION, PERITONITIS AND DRUG STATUS

Variable	N (608)	% (100)
Transfusion within past 60 days		
No	539	88.7
Yes, in preparation for transplant	22	3.6
Yes, precipitated by hemorrhage or surgery	10	1.6
Yes, other	37	6.1
Peritonitis within past 30 days		
No	516	84.9
Yes	91	15.0
Unknown	1	.2
Folate supplement ≥.5 mg per day		
No	166	27.3
Yes - in multivitamin supplement	284	46.7
Yes - as separate supplement	158	26.0
Androgens within past 30 days		
No	540	88.8
Yes, oral	20	3.3
Yes, parental	48	7.9
Iron therapy within past 60 days		
No	542	89.1
Yes, oral	61	10.0
Yes, parental	1	.2
Unknown	4	.7
Surgically Anephric		
No	594	97.7
Yes	12	2.0
Unknown	2	.3

patients took folate as a separate supplement. No patients reported taking recombinant erythropoietin and only 11% of patients had taken androgens in the preceding month. Iron therapy had been administered within the last 2 months in 10% of patients with almost every patient (61/62) using an oral administration. One patient reported using parenteral iron therapy. Only 12 patients (2%) were considered surgically anephric.

Overall, the mean hematocrit level for the 608 patients was 29.4% with a maximum of 58% and minimum of 10%. Few factors were found to influence hematocrit level in this population. No significant difference (p > .1) in hematocrit level was found between patients with or without: an episode of peritonitis within the past 60 days, folate supplementation of ≥ .5mg per day, androgen use within the past 30 days, iron therapy within the past 60 days, or prior therapy for

EXHIBIT 3

MEAN AND QUANTILE LEVELS OF HEMATOCRIT
BY SELECTED VARIABLE

Variable	N	Mean	Quantiles				
			0%	25%	50%	75%	100%
All patients	608	29.4	10	25	29	33	58
Primary Disease Type*							
Polycystic kidney disease	36	32.2	22	28	32	36	49
Other	572	29.2	10	25	29	33	58
Sex*							
Male	321	30.5	10	26	30	35	58
Female	287	28.1	17	24	28	31	49
Surgically Anephric*							
No	594	29.4	10	25	29	33	58
Yes	12	24.8	16	20	24	29	39
Transfusion ≤ 60 days*							
No	539	29.7	10	25	29	34	52
Yes	69	26.4	17	22	26	29	58
Race*							
White	457	29.8	10	25	29	34	58
Other	151	28.1	15	24	28	31	52

*Significant difference p<.01

end-stage renal disease. A significant rise in hematocrit level was not seen during the early months of CAPD/CCPD therapy use in this population. Mean hematocrit levels in patients who had been on CAPD or CCPD for < 3 months, 3–6 months, 6–9 months, and 9–12 months were 28.1%, 30.2%, 29.9%, and 29.2%, respectively.

Five factors were found to be significantly associated with lower hematocrit levels: female sex, non-white race, absence of kidney tissue, and report of a transfusion within the past 60 days, and one factor, primary renal disease diagnosis of polycystic kidney(s), was associated with elevated hematocrit levels. Quantile and mean values of hematocrit for these five variables as well as the entire cohort are given in Exhibit 3. All five variables significantly affected hematocrit levels when jointly considered ($p < .01$), and when examined separately ($p < .01$).

Discussion

In the surveyed population, we did not see differences in hematocrit related to time on CAPD, peritonitis within the past 30 days, folate supplementation, androgen therapy, or iron therapy. However, only small percentages of the patients had been exposed to peritonitis 30 days prior to the survey, were not taking folate supplements or were taking iron therapy or androgens. Large scale prospective studies would be needed to show an impact of these factors, if any, on hematocrit in the CAPD/CCPD population. Increases in red cell mass over the first few months of CAPD have been reported in longitudinal studies which would be more sensitive than a single cross sectional survey (3–7). Effects of peritonitis, if any, might better be seen in patients who had frequent recurring episodes and associated problems in maintaining nitrogen balance and adequate nutrition. Randomized prospective trials would most likely be necessary to prove effects of folate, androgens or iron therapy in this population. Folate clearances are much lower on a weekly basis with CAPD than with hemodialysis and adequate dietary intakes may be able to keep up with dialysis losses. However, low serum folate levels have been documented in some patients on CAPD without supplement and daily doses of 0.5 to 1 mg have been recommended [12].

We did note significantly higher hematocrits in males, whites, and patients with polycystic kidney disease. This result in males is not surprising as males normally tend to have higher hematocrit levels than females. Patients with cystic kidney diseases may have better preservation of erythropoietin production and occasionally can have high hematocrits suggesting excessive production [13].

We found significantly lower hematocrits in patients who were surgically anephric and in patients who had received transfusions in the past 60 days. Surgically anephric patients have very deficient erythropoietin production. Transfusions may have partially corrected only very low hematocrits and may have suppressed endogenous erythropoietin production.

Mean differences in hematocrits related to the above factors were quite small. Perhaps the most important finding is to document a mean hematocrit level of 29.4% maintained in the majority of patients without transfusions. Some CAPD patients, especially the 50% below the median hematocrit of 29% might have long-term benefits from recombinant erythropoietin therapy.

References

1. Fisher JW. Mechanism of the anemia of chronic renal failure. Nephron 1980; 25(3):106–111.
2. Editorial. The anemia of chronic renal failure. Lancet 1983; 1:965–966.
3. De Paepe MBJ, Schelstraete KHG, Ringoir SM, Lameire NH. Influence on continuous ambulatory peritoneal dialysis on the anemia of end stage renal disease. Kidney Int 1983; 23;744–748.
4. Saltissi D, Coles GA, Napier AF, Bentley P. The hematological response to continuous ambulatory peritoneal dialysis. Clin Neph 1984 Jul; 22(1):21–27.
5. Mehta BR, Mogridge C, Bell JD. Changes in red cell mass, plasma volume and hematocrit in patients of CAPD. Trans Am Soc Artif Organs 1983 Apr; 29:50–52.
6. Summerfield GP, Gyde OHB, Forbves AMW, Goldsmith HJ, Bellingham AJ. Haemoglobin concentration and serum erythropoietin in renal dialysis and transplant patients. Scand J Haematol 1983; 30:389–400.
7. Lamperi S, Carozzi S, Icardi A. In vitro and in vivo studies of erythropoiesis during continuous ambulatory peritoneal dialysis. Peritoneal Dial Bull 1983 Apr-Jun; 3(2):94–96.
8. Zappocosta AR, Caro J, Erslev A. Normalization of haemotocrit in patients with end stage renal disease on continuous ambulatory peritoneal dialysis. Am J Med 1982; 72:53–57.
9. McGonigle RJS, Wallin JD, Shadduck RK, Fisher JW. Erythropoietin deficiency and inhibition of erythropoiesis in renal insufficiency. Kidney Int 1984 Feb; 25(2):437–444.
10. Kurtz SB, Wong VH, Anderson CF, Vogel JP, McCarthy JT, Mitchell JC, Kumar R, Johnson WJ. Continuous ambulatory peritoneal dialysis. Three years' experience at the Mayo Clinic. Mayo Clin Proc 1983; 58:633–639.
11. Eschbach JW, Egrie JC, Downing MR, Browne JK, Adamson JW. Correction of the anemia of end-stage renal disease with recombinant human erythro-poietin: results of a phase I-II clinical trial. Am Soc Neph 1986 Dec 7–10; 19:41A. abstract.
12. Blumberg A, Hanek A, Saunder G. Vitamin nutrition in patients on CAPD. Clin Nephrol 1983; 20:244–250.
13. Donati RM, Lange RD, Gallagher NI. Nephrogenic erythrocytosis. Arch Intern Med 1963; 112:960.

C. Timing and Characteristics of Multiple Peritonitis Episodes

Introduction

Peritonitis defined by the National CAPD registry as turbid dialysate with white blood count greater than 100 cells/mm^3 is the major complication from continuous ambulatory peritoneal dialysis (CAPD). Peritoneal infections can be recurrent and are the most frequently cited cause for electively terminating CAPD without transplantation. This report will focus on multiple incidents of peritonitis, culture results and associated reasons for terminating therapy. In addition, a partial logistic likelihood model will be used to analyze the tri-annual follow-up periods to determine risk factors for recurrent peritonitis.

Methods

The cohort of all Class 1 patients initiating CAPD between 1/1/84 and 6/30/86 was selected. Tri-annual, continuous follow-up was included only through August 1986 when a change in follow-up forms was implemented. A total of 6,335 patients with 17,653 follow-up periods are included in the following analyses. Fifty-four percent of the patients are male, 76% are white, 48% had prior ESRD therapy and 29% entered with a diagnosis of diabetic glomulerosclerosis. The median patient age at entry was 54 with 4.2% under age 21 and 23.9% over the age of 64.

A partial logistic likelihood approach [1,2] has been used to estimate the probability Pij of an individual i developing a peritonitis episode in a tri-annual follow-up period j by letting;

$$\ln \frac{P_{ij}}{1-P_{ij}} = \ln \lambda_j + \underline{\beta} \ Z_{ij}.$$

84

The probability of infection as related to both fixed covariates (age, sex, etc) and time-varying covariates (infection history) is parameterized by β with covariate information included in Z_{ij}. The parameter λ_j represents the baseline risk of infection in the jth period.

Results

A total of 6,528 peritonitis episodes were reported with a maximum of 12 infections occurring in any individual. Nearly half of the peritonitis events $(2990/6528 = 45.8\%)$ were initial episodes; there were 1557 (23.9%) second, 891 (13.6%) third, and 499 (7.6%) fourth episodes recorded. Of the 499 patients with 4 peritonitis episodes, only 88 patients proceeded to have 7 or more infections during this period. Exhibit 1 displays the cumulative peritonitis distributions for times to first through fourth peritonitis episodes. The time to second peritonitis episode is measured from the first peritonitis date and a similar definition is used for subsequent episodes. Note that patients with multiple peritonitis episodes are included in multiple curves so that these distributions are not statistically independent. We observe that times to infection are shorter for the patients with successive peritonitis episodes.

EXHIBIT 1

CUMULATIVE PROBABILITY OF EXPERIENCING
AN EPISODE OF PERITONITIS BY EPISODE NUMBER

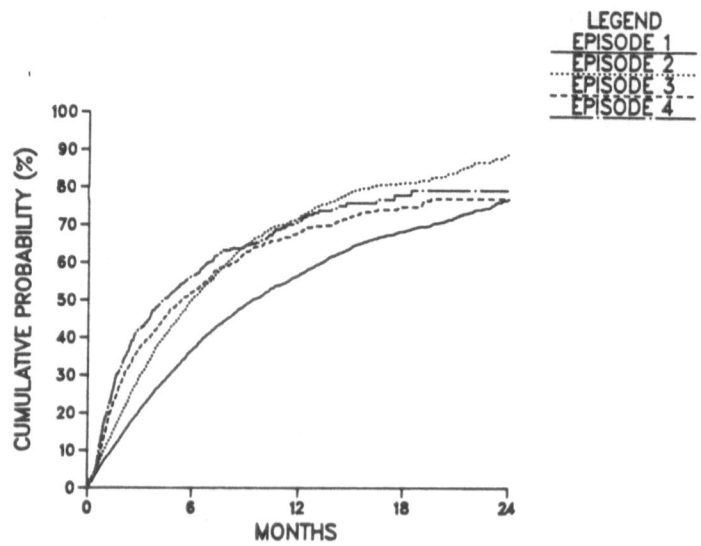

EXHIBIT 2

PERITONITIS CULTURE RESULTS FROM THE FIRST FOUR EPISODES

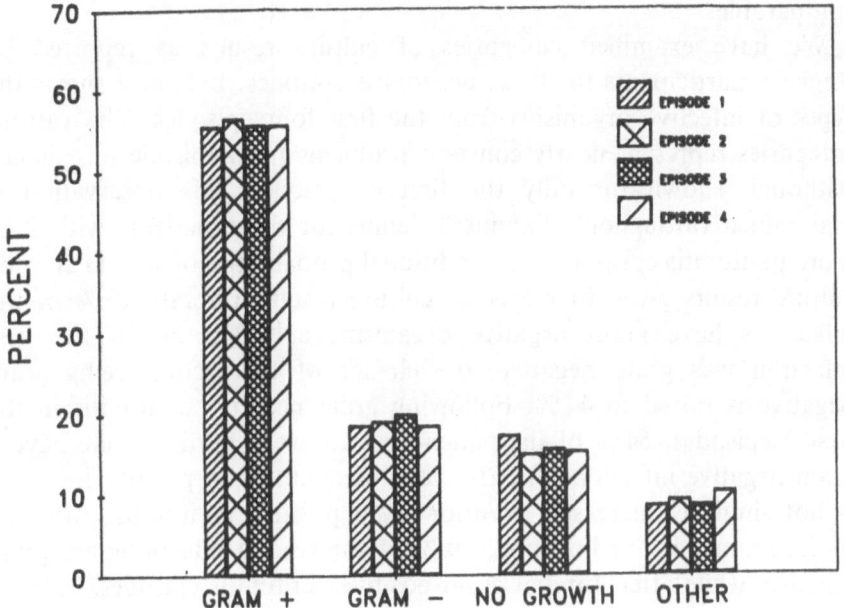

EXHIBIT 3

CONDITIONAL PROBABILITIES OF
SECOND PERITONITIS CULTURE CATEGORIZATIONS
BY FIRST EPISODE CULTURE CATEGORIES

First Episode	Gram +	Gram -	Second Episode No Growth	Other	Total
Gram +					
Frequency	621	116	100	47	884
Percent	70.3	13.1	11.3	5.3	100
Gram -					
Frequency	100	132	34	36	302
Percent	33.1	43.7	11.3	11.9	100
No Growth					
Frequency	122	38	89	24	273
Percent	44.7	13.9	32.6	8.8	100
Other					
Frequency	37	12	12	37	98
Percent	37.8	12.2	12.2	37.8	100
Total					
Frequency	880	298	235	144	1557
Percent	56.5	19.1	15.1	9.2	

Median time to first peritonitis is 9.4 months as opposed to 6.0, 5.4 and 4.3 months for the second through fourth episodes. Note that because of changing patient population groups, these medians are not directly comparable.

We have examined categories of culture results as reported by Registry participants for these peritonitis episodes. Exhibit 2 shows the types of infective organisms from the first four episodes. The various categories represent nearly constant problems from episode to episode. Although shown for only the first 4 episodes, this observation is maintained throughout. Exhibit 3 details for those patients with 2 or more peritonitis episodes, the conditional probabilities of second episode culture results given first episode culture results. Overall, 19% of the infections have gram negative organisms cultured; but if the first infection was gram negative, the chance of the second being gram negative is raised to 44%. Following gram negative peritonitis in the first 2 episodes, 64% of the patients who have a third episode have a gram negative infection. The risk of subsequent gram positive infection is not similarly increased by prior gram positive peritonitis. After an initial gram positive infection, 70% of the second infections are gram positive, while after 2 initial gram positive peritonitis episodes, 71% of third episodes are gram positive. Fungal infections are present in only 2.7% of the first episodes but following an initial fungal infection, 50% of recurrent infections culture positive for fungus. The median time to these second fungal infections was 2 months.

Exhibit 4 details for patients transferring to hemodialysis or IPD, or leaving dialysis without return of kidney function, their reasons for

EXHIBIT 4

REASONS FOR TRANSFER TO HEMODIALYSIS, IPD OR
EXITING DIALYSIS WITH NO RETURN OF KIDNEY FUNCTION
BY NUMBER OF PERITONITIS EPISODES (PERCENT)

| Reason for Transfer | # of Peritonitis Episodes | | | | | |
	0 (n=491)	1 (n=285)	2 (n=160)	3 (n=119)	≥4 (n=142)	Total (n=1197)
CAPD not able to meet fluid/biochemical standards	11	5	5	6	2	7
Other medically indicated reasons	18	9	7	5	6	12
Non compliance with technical excessive peritonitis	4	31	43	46	55	26
Patient/family choice	20	12	7	9	6	14
Catheter complications	11	12	9	5	6	10
Other or unknown	36	31	29	29	26	32

terminating CAPD by their number of peritonitis episodes. Peritonitis or noncompliance with technique is the leading overall reason for CAPD transfer being the cause of transfer in 26% of the patients. There is a steady increase in this cause as the number of episodes of peritonitis increases such that > 40% of therapy changes in patients with 2 or more episodes are attributed to this problem. Patient and family choice and other medically indicated reasons are the alternatives usually selected as cause for leaving in the patient who has not experienced peritonitis.

Exhibit 5 describes the reasons for terminating CAPD, i.e., transfer, transplantation, or death, by number of peritonitis episodes experienced. CAPD is seen to end in a transfer to other replacement therapy more frequently after multiple episodes of peritonitis. Transplantation, when it occurs, happens in 68% (437/643) of patients prior to a peritonitis episode.

Exhibit 6 shows the number of patients developing peritonitis, the number at risk in each 4 month follow-up period, and the percentage of patients developing an infection. Note that the risk in each period ranges from .26 to .29. A single parameter reflecting a constant period effect was used in the partial logistic model. Sex, race and diagnosis of diabetic glomerulosclerosis were separately examined and only race was found to be significantly related to peritonitis risk. Each of the other variates resulted in estimated risk of peritonitis which varied less than 1% for the different categorizations. When age was grouped as under 21, 21–64 and over 64, the youngest age was found to have an increased risk of peritonitis. It was hypothesized that peritonitis in a given period would predispose to an increase risk of peritonitis in the next 4 month period. Such an effect was observed to be highly statistically significant ($p < .0001$). An alternative formulation whereby an individual was

EXHIBIT 5

CAPD TERMINATION BY PERITONITIS
EPISODE FREQUENCY (PERCENT)

| | # of Peritonitis Episodes | | | | | |
	0	1	2	3	≥4	Total
Transfer	491(32)	285(47)	160(54)	119(62)	142(64)	1197(42)
Transplant	437(29)	122(20)	34(11)	21(11)	29(13)	643(23)
Death	600(39)	197(33)	103(35)	51(27)	50(23)	1001(35)
Total	1528(100)	604(100)	297(100)	191(100)	221(100)	2841(100)

EXHIBIT 6

SUMMARY OF PERITONITIS RESULTS
FOR 4 MONTH FOLLOW-UP PERIODS

		At Risk	Number with Peritonitis	Crude Peritonitis Rate
Period	1	6327	1635	.26
	2	4359	1240	.28
	3	2833	807	.28
	4	1860	526	.28
	5	1114	321	.29
	6	664	176	.27
	7	348	101	.29
	8	125	35	.28

EXHIBIT 7

MODEL SUMMARY

Parameter	Definition	Estimate	SE	Implication
		.286	.022	Baseline Risk of .22
$\beta 1$	Age <21	.186	.084	Increase Baseline Risk to .26
$\beta 2$	Race-non white	.346	.039	Increase Baseline Risk to .29
$\beta 3$	Peritonitis in prior period	.906	.041	Increase Baseline Risk to .41

permanently assigned to the elevated risk category after their original peritonitis episode, though significant, was substantially less informative (i.e., lower likelihood) than the preceding model. Exhibit 7 shows the complete model, parametric estimates and their impact. Note that peritonitis in the previous period causes a 19% elevation in the baseline risk of peritonitis in the subsequent period. Age and race effects though significant are limited to a few percentage point increase in the probability of peritonitis.

Discussion

It is important to evaluate the effects of duration of CAPD on peritonitis rates and the effects of a peritonitis episode on the probabilities for a subsequent episode; this is essential for understanding comparisons of peritonitis rates from one program to another with different populations and in designing studies to demonstrate the impact of connection devices on peritonitis rates. Studies to evaluate new devices consist of a variety of methodological designs [3–16]. The proportions of more experienced patients or the proportions of patients who have experienced peritonitis in any population group might influence respective peritonitis rates.

In this study the overall crude peritonitis rate during each consecutive follow-up period remained nearly constant. On the other hand, the time to first peritonitis is longer than the time between subsequent episodes. Thus, during each follow-up the transfers of patients from the therapy and departures for other reasons must have maintained the distributions of the populations at risk in fairly fixed proportions. The studies suggest that historical controls are not that unreasonable provided that the population remains relatively constant in terms of the proportions of patients with previous peritonitis experiences and those that are black and/or less than 21 years of age. On the other hand, transfers or departures from therapy during the historical control period could change the risks of developing peritonitis in the remaining population. A previous prospective randomized controlled study of a new connection device followed both a control and an eventual study population during a prolonged historical control period before randomization to the new device [16]. Both groups showed a reduction in peritonitis rate following the randomization and the beginning of the study period. The control group continued to use the standard technique during the study period. The decrease in peritonitis rate in controls may have been, at least in part, due to the vigorous retraining of the control population to match the training exposure of the group assigned to the new device. Concerns have been expressed in the literature concerning the use of historical controls only [17].

Once peritonitis occurs, the median time to a subsequent episode of peritonitis is shorter than the time to the original episode. Thus, it is important to remember that even prospective comparisons of parallel groups could be influenced by differences in drop out rates resulting in changes in the proportions of patients with different cumulative peritonitis experiences. Studies looking at the probability of developing a first peritonitis episode consisting entirely of new patients without any previous peritonitis experience may yield quite different results from populations that monitor peritonitis rates in groups consisting of patients with different degrees of peritonitis experience.

This study clearly demonstrates that increases in the number of peritonitis episodes result in higher percentages of transfers related to the problem of excessive peritonitis.

This study does not attempt to distinguish which recurrences might be relapses. Certainly the reporting centers thought that each episode reported was new and distinct, but as the time interval shortens between episodes this is very difficult to determine. This is particularly so since the culture results are very similar regardless of the number of the episode. The high probabilities for a subsequent episode to have organisms similar to the previous episode may in part relate to relapses. This is particularly so with the problem of fungal peritonitis. The observations of increased tendency for subsequent gram negative infection following initial gram negative infection indicates the increasing importance of early broad spectrum antibiotic coverage in these cases.

Many patients in our study were using newer connection devices-most likely increasing percentages in later follow-up periods. Should newer connection devices reduce the incidence of peritonitis, it is possible that the time intervals between progressive episodes would have been different (presumably even shorter) if all patients used only the standard manual technique.

References

1. Arjas E and Haara P. A marked point process approach to censored failure data with complicated covariates. Scand J Stat 1984; 11:193.
2. Slud EV. Efficiences of partial-likelihood-based inferences concerning survival regression models. Submitted for publication.
3. Maiorca R, Cantaluppi A, Cancarini GC, et al. Prospective controlled trial of a Y-connector and disinfectant to prevent peritonitis in continuous ambulatory peritoneal dialysis. Lancet 1983; 2:642.
4. Maiorca R, Cantaluppi A, Cancarini GC, et al. Y connector system for presentation of peritonitis in CAPD. Proc EDTA 1983; 20:223.
5. Cantaluppi A, Scalamogna A, Castelnovo C, et al. Peritonitis prevention in continuous ambulatory peritoneal dialysis: Long-term efficacy of a Y-connector and disinfectant. Peritoneal Dial Bull 1986 Apr-Jun; 6(2):58.
6. Verger C, Luzar MA. In vitro study of CAPD Y-line systems. Proceedings of the Sixth Annual CAPD Conference, Kansas City, Missouri, February 1986. Advances in Continuous Ambulatory Peritoneal Dialysis. Toronto: University of Toronto Press, 1986:160.
7. Buoncristiani U, Quintaliani G, Cozzari M, Carobi C. Current status of the Y set. Proceedings of the Sixth Annual CAPD Conference, Kansas City, Missouri, February 1986. Advances in Continuous Ambulatory Peritoneal Dialysis. Toronto: University of Toronto Press, 1986:165.
8. Maiorca R, Cancarini GC, Colombrita D, Camerini C. Further experience with Y-system in continuous ambulatory peritoneal dialysis. Proceedings of the Sixth Annual CAPD Conference, Kansas City, Missouri, February 1986. Advances in

Continuous Ambulatory Peritoneal Dialysis. Toronto: University of Toronto Press, 1986:172.

9. Maiorca R, Cancarini GC, Manili L, Camerini C. Effectiveness of an inline disinfection and wash-out (Y-system) in reducing peritonitis rates in CAPD. A long-term experience. Proceedings of the Sixth Annual CAPD Conference, Kansas City, Missouri, February 1986. Advances in Continuous Ambulatory Peritoneal Dialysis. Toronoto: University of Toronto Press, 1986:176.

10. Cantaluppi A, Scalamogna A, Castelnovo C, Graziani G. Long-term efficacy of a Y-connector and disinfectant to prevent peritonitis in continuous ambulatory peritoneal dialysis. Proceedings of the Sixth Annual CAPD Conference, Kansas City, Missouri, February 1986. Advances in Continuous Ambulatory Peritoneal Dialysis. Toronto: University of Toronto Press, 1986:182.

11. Hamilton RW. The sterile connection device: A review of its development and status report 1986. Sixth Annual CAPD Conference, Kansas City, Missouri, February 1986. Advances in Continuous Ambulatory Peritoneal Dialysis. Toronto: University of Toronto Press, 1986:186.

12. Perras, ST, Zappacosta AR. Reduction of peritonitis with patient education and the travenol CAPD germicidal exchange device. ANNA J 1986; 13:219.

13. Trooskin SZ, Donetz AP, Baxter J, et al. Infection-resistant continuous peritoneal dialysis catheters. Nephron 1987 Jul; 46(3):263.

14. Winchester JF, Ash SR, Bousquet G, et al. Successful peritonitis reduction with a unidirectional bacteriologic CAPD filter. Trans Am Soc Artif Intern Organs 1983 Apr; 29:611–616.

15. Slingeneyer A, Mion C. Peritonitis prevention in continuous ambulatory peritoneal dialysis: Long-term efficacy of a bacteriological filter. Proc Eur Dial Transplant Assoc 1983; 19:388–396.

16. Multi-center Study Group: A randomized multicenter clinical trial to evaluate the effects of an ultraviolet germicidal system on peritonitis rate in continuous ambulatory peritoneal dialysis. Peritoneal Dial Bull 1985 Jan-Mar; 5(1):19–24.

17. Nolph KD. A reminder of the lessons learned from the multicenter UV trial. Letter to the Editor. Peritoneal Dial Bull 1985 Jul-Sep; 5(3):203–206.

D. Geographical Distribution of Registry Coverage

Introduction

Coverage of the CAPD patient population in the United States by the National CAPD Registry has grown considerably since the Registry began in1981, as reported elsewhere in this publication. However, an assessment of the consistency of Registry coverage across the U.S. has never been performed. Also lacking is an understanding of the differences between participating and non-participating institutions. The report which follows details the extent of CAPD/CCPD patient and center coverage by describing Registry coverage within state and region. In addition, patient population and facility characteristics of participating centers are compared with nonparticipating centers that offer CAPD.

Subjects and Methods

Data provided by the Health Care Financing Administration (HCFA)[1] were used to estimate the number of CAPD/CCPD patients and peritoneal dialysis sites in the United States. The HCFA database was current through December 31, 1985 and contained information on 1430 renal facilities. Of these, 20 were located in U.S. territories and were excluded from all analyses. Fifteen Veterans Administration hospitals were also excluded as HCFA does not routinely report on VA hospitals. Of the remaining 1395 sites, 905 (65%) offered CAPD (or had at least 1 CAPD/CCPD patient) and were included in the analysis.

The National CAPD Registry had 492 centers as of February 28, 1987. Of these, 36 were VA hospitals and were excluded from all analyses. Twelve more were unable to be matched to a center in the HCFA database; 10 were not in the HCFA database, 1 was missing all identifying information except facility name, and the other had not submitted data to the Registry Coordinating Center for more than one year. These centers were also excluded. The remaining 444 centers were matched to centers in the HCFA database. There were 10 instances of two Registry centers mapping to a single HCFA center, and 3 instances of two HCFA centers mapping to a single Registry center. These duplications are due to centers who report separately to the Registry but report as one to HCFA, or vice versa. For example, a single center with two sites for seeing patients (e.g., adults versus pediatrics) might report to the Registry as two centers and report to HCFA as one. Multiple centers were collapsed leaving 437 Registry centers for the analysis. Of these 437 centers, 341 were in the Registry as of December 31, 1985, and the analysis of the extent of Registry coverage was based on these 341 centers and their 6,094 patients who were receiving CAPD on December 31, 1985.

For the comparison of patient population and facility characteristics between participating and non-participating centers, the 905 HCFA centers that offered CAPD (or had at least 1 CAPD/CCPD patient) were broken into 3 groups: N = 341 centers in the Registry as of Dec. 31, 1985 (Old Registry); N = 96 centers entering the Registry after Dec. 31, 1985 (New Registry); and the N = 468 centers that never participated in the Registry (Never Registry).

Coverage

Center coverage by the Registry within state was determined by dividing the number of centers offering CAPD within a state by the number of Registry centers within that state. Patient coverage within a state was similarly defined, and the process was repeated to determine coverage within region.

Results

The results of the analysis of Registry center and patient coverage within state are shown in Exhibits 1 and 2 respectively. Maps illustrating center coverage (Exhibit 3) and patient coverage (Exhibit 4) within state are also provided. Patient coverage was greater than center coverage in most states. Inconsistent results (e.g., coverage > 100 percent) were due to reporting differences. For example, a patient might have been registered with the Registry prior to being picked up by the HCFA database.

EXHIBIT 1

REGISTRY CENTER COVERAGE AS OF DECEMBER 31, 1985
WITHIN STATE

State	# of Registry Centers	# of HCFA Centers	% Registry Coverage
Alabama	5	23	21.7
Alaska	0	0	0.0
Arizona	8	16	50.0
Arkansas	2	13	15.4
California	67	118	56.8
Colorado	6	9	66.7
Connecticut	13	16	81.3
Delaware	1	2	50.0
District of Columbia	2	8	25.0
Florida	16	58	27.6
Georgia	10	37	27.0
Hawaii	1	7	14.3
Idaho	1	1	100.0
Illinois	9	43	20.9
Indiana	9	12	75.0
Iowa	3	8	37.5
Kansas	2	5	40.0
Kentucky	4	10	40.0
Louisiana	3	16	18.8
Maine	0	4	0.0
Maryland	6	21	28.6
Massachusetts	5	20	25.0
Michigan	15	27	55.6
Minnesota	2	8	25.0
Mississippi	2	10	20.0
Missouri	9	21	42.9
Montana	3	4	75.0
Nebraska	2	3	66.7
Nevada	3	4	75.0
New Hampshire	.1	4	25.0
New Jersey	4	19	21.1
New Mexico	3	8	37.5
New York	15	58	25.9
North Carolina	5	14	35.7
North Dakota	0	4	0.0
Ohio	14	27	51.9
Oklahoma	7	9	77.8
Oregon	6	9	66.7
Pennsylvania	20	63	31.7
Rhode Island	2	4	50.0
South Carolina	1	14	7.1
South Dakota	1	2	50.0
Tennessee	7	19	36.8
Texas	18	56	32.1
Utah	0	6	0.0
Vermont	1	1	100.0
Virginia	10	27	37.0
Washington	2	9	22.2
West Virginia	3	9	33.3
Wisconsin	12	18	66.7
Wyoming	0	1	0.0
Total	341	905	37.7

EXHIBIT 2

REGISTRY PATIENT COVERAGE AS OF DECEMBER 31, 1985
WITHIN STATE

State	# of Registry Patients	# of HCFA Patients	% Registry Coverage
Alabama	114	264	43.2
Alaska	0	0	0.0
Arizona	166	242	68.6
Arkansas	27	152	17.8
California	649	899	72.2
Colorado	166	165	101.0
Connecticut	123	217	56.7
Delaware	30	34	88.2
District of Columbia	50	104	48.1
Florida	223	459	48.6
Georgia	111	417	26.6
Hawaii	13	45	28.9
Idaho	18	17	106.0
Illinois	149	376	39.6
Indiana	439	618	71.0
Iowa	48	153	31.4
Kansas	33	138	23.9
Kentucky	158	211	74.9
Louisiana	44	133	33.1
Maine	0	27	0.0
Maryland	72	223	32.3
Massachusetts	162	264	61.4
Michigan	447	672	66.5
Minnesota	80	125	64.0
Mississippi	22	157	14.0
Missouri	232	341	68.0
Montana	46	56	82.1
Nebraska	29	128	22.7
Nevada	41	46	89.1
New Hampshire	0	34	0.0
New Jersey	83	465	17.8
New Mexico	35	87	40.2
New York	354	856	41.4
North Carolina	212	493	43.0
North Dakota	0	8	0.0
Ohio	289	564	51.2
Oklahoma	115	137	83.9
Oregon	140	203	69.0
Pennsylvania	307	685	44.8
Rhode Island	26	31	83.9
South Carolina	6	130	4.6
South Dakota	8	9	88.9
Tennessee	174	311	55.9
Texas	238	681	34.9
Utah	0	42	0.0
Vermont	18	21	85.7
Virginia	90	285	31.6
Washington	13	69	18.8
West Virginia	73	126	57.9
Wisconsin	221	264	83.7
Wyoming	0	2	0.0
Total	6094	12186	50.0

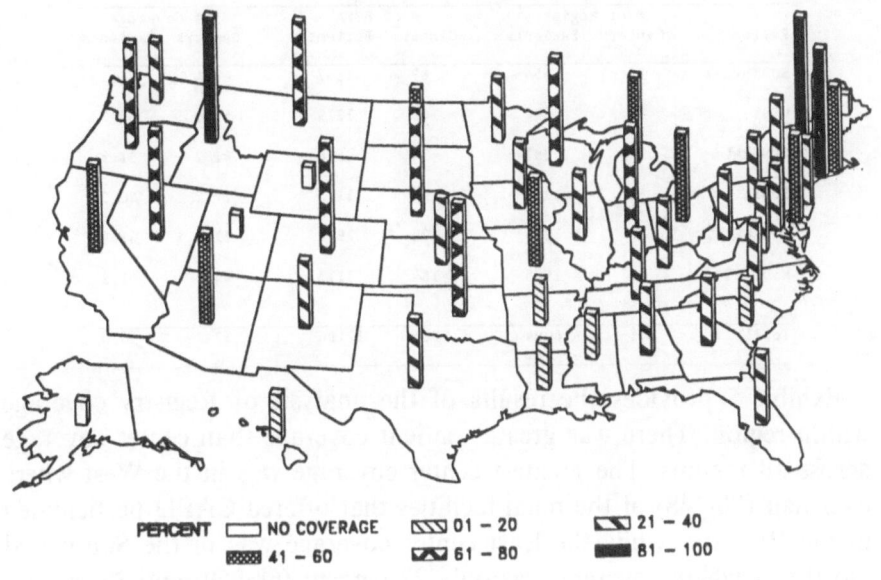

EXHIBIT 3

PERCENT OF HCFA PERITONEAL DIALYSIS SITES
PARTICIPATING IN THE CAPD REGISTRY WITHIN STATE

PERCENT ☐ NO COVERAGE   ▨ 01 – 20   ◩ 21 – 40
▩ 41 – 60   ▨ 61 – 80   ■ 81 – 100

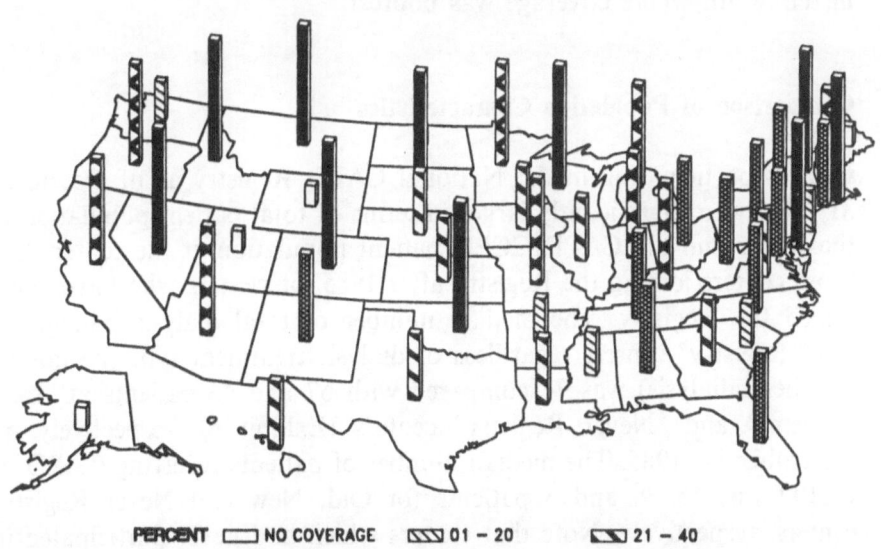

EXHIBIT 4

PERCENT OF HCFA CAPD/CCPD PATIENTS
IN THE CAPD REGISTRY WITHIN STATE

PERCENT ☐ NO COVERAGE   ▨ 01 – 20   ◩ 21 – 40
▩ 41 – 60   ▨ 61 – 80   ■ 81 – 100

EXHIBIT 5

REGISTRY CENTER AND PATIENT COVERAGE
AS OF DECEMBER 31, 1985 WITHIN REGION

Region	# of Registry		# of HCFA		% Coverage	
	Centers	Patients	Centers	Patients	Centers	Patients
SOUTHWEST	36	554	89	1147	40.4	48.3
WEST	80	874	148	1279	54.1	68.3
CENTRAL	14	282	34	548	41.2	51.5
SOUTH	68	1254	250	3138	27.2	40.0
NORTHEAST	70	1225	220	2961	31.8	41.4
MIDWEST	73	1905	164	3113	44.5	61.2
Total	341	6094	905	12186	37.7	50.0

Exhibit 5 provides the results of the analysis of Registry coverage within region. There was greater patient coverage than center coverage across all regions. The greatest center coverage was in the West where over half (80/148) of the renal facilities that offered CAPD participated in the Registry, while the least center coverage was in the South and Northeast where coverage was only 27 percent (68/250) and 32 percent (70/220) respectively. The greatest patient coverage was in the West, 68 percent (874/1279), and Midwest, 61 percent (1905/3113), and the least patient coverage was again in the South, 40 percent (1254/3138), and Northeast, 41 percent (1225/2961). It should be noted that the largest pool of centers and patients available to participate in the Registry was in the South where coverage was poorest.

Comparison of Population Characteristics

Centers participating in the National CAPD Registry as of December 31, 1985 were significantly larger in terms of total patient population at the center and the CAPD/CCPD patient population at the center than those centers joining the Registry after 1985, or centers who have never joined the Registry. The median number of total dialysis patients at 'Old Registry' centers regardless of dialysis treatment type (peritoneal and hemodialysis) was 74 compared with 57 and 46 patients at 'New Registry' and 'Never Registry' centers (Exhibit 6), respectively on December 31, 1985. The median number of patients receiving CAPD or CCPD was 15, 9, and 3 patients for Old, New and Never Registry centers, respectively. Note that centers which had never participated in the Registry were the smallest, both in terms of total patient population

EXHIBIT 6

COMPARISON OF PATIENT POPULATION CHARACTERISTICS
BY REGISTRY PARTICIPATION CATEGORY

Characteristic	Old Registry n=341	New Registry n=96	Never Registry n=468
Median # of Patients	74	57	46
Median # CAPD/CCPD Patients	15	9	3
% CAPD/CCPD Patients	22	14	8

receiving dialysis at the center as well as the total number of patients receiving CAPD or CCPD at the center.

'Old Registry' centers tended to have a higher proportion of patients treated by CAPD or CCPD compared to centers who joined the Registry after 1985 or centers who never joined the Registry. Twenty-two percent of ESRD patients at 'Old Registry' centers utilized CAPD or CCPD while only 14% of patients at 'New Registry' centers and 8% of 'Never Registry' centers were CAPD/CCPD patients.

Comparison of Facility Characteristics

Centers were classified as hospitals or free-standing renal facilities and were also classified by type of ownership as for-profit, not-for-profit, or

EXHIBIT 7

FACILITY CHARACTERISTICS
BY REGISTRY PARTICIPATION CATEGORY

Facility Type	Old Registry + New Registry n %	Never Registry n %	Total n %
Hospital	241 (55)	184 (39)	425 (47)
Free Standing	196 (45)	284 (61)	480 (53)
Total	437 (100)	468 (100)	905 (100)
Type of Ownership			
Government	58 (13)	40 (9)	98 (11)
Not For Profit	228 (52)	190 (41)	418 (46)
For Profit	151 (35)	238 (51)	389 (43)
Total	437 (100)	468 (100)	905 (100)

government. Facility type and type of ownership were compared across the three categories of Registry participation defined above. The distribution of facility type and type of ownership were very similar for centers parti- cipating prior to Dec. 31, 1985 and those joining after Dec. 31, 1985 and they were collapsed in the following discussion.

Exhibit 7 presents the results of the comparison of participating and non-participating centers with respect to type of ownership and facility type. Registry centers were more likely to be located at a hospital than non-Registry centers, as 55% (241/437) of the Registry centers were hospital based as opposed to 39% (184/468) of non-Registry centers. In addition, Registry centers tended to be not-for-profit (52%) or government owned (13%), whereas non-Registry centers were more likely to be for-profit (51%, 238/468). It should be noted, however, that 79 percent (378/480) of free-standing renal facilities were for-profit and 96 percent (414/425) of hospitals were either government or not-for-profit.

Discussion

This study was essentially explorative and descriptive. There were, however, a few findings worth noting. The Registry appears to be broadening its coverage by attracting smaller centers (in terms of patient population) as the larger centers tended to be early participants. The consistency of coverage across the U.S. provided by the National CAPD Registry is fairly uniform, although the South appears to be a region with a lower than expected participation rate. Unfortunately, it is this region of underrepresentation that offers the Registry the largest pool of potential centers and patients.

There are, also, considerable differences in the participation rates of for-profit and not-for-profit institutions, and, in a related finding, in the participation rates of hospitals and free-standing renal facilities. Although the relationship is not completely understood, the reader should note that participation in the National CAPD Registry is on a voluntary basis.

The relationship between regional coverage and type of ownership was not explored in this study but may be of interest in the future.

Reference

1. End-Stage Renal Disease (ESRD) Survey. Patient Management and Medical Information Systems. Bureau of Data Management and Strategy, Health Care Finance Administration, 1985.

E. Characteristics and Treatment Course of Long-term CAPD/CCPD Patients

Introduction

Peritoneal dialysis, which has been used as an acute therapy since the 1960's, was first attempted on a continuous basis by Popovich and Moncrief in 1976 [1]. In October 1981, the National CAPD Registry began collecting information regarding the number of patients receiving CAPD and/or CCPD therapy, their characteristics, the extent of some of the more important treatment-related complications, and selected outcomes to therapy. With continued follow-up by the Registry, the cohort of patients who have continuously remained on CAPD or CCPD for 3 or more years has steadily grown. These so called 'long-term' CAPD/CCPD users are of potential clinical significance and form the basis of the report which follows.

Subjects and Methods

All Class I Registry patients who were registered in 1984 or before were considered in this analysis. Patients who had received CAPD and/or CCPD for 3 or more years are designated as 'long-term' users while patients who had utilized CAPD and/or CCPD for less than 3 years are referred to as 'short-term' users. Patients who registered after 1984 were not included in this latter group as they would not have had the opportunity to remain on CAPD/CCPD for 3 or more years. In addition, only patients who had continuous follow-up by the Registry were included.

Complication rates per patient year and probability distribution of time to first peritonitis were calculated as described in Section 3 of this report.

EXHIBIT 1

NUMBER OF PATIENTS RECEIVING
CAPD/CCPD FOR 3 OR MORE YEARS
BY YEAR REGISTERED AND DURATION OF THERAPY

| CAPD/CCPD Duration | Year Registered | | | 1984 | Total |
	1981	1982	1983		
≥ 3, < 4 Years	49	130	177	422	778
≥ 4, < 5 Years	33	110	223	15	381
≥ 5, < 6 Years	28	149	10	0	187
≥ 6 Years	32	0	0	0	32
Total	142	389	410	437	1,378

EXHIBIT 2

PATIENT CHARACTERISTICS OF PATIENTS ON CAPD/CCPD
FOR 3 OR MORE YEARS AND LESS THAN 3 YEARS

Characteristics	CAPD/CCPD ≥ 3 years (n=1378)	CAPD/CCPD < 3 years (n=5783)
Sex (%)		
Male	54	55
Female	46	45
Race (%)		
White	74	77
Black	18	17
Other	8	6
Primary Renal Disease Type (%)		
Diabetic Glomerulosclerosis	18	27
Chronic Glomerulonephritis	22	17
Hypertensive Renal Disease	15	15
Interstitial Nephritis/chronic		
Pyelonephritis	7	8
Polycystic Kidney(s)	8	6
All other types	28	27
Therapy Type (%)		
CAPD	97	95
CCPD	3	5
CAPD and CCPD	<1	<1
Age (%)		
≤20	5	7
>20	95	93
Median Age	52 years	53 years
Prior ESRD Therapy (%)		
Yes	61	60
No	39	40

Results

Nineteen percent (1378/7161) of patients were reported to have been continuously receiving CAPD or CCPD for 3 or more years. Exhibit 1 details the distribution of these patients by year registered and duration of CAPD/CCPD use. Over half the 'long-term' patients have used CAPD/CCPD for at least 3 but less than 4 years. Thirty-two patients have continuously received CAPD/CCPD for at least 6 years.

Exhibit 2 provides a summary of the patient characteristics of the 1378 'long-term' (≥ 3 years) CAPD/CCPD users compared with the 5783 'short-term' (< 3 years) CAPD/CCPD users. Sex, race, therapy type, age, and prior ESRD therapy distributions among 'long-term' patients are similar to the distributions of 'short-term' patients. Primary renal disease diagnoses were notably different in the two groups. The 'long-term' cohort tended to have a lower percentage of diabetics (18% vs. 27%) and a corresponding higher percentage of patients whose primary renal disease type was diagnosed as Chronic Glomerulonephritis (22% vs. 17%).

Previous Registry reports have noted a trend of increasing numbers of patients diagnosed with Diabetic Glomerulosclerosis. To explore the effect of this trend on the distribution of diagnoses, 'long-term' and 'short-term' users were examined by year of registration. Within each

EXHIBIT 3

PERCENT OF PATIENTS WITH DIABETIC GLOMERULOSCLEROSIS
BY YEAR REGISTERED AND CAPD/CCPD DURATION

| CAPD/CCPD Duration | Year Registered | | | |
	1981	1982	1983	1984
< 3 Years	21	24	29	29
≥ 3 Years	16	17	20	19

PERCENT OF PATIENTS WITH CHRONIC GLOMERULONEPHRITIS
BY YEAR REGISTERED AND CAPD/CCPD DURATION

| CAPD/CCPD Duration | Year Registered | | | |
	1981	1982	1983	1984
< 3 Years	20	20	18	15
≥ 3 Years	17	23	25	20

year, 'long-term' users had a lower percentage of diabetics as compared with 'short-term' users (Exhibit 3).

Complication rates per patient year and probability distributions of the occurrence of a first event are not strictly comparable, as patients who terminate CAPD/CCPD prior to 3 years provide information only while on CAPD/CCPD. For example, patients who leave CAPD/CCPD to receive a kidney transplant (a favorable outcome) prior to three years can cause a bias in the calculation of rates and probability distributions on cohorts defined by time on CAPD/CCPD. The observations which follow are descriptive and are not intended for statistical comparisons.

'Long-term' patients experienced 1.0 peritonitis episodes per patient year (Exhibit 4). This rate was fairly constant regardless of whether the patient had been receiving CAPD/CCPD for 3, 4, 5, or 6 years. Of the thirty-two patients who have used CAPD/CCPD for 6 years, 44% (14/32) experienced an episode of peritonitis during their first year of therapy and 66% (21/32) reported a peritonitis episode in the last year. The peritonitis rate for 'short-term' patients was 1.6 episodes per patient year. Exit site/tunnel infections and catheter replacement rates were similar for the two cohorts.

EXHIBIT 4

SUMMARY OF COMPLICATION REPORTS
BY DURATION OF CAPD/CCPD USE

	Duration of CAPD/CCPD	
	≥ 3 years (n=1378)	< 3 years (n=5783)
Complication Rates Per Patient Year		
Peritonitis	1.0	1.6
Exit Site/Tunnel Infection	.5	.6
Catheter Replacement	.2	.3
Probability of First Peritonitis		
6 months	31	44
(95% C.I.)	(29,33)	(43,46)
12 months	51	64
(95% C.I.)	(48,53)	(62,66)
18 months	61	75
(95% C.I.)	(59,64)	(72,77)
24 months	71	83
(95% C.I.)	(69,74)	(81,85)
Median time to first peritonitis episode	11.7 months	7.3 months

Exhibit 4 lists the 6, 12, 18, and 24 month probabilities of experiencing a first episode of peritonitis and the corresponding 95% confidence intervals. In general, 'short-term' patients are expected to have experienced a first episode of peritonitis sooner than 'long-term' patients. The median time to first peritonitis is 11.7 months for 'long-term' patients and 7.3 months for 'short-term' patients. Recall, however, that the probability distribution estimated for short-term patients is biased because patients who leave CAPD/CCPD prior to experiencing a peritonitis episode contribute information only while receiving CAPD/CCPD.

Of the 1378 'long-term' patients, 56% (776) were continuing on CAPD/CCPD at last contact. Two hundred-eight reported transferring to hemodialysis, IPD or off all dialysis (Exhibit 5). The primary reason for these patients discontinuing CAPD/CCPD is tabulated in Exhibit 6.

EXHIBIT 5

LAST REPORTED STATUS OF PATIENTS ON CAPD/CCPD
FOR 3 OR MORE YEARS BY NUMBER OF YEARS ON THERAPY

Last Reported Status	Years on CAPD/CCPD				Total
	3	4	5	6	
Continuing on CAPD/CCPD	385	218	143	30	776
Transferred to Hemodialysis, IPD, or off Dialysis	136	57	14	1	208
Transplanted	56	14	1	0	71
Died	173	83	27	1	284
Transferred to a non-Registry Center	24	9	1	0	34
Status Unknown	4	0	1	0	5

EXHIBIT 6

PRIMARY REASON FOR TERMINATING CAPD/CCPD AND
TRANSFERRING TO HEMODIALYSIS, IPD, OR OFF ALL DIALYSIS

Primary Reason	N	% (n=208)
Excessive Peritonitis	67	32
Catheter Complication	12	6
Exit Site/Tunnel Infection	12	6
Patient/Family Choice	13	6
Fluid/Biochemical Inadequacy	9	4
Other Medical Reasons	33	16
Other	18	9
Unknown	44	21

Excessive peritonitis, as in the general CAPD Registry population, is the most common reason for transferring to another modality after having remained on CAPD/CCPD for 3 or more years.

Discussion

On April 29, 1988, at the Toronto Western Hospital, results in four patients who had been maintained on CAPD for more than 10 years were presented. A fifth patient was almost at the ten year mark. The NIH CAPD Registry began in 1981 and thus has had the opportunity to follow patients for a little over six years. The Registry has followed the course of 32 patients over six years or more of CAPD/CCPD therapy. A total of 1,378 patients have been continuously followed three years or more. Although, as we have documented, the majority of patients abandoned the therapy before three years for reasons of death, transfer, kidney transplantation or occasionally recovery of renal function, it is important to note that some patients persist on CAPD/CCPD beyond three years and even up to six years.

It is of interest to compare patients who remain on therapy three years or more to those who do not. The long-term patients included a smaller percentage of patients with diabetic nephropathy than the short-term cohorts registered over the same periods. This was true year by year for the registration years included in the study. Previous reports have shown diabetes to be associated with a slight increased risk of peritonitis but not for an increased risk of transfer. It is known that patients with diabetic nephropathy are at increased risk of death and this may explain why higher percentages of the short-termers had diabetes. We have also found that the long-term patients have lower peritonitis rates, reduced probabilities for developing the first episode of peritonitis, and a longer median time to first peritonitis than their short-term cohorts. The association between peritonitis rate and transfer has been documented elsewhere in this report and in previous reports. It is of note that sex, race, age, and prior ESRD therapy could not distinguish long-term patients from their short-term cohorts.

For patients who persisted on CAPD/CCPD for three years or more the most common reason for stopping therapy was death. Elsewhere in the report we have shown that most deaths are not related to the therapy per se and are often related to cardiovascular causes. Transfer was the second most common reason for eventual departure form CAPD/CCPD with excessive peritonitis as the most frequently indicated reason. Thus, although the peritonitis rates are relatively low with many years on therapy, the number of cumulative episodes and/or a very severe episode may trigger the decision to transfer.

Note that only 4% of the long-term patients who eventually transferred did so for reason of fluid or biochemical inadequacy. This is compatible with many clinical reports suggesting that most patients on CAPD/CCPD for several years have stable membrane transport parameters or slight increases in membrane permeability without major clinical consequences [2–4].

It is important to remember that this analysis focuses on patients registered prior to 1985. With the introduction of new devices that may reduce peritonitis rates, it is possible that higher percentages of patients will remain on CAPD/CCPD long-term and their distinguishing characteristics may be different than those reported in this study.

References

1. Popovich RP, Moncrief JW et al. The definition of a novel portable/ wearable equilibrium peritoneal dialysis technique. Abstr Am Soc Artif Intern Organs 1976; 5:64.
2. Krediet RT, Boeschoten EW, Zuyderhoudt FMJ, Arisz L. Peritoneal trans- port characteristics of water, low-molecular weight solutes and proteins during long-term CAPD. Peritoneal Dial Bull 1986 Apr-Jun; 6(2):61–65.
3. Ota K, Mineshima M, Watanabe N, Naganuma S. Functional deterioration of the peritoneum: does it occur in the absence of peritonitis? Neph Dial Transplant 1987; 2:30–34.
4. Randerson DH, Farrell PC. Long-term peritoneal clearance in CAPD. In: Atkins RC, Thomson NM, Farrell PC, eds. Peritoneal Dialysis. Edinburgh, London, Melbourne, and New York: Churchill Livingstone, 1981:22–29.

Special Reports—1987

A. Update on Children Who Use CAPD/CCPD *

Introduction

During the past few years, there has been an increasing interest in the experience of pediatric patients who have been enrolled in the National CAPD Registry. The results of a preliminary assessment of data routinely collected by the National CAPD Registry were presented in the 1986 report [1]. That report contained data which suggested that pediatric patients did not do as well as the pediatric nephrologists who care for them had expected, e.g. age < 20 years at CAPD initiation was found to be associated with increased risk of developing peritonitis and with early first hospitalization (relative risks 1.2 and 1.6, respectively).

Since that report, the number of pediatric clinical centers participating in the Registry has increased substantially, as have the number of pediatric patients in our files. The increase in the number of patients available for analysis provides the opportunity to examine the pediatric population more thoroughly. Accordingly, the analysis which follows details the characteristics, complications and outcomes of therapy for children receiving CAPD/CCPD, as a whole and by age group.

Subjects and Methods

Six hundred fifty-eight patients under the age of 21 at the time of CAPD/CCPD initiation, who had no prior CAPD/CCPD experience before being registered were available for analysis. Patient age was based

* The material contained in this report has been submitted for publications as follows: Alexander S, Lindblad AS, Nolph KD, Novak JW. Pediatric CAPD/CCPD in the United States. A review of the experiences of the National CAPD Registry's pediatric population for the period January 1, 1981 through August 31, 1986.

on age at first CAPD/CCPD exchange. Complication rates per patient year were calculated using standard epidemiologic techniques [2] and probability distributions for various complications and outcomes were estimated using the methods of Kaplan and Meier [3]. Covariate contributions were assessed using Cox's proportional hazard's model [4].

Results

Patients were grouped, by age, into 5 categories as follows: < 1 year, 1–4 years, 5–9 years, 10–14 years, and 15–20 years. Age distribution according to first treatment for end stage renal disease (ESRD), first CAPD/CCPD exchange and at last contact are given in Exhibit 1. Thirty- nine percent of patients began treatment for ESRD under the age of 10; 11% of patients who began CAPD/CCPD as a pediatric patient have since reached their 21st birthday.

Patient characteristics are detailed in Exhibit 2. Reports to the Registry suggest that pediatric patients are more likely than their adult counterparts to be placed on CCPD or a combination of CAPD/CCPD—as opposed to CAPD alone. Males dominate the pediatric cohort in the younger age groups (< 10 years), while females account for more of the patients in the 15–20 year old age group. While white patients account for 77% of the adults registered, only 72% of the pediatric patients were white. As might be expected, the percent of

EXHIBIT 1

ACE CROUP DISTRIBUTION OF CLASS 1 PEDIATRIC PATIENTS
ACCORDING TO TIMING OF AGE CALCULATION

Age Group	Age At Time Of:		
	First Treatment for ESRD N (%)	First CAPD/ CCPD Exchange N (%)	Last Contact N (%)
< 1 year	40 (6)	35 (5)	8 (1)
1–4 years	88 (13)	77 (12)	85 (13)
5–9 years	129 (20)	115 (17)	99 (15)
10–14 years	211 (32)	191 (29)	167 (25)
15–20 years	190 (29)	240 (36)	227 (34)
> 20 years	*	*	72 (11)
TOTAL	658 (100)	658 (100)	658 (100)

EXHIBIT 2

SELECTED PATIENT CHARACTERISTICS

	Age at First CAPD/CCPD Exchange						
Characteristic	<1 yr. (n=35)	1-4 yrs. (n=77)	5-9 yrs. (n=115)	10-14 yrs. (n=191)	15-20 yrs. (n=240)	Total Registry Pediatrics (n=658)	Total Registry Adults (n=11,834)
% CAPD	83	80	80	82	89	84	95
% Male	63	61	58	52	43	52	55
% White	66	73	77	70	71	72	77
% Prior ESRD Therapy	26	36	38	55	59	50	56

EXHIBIT 3

COMPLICATION RATES PER PATIENT YEAR FOR CLASS 1 PEDIATRIC PATIENTS
RECEIVING CAPD BY AGE AT CAPD INSTITUTIONS

Age Group:	Peritonitis	Exit Site/Tunnel	Catheter Replacement	Total Days Hospitalized	Days CAPD Hospitalized
< 1	1.7	.3	.4	28.9	9.6
1-4	1.5	.7	.7	26.0	13.2
5-9	1.4	.7	.4	28.7	11.6
10-14	1.6	.8	.4	20.1	9.6
15-20	1.4	.9	.3	16.1	6.5
Total Registry	1.3	.6	.3	20.7	8.1

patients treated with prior ESRD therapies is lower among pediatric patients than among adults.

Complication rates per patient year are summarized in Exhibit 3. In general, pediatric patients are reported to have more peritonitis, exit site/tunnel infections, and catheter replacements than Registry patients at large, and, total days hospitalized and total days hospitalized for CAPD related events are greater for pediatric patients than for adults.

Probability distributions of time to first event were calculated for each age group; and, one year probabilities and 95% confidence intervals for those probabilities are presented in Exhibit 4. Here again, it appears that pediatric patients tend to develop initial complications earlier in the course of their therapy than do adult Registry patients. The probability of a pediatric patient experiencing his/her first episode of peritonitis and exit site/tunnel infection at one year is .65 and .40, respectively; comparable probabilities for the adult cohort are .59 and .30, respec-

EXHIBIT 4

SELECTED PATIENT COMPLICATIONS

	Age at First CAPD/CCPD Exchange						
Complication	<1 yr. (n=35)	1-4 yrs. (n=77)	5-9 yrs. (n=115)	10-14 yrs. (n=191)	15-20 yrs. (n=240)	Total Registry Pediatrics (n=658)	Total Registry Adults (n=11,834)
First Peritonitis:							
1 year probability	.63	.59	.61	.67	.67	.65	.59
(95% C.I.)	(.37, .83)	(.39, .77)	(.55, .74)	(.57, .77)	(.57, .75)	(.59, .70)	(.57, .60)
First Exit Site/ Tunnel Inf.:							
1 year probability	.24	.30	.43	.41	.42	.40	.30
(95% C.I.)	(.09, .51)	(.17, .49)	(.28, .59)	(.30, .54)	(.33, .52)	(.34, .46)	(.29, .32)
First Catheter Replacement:							
1 year probability	.22	.20	.42	.24	.34	.30	.18
(95% C.I.)	(.08, .48)	(.05, .53)	(.25, .56)	(.14, .38)	(.25, .45)	(.24, .35)	(.17, .19)

tively. The probability of having at least one catheter replaced within the first year of treatment for pediatric patients is almost double that for adults (.30 vs. .18, respectively). However, it is noteworthy that patients under the age of 5 years appear to have experienced rates with CAPD/CCPD complications (i.e. peritonitis, exit site/tunnel infection, catheter replacement) which are more comparable to the adult cohort, than to those of older children and teenagers (> 5 years). This observation might be explained by concentrated adult involvement in the maintenance and operation of CAPD/CCPD procedures in younger children.

The risk of first peritonitis as a function of the number of pediatric patients at an institution was investigated. Only nine percent of centers joining the Registry prior to December 1, 1985 with pediatric patients, registered more than 10 patients who were 20 years of age or younger. However, those centers account for 42 percent of the pediatric cohort studied. Similarly, 4% of centers registered more than 20 patients, and those centers account for 27 percent of patients studied here (see Exhibit 5). Using a Cox proportional hazard's model, a reduced risk of developing first peritonitis was demonstrated for patients coming from centers who had registered more than 10 patients; and, that risk decreased further for patients coming from centers with more than 20 patients registered. Differences in pediatric patient load did not affect the probabilities of exit site/tunnel infections, catheter replacements, death, transfer, or transplantation.

Probabilities of terminating CAPD/CCPD due to transplantation,

EXHIBIT 5

PERCENT OF PEDIATRIC PATIENTS (n=510)
AND PERCENT OF CENTERS (n=170)
BY NUMBER OF PEDIATRIC PATIENTS REGISTERED

	Number of Pediatric Patients Registered	
	≤ 10 Ped. Patients	> 10 Ped. Patients
Percent Centers	91	9
Percent Patients	58	42
	≤ 20 Ped. Patients	> 20 Ped. Patients
Percent Centers	96	4
Percent Patients	73	27

Note: Only centers entering the Registry before December 1, 1985 were included.

EXHIBIT 6

SELECTED PATIENT OUTCOMES

Outcome	Age at First CAPD/CCPD Exchange						
	<1 yr. (n=35)	1-4 yrs. (n=77)	5-9 yrs. (n=115)	10-14 yrs. (n=191)	15-20 yrs. (n=240)	Total Registry Pediatrics (n=658)	Total Registry Adults (n=11,834)
Dying while on Registry:							
1 year probability	.22	.12	.06	.03	.03	.06	.17
(95% C.I.)	(.06, .52)	(.05, .28)	(.01, .32)	(.01, .07)	(.01, .10)	(.04, .10)	(.16, .18)
Transferring to Hemo, IPD, or off Dialysis:							
1 year probability	.05	.12	.09	.16	.24	.16	.20
(95% C.I.)	(.01, .42)	(.03, .33)	(.04, .20)	(.10, .25)	(.16, .29)	(.13, .21)	(.19, .21)
Transplanted:							
1 year probability	.17	.27	.31	.32	.23	.27	.09
(95% C.I.)	(.06, .39)	(.16, .42)	(.21, .43)	(.24, .42)	(.17, .29)	(.23, .32)	(.08, .10)

death, and transfer to an alternate dialysis technique are given in Exhibit 6. More than one quarter of the pediatric cohort is expected to have received a kidney transplant by the end of one year of CAPD/CCPD therapy, as opposed to less than 10% of the adult Registry population. Similarly, the probability of a pediatric death at one year is less than half that reported for adult patients registered. However, observed one year death probabilities are higher for children under 1 year of age, although the small number of patients in that group severely limits the reliability of the estimate (95% confidence interval width .46).

References

1. Report of the National CAPD Registry of the National Institutes of Health. January, 1986.
2. Kahn HA. An Introduction to Epidemiologic Methods. New York: Oxford University Press, 1983.
3. Kaplan E and Meier P. Nonparametric estimation from incomplete observations. J Am Stat Assoc 1958; 53:457–458.
4. Cox DR. Regression models and life tables. J Stat Soc B 1972; 34: 187–200.

B. First Exchange Device and Peritonitis among CAPD Patients

Introduction

Peritonitis is considered to be a major problem associated with CAPD replacement therapy. The National CAPD Registry has reported that 62% of patients using CAPD experienced their first episode of peritonitis during the first year of therapy [1]. An in depth analysis of risk factors associated with the development of the first episode of peritonitis has previously been reported on by the Registry [2]. Age, race, primary renal disease diagnosis, prior ESRD therapy, and living arrangement were identified as being associated with earlier episodes of this complication.

In 1984, the Registry began collecting data on types of exchange devices used by patients. As those data are now sufficiently mature, it is of interest to examine the potential effects of the type of exchange device on the incidence and timing of peritonitis episodes.

Subjects and Methods

A cohort of 4,538 patients form the basis of the analysis. All entered the Registry after 1983, began CAPD at the time of registration, and used a known type exchange device at the time of treatment initiation. Five types of exchange device were identified among study patients: manual system, in-line filter system, sterile weld device, ultra-violet system and unspecified other. Patients were grouped by exchange device based on the information provided to the Registry with patient's first status report. Patients for whom exchange device was unknown were excluded. Peritonitis data were analyzed only for initial exchange devices. As the exact date of transfer to a second exchange device was not recorded, peritonitis episodes occurring during the reporting period in which a change was reported were attributed to the initial exchange device. Equipment transfer rates and type of equipment chosen as the second exchange device were based on information provided at the time the change was reported.

Peritonitis rates per patient year were calculated over all and for eachtype of peritonitis for each exchange device. The probability distribution of remaining free of the first episode of peritonitis was estimated using the life table methods of Kaplan and Meier [3].

EXHIBIT 1

PERCENT OF PATIENTS WITH SELECTED PATIENT
CHARACTERISTICS BY EXCHANGE DEVICE

Patient Characteristics	Manual (n=3,178)	In-Line Filter (n=50)	Sterile Weld (n=38)	Ultra-Violet (n=1046)	Other (n=226)
Dialysis Method					
CAPD	98	86	100	99	87
CCPD	1	14	0	1	10
Both	1	0	0	0	3
Prior ESRD Therapy					
Yes	35	42	35	41	32
No	65	58	65	59	68
Diabetic Glomerulosclerosis					
Yes	22	22	22	36	40
No	78	78	78	64	60
Age					
< 20	5	6	0	3	4
20-39	24	12	21	25	23
40-59	38	36	28	35	41
60-69	22	34	32	24	22
≥ 70	11	12	19	14	10
Median age (yrs)	52	59	60	54	54
Living Arrangement					
With Family	87	89	86	86	91
Not With Family	13	11	14	14	9
Sex					
Male	54	58	60	54	54
Female	46	42	40	46	46
Race					
White	75	74	70	79	76
Black	19	22	20	12	19
Other	6	4	10	9	5

Results

Patient Characteristics

The majority of patients (70%) included in this study began CAPD/CCPD using the manual connection system. The ultra-violet system was used by 23% of patients, while the in-line filter system and sterile weld device together accounted for less than 2% of the equipment used at CAPD/CCPD initiation. Unspecified other exchange devices were used by 5% of the population studied (see Exhibit 1).

Patient characteristics are also presented in Exhibit 1. Age and sex distributions appear comparable among the manual, ultra-violet and other systems, patients using the in-line filter system and sterile weld device tend to be older than patients using either the manual or ultra-violet system. The median age of patients using the in-line filters is 59 years, while the median age for patients using the manual system is 52 years.

A comparison of transfers in exchange devices is given in Exhibit 2. Eighty-nine percent of patients who began CAPD/CCPD using the manual system remained on that system through last follow-up. Similarly, 96% and 95% of patients beginning therapy using the ultra-violet system and sterile weld device, respectively, had not transferred to another form of equipment at last report. Note that 50% of patients initially using the in-line filter system and 42% of patients using 'other' systems switched to a new exchange device. The manual system was the

EXHIBIT 2

PERCENT OF PATIENTS BY FIRST AND SECOND
EXCHANGE DEVICE REPORTED

First Reported Exchange Device	Second Reported Exchange Device				
	Manual	In-Line Filter	Sterile Weld	Ultra-Violet	Other
Manual (n = 3,178)	(89)	1	1	7	2
In-Line Filter (n = 50)	50	(50)	0	0	0
Sterile Weld (n = 38)	0	0	(95)	5	0
Ultra-violet (n = 1,046)	3	0	0	(96)	1
Other (n = 226)	31	1	0	10	(58)

NOTE: Percentages in parentheses pertain to patients who remained on the first type of device through last follow-up.

apparent equipment of choice following termination of the in-line filter system or unspecified other equipment. Note that patients using 'other' exchange devices were scored as a transfer only when they switched to the manual, in-line filter, sterile weld or ultra-violet exchange devices.

Peritonitis Rates

Peritonitis rates per patient year were calculated for each exchange device and by offending organism (see Exhibit 3). Rates were not compared statistically due to the correlation between multiple events within a patient. Note that estimates of peritonitis rates associated with use of the in-line filter system and sterile weld device are subject to substantial chance variation due to small sample sizes and limited patient years of follow-up. Additional follow-up should yield more reliable estimates. Available data indicate that patients using the in-line filter system at the time of CAPD/CCPD initiation, experienced more peritonitis episodes on a yearly basis than patients beginning

EXHIBIT 3

PERITONITIS RATE PER PATIENT YEAR BY FIRST EXCHANGE
DEVICE AND TYPE OF PERITONITIS

		Exchange Device			
	Manual	In-Line Filter	Sterile Weld	Ultra-Violet	Other
Number of Patients	3178	50	38	1046	226
Patient Years	2781	24	21	756	162
Peritonitis Organism					
Any fungal	.03	.00	.10	.03	.03
Gram +	.70	.65	.39	.62	.83
Gram −	.24	.29	.24	.18	.25
Both GR+ GR−	.03	.08	.00	.05	.03
Other organism	.02	.08	.05	.01	.00
Cultured:No growth	.22	.33	.29	.20	.19
No culture	.02	.04	.00	.03	.02
Total	1.26	1.47	1.07	1.12	1.35

CAPD/CCPD with any other device. This result was observed across all types of peritonitis with the exception of those involving gram positive and fungal organisms.

The ultra-violet and manual systems were similar with respect to the rate of fungal infections. Fewer gram positive and gram negative infections were seen among patients using the ultra-violet system; and, the sterile weld device had the lowest rate of gram positive infections per patient year of observation. However, we must repeat that caution should be used when interpreting these results, due to the small sample sizes that are involved.

Exhibit 4 illustrates the probability of remaining peritonitis free for patients using the manual and ultra-violet system. The median time to first peritonitis was 9.8 months for patients using the manual system and 11.7 months for patients using the ultra-violet system.

Discussion

Devices such as those mentioned in this study are designed to prevent intraluminal contamination; they were not intended to prevent perilumi-

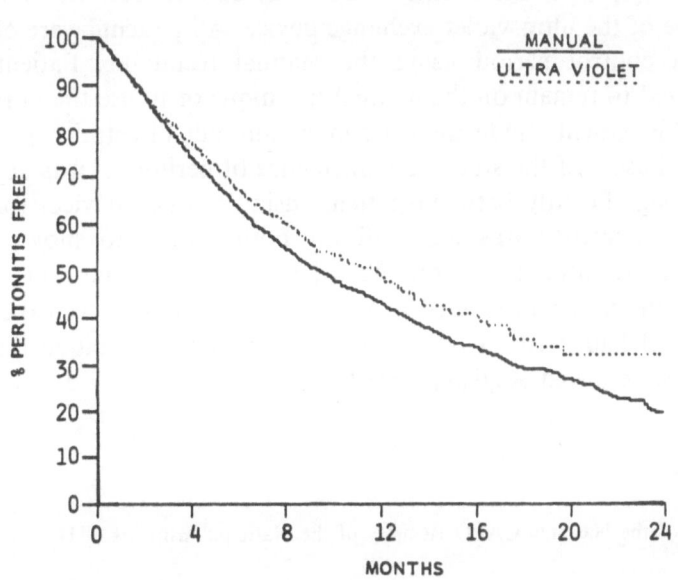

EXHIBIT 4

PROBABILITY OF REMAINING
PERITONITIS FREE BY TYPE OF EQUIPMENT

nal contamination associated with exit site or tunnel infections. Also, they are not expected to prevent peritonitis secondary to the migration of bacteria into the peritoneal cavity from visceral organs, by hematogenous spread or by ascending vaginal contamination. A recent report from one center analyzing an 8 year experience with peritonitis in a CAPD program suggested that 43.2% of infections might relate to contamination during exchanges and the intraluminal introduction of bacteria into the peritoneal cavity [4]. In that report, 20% of peritonitis episodes were attributed to exit site/tunnel infections, 10.5% to intrinsic contamination from visceral organs, 4.2% to product failure, 2.1% to recurrent infections, 17.9% to unknown, and 2.1% to other. Thus, a small scale study of the exchange devices evaluated here suggests that they may have little impact on observed peritonitis, since any effect might be masked by an above average incidence of infections, other than those involving intraluminal contamination.

Concern has also been expressed that diabetic patients who add insulin to their bags might also be adding a contaminant in the process. A recent report from the Registry suggests that diabetics do have a slightly increased risk of peritonitis, but it is not accounted for by the addition of insulin to bags [5]. In fact, diabetics adding insulin to bags tend to have lower rates of peritonitis than those who take subcutaneous insulin or no insulin.

The best way to evaluate the impact of exchange devices on peritonitis is via a prospective, randomized controlled study. There has only been one such study for the devices reported as being used in our Registry population [6]. This multicenter study was carried out with an earlier prototype of the ultra-violet exchange device. All patients were observed during a control period using the manual technique. Patients were randomized to remain on the manual technique or to use the ultra-violet device. All patients underwent a similar amount of retraining prior to starting phase 2 of the study. The incidence of peritonitis was not found to differ significantly between patients using the two devices for either period. A tendency was observed for both groups to show a lower peritonitis rate after the retraining experience. It is important to point out that the patients included in this study were from very experienced centers and had peritonitis rates with the manual technique that were well below reported Registry statistics.

References

1. Report of the National CAPD Registry of the National Institutes of Health. January, 1986.

2. Steinberg SM, Cutler SJ, Novak JW, Nolph KD: Prognostic factors associated with the first episode of peritonitis in patients treated with continuous ambulatory peritoneal dialysis (CAPD). Am Soc Artif Intern Organs J 1985; 8:238–243.
3. Kaplan E, Meier P: Nonparametric estimation from incomplete observa- tions. J Am Stat Assoc 1958; 53:457–458.
4. Prowant B, Nolph K, Ryan L, Twardowski A, Khanna R: Peritonitis in continuous ambulatory peritoneal dialysis: Analysis of an 8–year experience. Nephron 1986 Jun; 43(2):105–109.
5. Nolph KD, Cutler SJ, Steinberg SM, Novak JW: Special studies from the NIH USA CAPD Registry. Peritoneal Dial Bull 1986 Jan-Mar; 6(1):28–34.
6. A randomized multicenter clinical trial to evaluate the effects of an ultraviolet germicidal system on peritonitis rate in continuous ambulatory peritoneal dialysis. Peritoneal Dial Bull 1985 Jan-Mar; 5(1):19–23.

C. Follow-up of Transfer from CAPD/CCPD

Introduction

The National CAPD Registry has reported that 20% of patients beginning CAPD/CCPD will have transferred to other modalities within one year [1].While available Registry data do provide a variety of explanations for such transfers, they do not clearly distinguish among biochemical inadequacy of peritoneal dialysis, patients inability to cope with self-care procedures, patient preference for other dialysis or non-dialysis approaches, and availability of a transplant. Further, there are no follow-up data on CAPD dropouts to indicate whether or not they subsequently remain on hemodialysis, go to alternative treatments, return to peritoneal dialysis or undergo transplantation. Similarly, it has not been clear, whether those patients who failed transplantation return to peritoneal dialysis or go to hemodialysis.

The purpose of this study was to establish patterns of treatment after transfer from CAPD/CCPD, and to describe the subsequent clinical course of those patients who transfer off of CAPD/CCPD.

Subjects and Methods

Patients 20 years or older at CAPD/CCPD initiation and who were new to CAPD/CCPD at the time of registration were eligible for this study. Patients must have begun CAPD/CCPD after 1981 and discontinued CAPD/CCPD prior to September 1, 1985. Only patients from currently active centers, who were reported to have transferred to an alternative modality were sampled. Patients who died while on CAPD/CCPD or within two weeks of discontinuing CAPD/CCPD were also considered eligible for study, as a subset of this population represents early failures on alternative therapies.

Seven hundred patients meeting the inclusion/exclusion criteria detailed above were randomly selected from the Registry population. Information was abstracted from the clinical records of selected patients by clinical center personnel. Requested data, including intervening therapy and outcomes were collected on study specific forms which were returned to the Data Coordinat-ing Center where they were edited for errors.

Analysis of the collected data is essentially explorative and descriptive. The life table methods of Kaplan-Meier were used to evaluate time on first therapy following CAPD/CCPD [2].

Results

Five hundred thirty-two of the 700 questionnaires (76%) sent out were returned to the Data Coordinating Center; 480 (69%) had adequate patient status information. Patients were reported to have transferred to a different center in 25% of the returned questionnaires. Exhibit 1 compares the characteristics of those patients for whom responses to the questionnaire were received, with those patients for whom no response was received. Age distributions and percent of patients diagnosed with diabetic glomerulosclerosis are essentially the same for the two groups.

EXHIBIT 1

COMPARISON OF SELECTED CHARACTERISTICS FOR
PATIENTS FOR WHOM DATA FORMS WERE RECEIVED
WITH THOSE FOR WHOM DATA WERE NOT RECEIVED

| | Data Form | |
Characteristic	Received (N = 480)	Not Received (N = 220)
% Male	56	53
% White	81	77
% Prior ESRD therapy	55	58
% Diabetic glomerulosclerosis	28	28
% Age		
20 - 29 years	10	10
30 - 39 years	16	17
40 - 49 years	17	16
50 - 59 years	18	22
60 - 69 years	24	23
$\geq$ 70 years	15	12
Median Age	54 years	53 years

Differences in sex, race, and prior ESRD therapy were not greater than 4% in any one category. An informal telephone survey suggested that nonresponse was a center related phenomenon and not a patient outcome related phenomenon.

The 480 patients who form the basis of this analysis were distributed as follows:
— 178 transferred to hemodialysis;
— 90 received a kidney transplant;
— 23 transferred to medical management;
— 10 transferred to IPD;
— 179 died while on CAPD.

Transfers to Hemodialysis

In all, one hundred seventy-eight patients were reported to have discontinued CAPD/CCPD in favor of hemodialysis. Of these 178, 35% (62/178) subsequently died, 18 within two weeks of leaving CAPD/CCPD. Median follow-up on the cohort is 11 months.

Ninety-three percent of patients [164/178] received hemodialysis performed in-center; only 7 (4%) and 5 (3%) patients carried out hemodialysis in a self-care unit or at home, respectively. Twelve patients changed location: 9 went from receiving center hemodialysis to performing hemodialysis at home and 2 patients changed from center to a self-care unit; and, only one patient changed from a self-care unit to in-center dialysis.

Complications were assessed by requesting the total number of days spent in the hospital and the number of days of hospitalization which were attributed to hemodialysis related complications such as access related infections, hypotension, fluid overload, etc. Vascular access infections, weight maintenance, serum creatinine and serum phosphate levels were likewise assessed; they are summarized in Exhibit 2. As response rates were not uniform for all items, sample sizes are identified on an item by item basis.

Number of days hospitalized during treatment with hemodialysis was reported for sixty-seven patients. Hospital days per patient year were calculated for this cohort while on CAPD and while on hemodialysis. The group appears to have spent more total days in the hospital while receiving CAPD than while receiving hemodialysis (27.3 days per patient year vs. 7.7 days per patient year, respectively). The same result holds

EXHIBIT 2

SUMMARY OF HEMODIALYSIS RELATED COMPLICATIONS

Complication Type:	N	%
Vascular Access Infections (n = 125)	N	%
Infection Frequency		
0	113	90
1	8	6
2	2	2
3	0	0
4	1	1
5	0	0
6	1	1
Oral Phosphate Binder Dosage (n = 86)		
Dose as compared to CAPD Dose		
Increased	32	37
No change	40	47
Decreased	14	16
Days Hospitalized per Patient Year		
All Causes	17.7 days	
Hemodialysis Related Causes	7.0 days	
Median Weight Gain Between Hemodialysis Treatments (n = 104)	3 kg	
Median Difference Between Target Dry Weight and Patient's Usual Weight Post Dialysis (n = 95)	0 kg	
Median Serum Creatinine Level (n = 43)		
Hemodialysis: 3 pre and 3 post dialyses	11.6 mg/100 ml	
CAPD: Last 3 months	11.2 mg/100 ml	
Median Serum Phosphorous Level (n = 44)		
Hemodialysis: 3 pre and 3 post dialyses	5.4 mg/dl	
CAPD: Last 3 months	4.9 mg/dl	

for hospitalizations for dialysis related events. Fourteen days per patient year were spent in the hospital while on CAPD; 7 days were spent in hospital per patient year of observation while on hemodialysis. It is not clear if the reduction in hospitalization rates following transfer to hemodialysis represents a true advantage of hemodialysis in these patients, or if it represents the phenomenon of regression to the mean; as the number of days hospitalized while on hemodialysis is similar to rates reported for all Class I CAPD Registry patients. Note that hospitalization for these patients while on CAPD is greater than for all Registry patients: 27.3 vs. 19.4 days ppy for all causes; and, 14.0 vs. 7.7 days ppy for treatment related causes.

Twelve of 125 patients (10%) for whom data pertaining to hemodialysis experience was available were reported as having had at least one vascular access infection that required antibiotics; four of the twelve patients reported more than one such infection.

Information on oral phosphate binder dosage modifications was available for 86 patients. Dose of oral phosphate binder received during the last 3 months of hemodialysis was compared with the dose received during the last three months on CAPD/CCPD. Over one-third of the patients (37%) were receiving higher doses while on hemodialysis as compared with those received while on CAPD/CCPD, while 47% reported no change in dose and 16% reported a decrease in dose.

Weight gains between dialyses, target dry weight and usual post hemodialysis weights were requested. Median weight gain between dialyses was 3 kg and the median difference between usual post dialysis and target dry weight was nil. Median levels of serum phosphorous and serum creatinine while on CAPD were observed to be lower than the median of average of values taken prior to hemodialysis, and post hemodialysis, but this difference was not significant.

Reasons for discontinuing CAPD in favor of hemodialysis were solicited and have been summarized in Exhibit 3. Thirty-five percent of the patients were coded as terminating peritoneal dialysis due to peritonitis, while 20% of the patients for whom data are available changed modalities for reasons of preference. Catheter complications and failure to control fluid/biochemical standards were coded as primary reasons for 14% and 10% of patients, respectively.

Exhibit 4 summarizes the status of patients transferring to hemodialysis by the therapy received prior to CAPD. For 57% the transfer was a return to hemodialysis. Just under half of the patients were alive and

EXHIBIT 3

REASONS CAPD PATIENTS TRANSFER TO HEMODIALYSIS

Reason	N	%
Peritonitis	62	35
Failure to Control Fluid/ Biochemical Standard	18	10
Catheter Complication	25	14
Physical inability	11	6
Other Medical reasons	18	10
Patient Preference/Inability to Cope	35	20
Other	5	3
Unknown	4	2
Total	178	100

EXHIBIT 4

STATUS OF PATIENTS WHOSE FIRST THERAPY
FOLLOWING PERITONEAL DIALYSIS WAS HEMODIALYSIS
ACCORDING TO THERAPY PRIOR TO CAPD INITIATION

				STATUS				
Therapy Prior to CAPD	Total			Remaining on Hemo		Therapy Following Hemo.		
	N	%	Unknown	Alive	Dead	Trans.	CAPD	Med. Man.
No prior therapy	50	(28)	1	26	12	6	5	0
Hemodialysis	101	(57)	6	46	27	13	9	0
IPD	14	(8)	0	7	5	0	0	2
Medical management	11	(7)	0	6	3	1	1	0
Transplant	2	(1)	0	2	0	0	0	0
TOTAL	178	(100)	7	87	47	20	15	2

continuing hemodialysis at last contact. Patients reporting no ESRD treatment prior to beginning CAPD were as likely to leave hemodialysis in favor of CAPD as to receive a transplant. Although the numbers are small, return rates to CAPD among patients transferring to hemodialysis are comparable regardless of pre-CAPD therapy. In total, 8% returned to CAPD after an interval of hemodialysis treatment.

Probability estimates for selected time points of patient survival, transplantation, or transfer off of hemodialysis are given in Exhibit 5. Patients dying within 2 weeks of beginning hemodialysis are not considered as hemodialysis deaths. At two years 65% (52%–77%; 95% C.I.) of patients transferring to hemodialysis were observed to be alive and receiving hemodialysis. Transplants were observed in 18% (9%–33%; 95% C.I.) of patients and transfers to CAPD/CCPD, IPD or

EXHIBIT 5

CUMULATIVE PROBABILITIES AND 95% CONFIDENCE INTERVALS FOR SELECTED EVENTS
IN 178 PATIENTS TRANSFERRING TO HEMODIALYSIS

	Months							
	6 months		12 months		18 months		24 months	
Event	Prob.	95% C.I.	Prob.	95% C.I.	Prob.	95% C.I.	Prob.	95% C.I.
Survival	85	(76,91)	74	(64,83)	69	(58,79)	65	(52,77)
Transplantation	6	(3,13)	12	(7,22)	14	(7,26)	18	(9,33)
Transfer to CAPD/IPD/ Off Dialysis	10	(5,18)	10	(5,20)	14	(7,25)	16	(8,30)

medical management may be expected in 16% (8%–30%; 95% C.I.) of patients at two years.

Transplant

Ninety patients were reported to have received a renal allograft, after which replacement therapy with CAPD/CCPD was terminated. Nine of these patients, 10% have subsequently died, 4 within two weeks of terminating CAPD/CCPD. Median follow-up for these patients is nine months.

Data regarding complications of the transplantation were completed for over three quarters of the transplanted patients; they are summarized in Exhibit 6. Again, sample sizes for individual items are variable due to nonresponse. Complications resulting from immunosuppression were reported in 11 of 65 (17%) of transplanted patients; such complications included diabetes, hip necrosis, urinary tract infections, colostomy, hypertension, hepatitis, pneumonia, pyelonephritis and cyclosporin A toxicity. Post-operative peritonitis and exit site/tunnel infections occurred in 5/75 (7%) and 4/78 (5%) of patients, respectively.

The patient cohort appeared to have fewer days hospitalized overall and for CAPD/CCPD related complications while on CAPD. As a group the patients who left CAPD/CCPD to receive a transplant were hospitalized for 17 days per patient year for all causes and 7 days per patient year for CAPD/CCPD related causes. The Registry reports 19 and 8 days per patient year, respectively.

EXHIBIT 6

SUMMARY OF COMPLICATIONS AND PATIENT COURSE
FOLLOWING TRANSPLANTATION

	Fraction	Percent %
Immunosuppressive Related Complications	11/65	17
Post-operative Peritonitis	5/75	7
Post-operative Exit Site/Tunnel Infection	4/78	5
Post-operative Dialysis Required		
No Dialysis Required	55/72	76
Hemodialysis	11/72	15
CAPD/CCPD	5/72	7
Hemodialysis and CAPD/CCPD	1/72	1

EXHIBIT 7

STATUS OF PATIENTS WHOSE FIRST THERAPY
FOLLOWING PERITONEAL DIALYSIS WAS TRANSPLANTATION
ACCORDING TO THERAPY PRIOR TO CAPD INITIATION

Therapy Prior to CAPD	Total N	Total %	STATUS Graft Functioning Unknown	Alive	Dead	Therapy Following Graft Failure Hemo.	CAPD	Med. Man.
No prior therapy	49	(54)	1	40	4	2	2	0
Hemodialysis	27	(30)	0	20	3	3	1	0
IPD	9	(10)	0	6	0	2	0	1
Medical Management	5	(6)	0	5	0	0	0	0
TOTAL	90	(100)	1	71	7	7	3	1

Postoperative dialysis was required in 17/72 (24%) of transplanted patients. Hemodialysis was used for 11 of those patients (65%), 5 patients (29%) were treated postoperatively with CAPD and both modalities were used in one patient. Catheters were removed at a median of 30 days post transplant.

Patient status according to therapy type prior to receiving CAPD/CCPD is given in Exhibit 7. Transplant patients were more likely not to have had pre CAPD therapy (54%) (Exhibit 7) than were patients who transferred from CAPD to hemodialysis (28%) (Exhibit 4). Among transplanted patients, 30% had had prior hemodialysis (Exhibit 7) while 57% of patients transferring from CAPD to hemodialysis (Exhibit 4) had received pre-CAPD hemodialysis.

Eleven of the 90 transplanted patients (12%) experienced graft failure; seven of those patients chose to resume dialysis with hemodialysis and four returned to CAPD/CCPD. Overall, the probability of graft survival observed was 85% (69%–94%; 95% C.I.) at six months and 79% (60%–90%; 95% C.I.) at one year.

Transfer to Medical Management

Twenty-three patients transferred to medical management as their only treatment for end stage renal disease. Thirteen of those patients had experienced a return of kidney function; ten did not. Only four patients subsequently reported a return to dialysis; all were patients whose kidney function had returned. Three of the four chose hemodialysis and then received a transplant at 2, 5, and 7 months each and one chose CAPD.

Eleven patients in this cohort (49%) have died. Nine of the deaths occurred in the 10 patients terminating dialysis with no kidney function return. Cause of death in these patients was reported as; suicide [2], cancer [2], cardiovascular [2], uremia [1], unknown [2]. The one patient who is reported as alive has no follow-up available. Of the two deaths occurring in patients terminating dialysis due to a return of kidney function, one has died due to cardiac arrest; cause of death in the second patient is unknown.

Therapy type prior to receiving CAPD and reasons for discontinuing CAPD are given in Exhibit 8. The majority of patients, 65%, who transferred to medical management were previously untreated or had been on medical management prior to CAPD initiation. As might be expected, reasons for leaving CAPD varied for the two medical management cohorts. Five patients (50%) left dialysis with no return of kidney function due to preference. Peritonitis [2], physical inability [1] and other medical factors [2] were listed as causes of dialysis termination in the remaining five patients. Only three patients with a return in kidney function, who terminated dialysis in favor of medical management, did so due to complications: peritonitis [2], other medical reasons [1].

EXHIBIT 8

PRIOR THERAPY AND REASON FOR TERMINATING CAPD
BY TREATMENT FOLLOWING CAPD TERMINATION

	Medical Management No Kidney Function Return (n = 10)	Medical Management Kidney Function Returned (n = 13)	IPD (n = 10)
Prior Therapy:			
None	2	4	6
Hemodialysis	3	4	1
Transplant	0	0	0
IPD	0	1	3
Medical Management	5	4	0
Reason for Terminating CAPD:			
Peritonitis	2	2	0
Physical Inability	1	0	3
Patient Preference	5	0	4
K.F. Return	0	10	1
Other Medical Reason	2	1	2

Transfer to IPD

Ten patients were reported to have transferred from continuous to intermittent peritoneal dialysis. One of those patients later returned to CAPD. Data on the average number of days dialyzed, hours per session, and liters exchanged were reported on 6 patients. The majority of these patients [5/6] dialyzed 3 times per week. A range of 8–12 hours per session was reported, and an average of 18.8 liters were exchanged per session.

Six of the ten patients were previously untreated for ESRD at CAPD initiation and three had pre-CAPD experience with IPD. Patient preference [4], physical inability [3], other medicalreasons [2] and kidney function return [1] were given as reasons for discontinuing CAPD in favor of IPD.

EXHIBIT 9

CAUSE OF DEATH SUMMARY

		N	%
Total Deaths Reported		266	100
Cause of Death:			
RELATED TO ESRD TREATMENT:	33		
Peritoneal Dialysis Only		16	6
Peritoneal Dialysis and Hemodialysis		2	1
Peritoneal Dialysis and Unrelated to ESRD Therapy		2	1
Hemodialysis Only		6	2
Transplantation Only		7	2
UNRELATED TO ESRD TREATMENT:	201		
Cardiovascular		91	34
Pneumonia		8	3
Septicemia		9	3
Carcinoma		8	3
Suicide (or dialysis withdrawal)		8	3
Other		21	8
Unrelated cause not stated		56	21
UNKNOWN	32		12

Mortality

In all, two hundred sixty-six patients (55%; 266/480) are reported to have died. One hundred seventy-nine of these deaths were reported while the patient was still receiving CAPD/CCPD; 87 deaths were reported among patients who had terminated CAPD/CCPD. Of the 87 deaths, 34 (39%) occurred within two weeks of transfer off CAPD/CCPD. Two hundred fourteen (45%) were alive at last contact.

Information on cause of death was requested. Two hundred one of the deaths reported (76%) were attributed to causes other than end stage renal disease or its treatment; thirty-three of the deaths (12%) were related to treatment, and cause of death in thirty-two patients (12%) was unknown. A listing of the causes of death provided is given in Exhibit 9. One-third of all deaths were claimed as cardiovascular related. Pneumonia, septicemia, carcinoma and suicide each accounted for 3% of reported deaths. Eight percent of reported deaths (20/266)

EXHIBIT 10

CAUSE OF ESRD TREATMENT RELATED DEATHS

Related to:

Peritoneal Dialysis (n = 20)

    Peritonitis, Gastrointestinal bleed
    Peritonitis, also Hemodialysis related hypotension
    Peritonitis, also Hemodialysis related (cause not stated)
    Peritonitis, also related to heart failure
    Peritonitis, also related to other medical problems
    Peritonitis
    Peritonitis
    Peritonitis
    Peritonitis, Sepsis
    Septicemia
    Sepsis, pulmonary edema
    Congestive heart failure
    Cardiac arrest
    Hypokalemia
    6 Unknown

Hemodialysis (n = 6)

    Acute MI
    Cardiac arrest, secondary to hyperkalemia
    Uremia
    Renal failure
    Withdrawal from dialysis
    1 unknown

Transplantation (n = 7)

    Pulmonary embolism
    Heart attack
    Acute rejection, meningitis
    Hepatitis
    Sepsis
    2 unknown

---

were related to ESRD treatment with peritoneal dialysis. Four of the 20 peritoneal dialysis related deaths were also attributed to hemodialysis [2] or unrelated to ESRD treatment [2]. Six deaths were attributed to treatment with hemodialysis and seven deaths to transplantation. Causes as individually reported for all treatment related deaths are listed in Exhibit 10. Nine of the 20 cases of peritoneal dialysis related deaths claimed peritonitis as a primary or contributing factor.

Discussion

The results of this study must be cautiously interpreted as subgroups often contain limited sample sizes. However, several observations are worth noting. It has previously been suggested that CAPD/CCPD might allow reduced exposure to phosphate binders as compared with hemodialysis [3].This survey does not support that claim as only 35% increased the dose and 16% actually reduced the dose of phosphate binders while on hemodialysis. The observation that the most common cause of death in the CAPD/CCPD population surveyed was cardiovascular cannot be entirely unexpected in a population, given that the median age is 54 years and a 28% prevalence of diabetic glomerulosclerosis was observed. Unfortunately, the number of patients for whom responses were received does not allow us comment, on whether the incidence of cardiovascular death in non-diabetics less than 60 years of age is greater than what might be expected in a similar population without renal failure. However, we do note that an increased incidence of cardiovascular death in hemodialysis patients has been suggested elsewhere [4].

The results of this survey suggest that the movement of patients from one therapy to another is a common occurrence. Presumably, it is the patient who is not doing well (medically or psychologically) on one therapy that is more likely to transfer to another modality. Significantly, we observe that such patients are not likely to do well under the new therapy, either; and hence, patients requiring transfers might be looked upon as requiring more attention than patients who remain on CAPD therapy. However, while such transfers often trade one type of dialysis related problem for another, they also provide the potential for solving problems for some.

References

1. Report of the National CAPD Registry of the National Institutes of Health. January, 1986.

2. Kaplan E and Meier P. Nonparametric estimation from incomplete observations. J Am Stat Assoc 1958; 53:457–458.
3. Lindner A, Charra B, Sherrard DJ and Scribner BH. Accelerated atherosclerosis in prolonged hemodialysis. N Engl J Med 1974; 290:697–701.
4. Neu S and Kjellstrand CM. Stopping long-term dialysis. An empirical study of withdrawal of life-supporting treatment. N Engl J Med 1986; 314:14–20.

D. Pediatric Population Evaluation*

Introduction

CAPD/CCPD has become the preferred treatment for infants and very young children with ESRD in most of the Western industrialized countries including the United States. An analysis of the characteristics and some of the experiences of pediatric patients within the National CAPD Registry is reported elsewhere in this publication.

The purpose of this study was to further detail the experience of children treated with CAPD and CCPD, particularly in regard to some of the issues which are of unique interest to children, and therefore which are not addressed in the routine data collections of the Registry. The issues addressed in this survey include:
— The prevalence of certain primary renal disease diagnosis categories commonly found in children but infrequently found in adults;
— Physical growth and sexual development;
— Further examination of the reasons children discontinue CAPD/CCPD;
— Level of involvement of pediatric nephrologists in the care of pediatric patients.

Subjects and Methods

All Registry patients under 20 years of age at CAPD/CCPD initiation who were new to CAPD/CCPD at the time of registration were eligible

* The material contained in this report has been submitted for publications as follows: Alexander S, Lindblad AS, Nolph KD, Novak JW. Pediatric CAPD/CCPD in the United States. A review of the experiences of the National CAPD Registry's pediatric population for the period January 1, 1981 through August 31, 1986.

for inclusion in this special survey. Patients must have begun CAPD/CCPD after 1981 and prior to September 1, 1985. To minimize the number of patients who would be lost to follow-up after they were included in the study, only patients from currently active centers were considered. Four hundred eighty-five patients were identified in the Registry population who met the inclusion/exclusion criteria detailed above. Special purpose data forms were prepared and sent to participating clinical centers, and data were abstracted from hospital and clinic records by center personnel and then edited for errors by the staff of the Data Coordinating Center.

Results

Three hundred forty-eight (72%) of the 485 questionnaires distributed were returned to the Data Coordinating Center. Twenty-eight of the questionnaires did not contain usable information and hence, the analysis is based on 320 patients, or 66% of the target population.

The characteristics of patients for whom study data were received are compared with those from whom study data were not received (Exhibit 1). We note that the population for whom supplemental data were

EXHIBIT 1

SELECTED CHARACTERISTICS OF RESPONDERS
AND NONRESPONDERS TO THE QUESTIONNAIRE

Characteristics	Data Submitted (n = 320)	Data not Submitted (n = 165)
% Age		
< 1 year	6	4
1-4 years	12	12
5-9 years	19	15
10-14 years	32	27
15-19 years	30	43
Median Age	12 years	14 years
% Prior ESRD Therapy	46	51
% Male	48	58
% White	77	69

provided is younger and contains more females and whites than the
population for whom said data were not provided. Any resulting bias in
the analysis of outcomes remains unevaluated.

EXHIBIT 2

DISTRIBUTION OF PRIMARY RENAL DISEASE DIAGNOSES

Disease Type	N	%
Aplastic/hypoplastic/dysplastic kidney(s)	48	15
Chronic glomerulonephritis	39	12
Focal glomerulosclerosis	29	9
Pyelonephritis/interstitial nephritis due to congenital obstructive uropathy with or without vesico-ureteric reflux	20	6
Obstructive uropathy	17	5
Rapidly progressive glomerulonephritis	16	5
Hemolytic uremic syndrome	14	4
Systemic immunological disease with renal involvement	13	4
Cystinosis	11	3
Medullary cystic disease/juvenile nephronophthisis	9	3
Pyelonephritis/interstitial nephritis due to vesico-ureteric reflux without obstruction	7	2
Hypertensive renal disease	7	2
Syndrome of agenesis of abdominal musculature	6	2
Diabetic glomerulosclerosis	4	1
Polycystic kidney disease	4	1
Other pyelonephritis	3	1
Familial nephritis	3	1
Chronic pyelonephritis; nephrosclerosis	3	1
Bilateral cortical necrosis	2	<1
Nephrectomy, secondary to cancer	2	<1
Renal infarct	2	<1
Oxalosis	2	<1
Membranous nephropathy	2	<1
Juene's syndrome	2	<1
Other	8	3
Unknown or not stated	47	15

A summary of primary renal disease diagnoses for those for whom data were provided is given in Exhibit 2. Frequencies for the primary renal disease reported were widely distributed over the 29 categories: aplastic/ hypoplastic/dysplastic kidney(s) was the cause of 15% of the patients' renal failure; chronic glomerulonephritis and focal glomerulo-sclerosis were diagnosed in 12% and 9% of the sampled children, respectively; and, forty-seven patients (15%) were coded as disease type unknown or not stated.

Age at diagnosis of renal insufficiency and transplantation status 12 months after CAPD/CCPD initiation are summarized for the cohort in Exhibit 3. Fifty percent of study patients were under age ten years at the time renal insufficiency was first detected. The median time reported from detection to treatment initiation with CAPD/CCPD was 9 months.

EXHIBIT 3

AGE AT RENAL INSUFFICIENCY DIAGNOSIS
AND 12 MONTH TRANSPLANTATION STATUS

Age at Renal Insufficiency Diagnosis	Percent (%) n = 320
< 1 year	12
1-4 years	19
5-9 years	19
10-14 years	30
15-19 years	13
Date of diagnosis unknown	7
Transplantation Status - 12 months after CAPD Initiation	
Received a transplant < 12 months	21
Transferred off CAPD < 12 months	14
On cadaveric transplant waiting list; high cytoxic antibody titer (> 40% of panel)	8
On cadaveric transplant waiting list; low cytotoxic antibody titer	17
Living donor transplantation planned within the next 12 months	3
No active plans for transplantation at patient/family request	14
Medical complications prohibiting transplant	2
Previous graft failure, no transplantation planned	2
Not stated	18

Twenty-one percent of patients received a transplant within 12 months of peritoneal dialysis initiation; and, another 28 percent of the patients were either on transplant waiting lists or had a living donor transplant planned within the next 12 months. Only fourteen percent of the patients included in this survey had no active plans for a transplant due to patient or family request. Medical complications prevented two percent of patients from receiving a transplant.

Primary Care Physician

Pediatric nephrologists were found to be serving as primary attending physician for 66% of the patients for whom responses were received (Exhibit 4). 'Consultation by a pediatric nephrologist', defined as seeing the patient and/or reviewing medical records at least once a year, was used by 15% of the patients studied, while 19% had no pediatric nephrologist involvement excepting the possibility of an occasional telephone consultation. A breakdown of pediatric nephrologist involvement by patient age group reveals a decline in the involvement of pediatric nephrologists as a patient's age increases. Note that 89% of children under the age of five used a pediatric nephrologist as the primary care physician, while only 44% of children between the ages of 15 and 19 had reports of such care.

EXHIBIT 4

PEDIATRIC NEPHROLOGIST'S INVOLVEMENT BY PATIENT AGE

Pediatric Nephrologist's Involvement	Total N (%)	Age Group				
		< 1	1-4	5-9	10-14	15-19
Primary Attending Physician	203 (66)	16 (89)	33 (89)	45 (76)	67 (68)	42 (44)
Consultation* Only, Ped. Neph. on Staff	21 (7)	0 (0)	1 (3)	3 (5)	9 (9)	8 (8)
Consultation* Only, Ped. Neph. not on Staff	24 (8)	0 (0)	0 (0)	5 (8)	9 (9)	10 (11)
No Pediatric Neph. Involvement	59 (19)	2 (11)	3 (8)	6 (10)	13 (13)	35 (37)
TOTAL	307**(100)	18 (100)	37 (100)	59 (100)	98 (100)	95 (100)

*Patient seen and/or medical records reviewed at least once a year.
**Pediatric Nephrologist's involvement not stated in 12 patients.

EXHIBIT 5

PUBERTY ASSESSMENT - BOYS
NUMBER OF PATIENTS BY AGE AND PUBERTY STAGING

Age Group	Genital Development Stage* 1	2	3	4	5	Total Patients
≤ 9	30	0	0	0	0	30
10 - 12	10	2	2	1	0	15
13 - 15	5	1	3	2	1	12
16 - 18	0	0	1	2	8	11
≥ 19	0	0	1	0	6	7

*Genital Development Stage Criteria

1 - Pre-adolescent. Testes, scrotum and penis are about the same size and proportion as in early childhood.
2 - Enlargement of scrotum and testes. Skin of scrotum reddens and changes in texture. Little or no enlargement.
3 - Enlargement of penis, which occurs at first mainly in length. Further growth of testes and scrotum.
4 - Increased size of penis with growth in breadth and development of glans. Testes and scrotum larger; scrotal skin darkened.
5 - Genitalia adult in size and shape.

Age Group	Pubic Hair Stage** 1	2	3	4	5	Total Patients
≤ 9	29	1	0	0	0	30
10 - 12	11	2	1	1	0	15
13 - 15	3	2	4	2	1	12
16 - 18	0	0	0	4	6	10
≥ 19	0	0	0	1	6	7

**Pubic Hair Stage Criteria

1 - The vellus over the pubes is not further developed than that over the abdominal wall, i.e. no pubic hair.
2 - Sparse growth of long, slightly pigmented downy hair, straight or slightly curled, chiefly at the base of the penis or along labia.
3 - Hair considerably darker, coarser and more curled. The hair spreads sparsely over the junction of the pubes.
4 - Hair now adult in type, but area covered is still smaller than in the adult. No spread to the medial surface of thighs.
5 - Adult in quantity and type with distribution of the horizontal (or classically "feminine") pattern. Spread to medial surface of thighs but not up linea alba or elsewhere above the base of the inverse triangle (spread up linea alba occurs late and is rated stage 6).

EXHIBIT 6

PUBERTY ASSESSMENT - GIRLS
NUMBER OF PATIENTS BY AGE AND PUBERTY STAGING

Age Group	Breast Development Stage* 1	2	3	4	5	Total Patients
≤ 9	14	1	0	0	0	15
10 - 12	11	4	2	0	0	17
13 - 15	4	3	2	3	5	17
16 - 18	0	1	3	2	6	12
≥ 19	0	1	1	3	4	9

*Breast Development Stage Criteria

1 - Pre-adolescent: elevation of papilla only.
2 - Breast bud stage: elevation of breast and papilla as small mound. Enlargement of areola diameter.
3 - Further enlargement and elevation of breast and areola with no separation of contours.
4 - Projection of areola and papilla to form a secondary mound above the level of the breast.
5 - Mature stage: projection of papilla only, due to recession of the areola to the general contour of the breast.

Age Group	Pubic Hair Stage** 1	2	3	4	5	Total Patients
≤ 9	13	1	0	0	0	14
10 - 12	11	3	2	0	0	16
13 - 15	7	0	2	4	4	17
16 - 18	1	1	2	2	6	12
≥ 19	1	0	1	1	6	9

**Pubic Hair Stage Criteria

1 - The vellus over the pubes is not further developed than that over the abdominal wall, i.e. no pubic hair.
2 - Sparse growth of long, slightly pigmented downy hair, straight or slightly curled, chiefly at the base of the penis or along labia.
3 - Hair considerably darker, coarser and more curled. The hair spreads sparsely over the junction of the pubes.
4 - Hair now adult in type, but area covered is still smaller than in the adult. No spread to the medial surface of thighs.
5 - Adult in quantity and type with distribution of the horizontal (or classically "feminine") pattern. Spread to medial surface of thighs but not up linea alba or elsewhere above the base of the inverse triangle (spread up linea alba occurs late and is rated stage 6).

Sexual Maturation

Sexual maturational assessments were available for 146 patients. As this response represents only 30% of the pediatric population and 46% of the returned questionnaires, interpretation of the observations which are summarized in Exhibits 5, 6, and 7 require unusual caution. Puberty onset is defined as reaching at least Stage 2 in pubic hair or genital development. Using this criteria, 67% (10/15) boys age 10–12 at the time of maturational assessment had not reached puberty. Nine of these 15 boys were at least age 11 and of these nine, 5 (55%) had yet to reach puberty. By age 16 or older, all 18 boys had progressed to at least Stage 3; at the same age 14 boys (78%) were considered fully mature (Exhibit 5). Ten girls were coded as having reached Stage 2 of maturity; median age at the time of maturational assessment for these girls was 12 years (Exhibit 6). Thirty-four percent (15/44) of the girls 12 or older, for whom maturational data were available, were reported to have reached menarche (Exhibit 7). Median age of menarche was 15 years.

Anthropometric Measurements

Measures of height, weight, head circumference (for children $\leq$ 3 years), triceps skinfold thickness and midarm circumference were requested at CAPD initiation and following one year of peritoneal dialysis. Responses to these data items were sparse, probably because data for the requested time points were not available. It is important to note that the one year results reported are based on children who completed at least one year of therapy with CAPD/CCPD. Patients who received a

EXHIBIT 7

MENARCHE STATUS
NUMBER OF PATIENTS BY AGE

Age at Assessment	Menarche Status		
	Yes	No	Total
$\leq$ 11	0	27	27
12–14	6	12	18
15–17	6	8	14
> 17	3	9	12
Total Patients	15	56	71

transplant prior to one year of replacement therapy are excluded, as are patients who transferred to hemodialysis, IPD, or who otherwise discontinued CAPD/CCPD prior to one year of therapy. Measurements obtained were compared with the 50th percentile of normals of comparable age and sex [1,2] and the percentage difference between CAPD patients and normals was determined. Percent difference was defined as:

$$\frac{\text{Individual Measurement} - \text{50th Percentile Normal}}{\text{50th Percentile Normal}} .$$

As all differences were negative, the data presented are shown as mean percent deficits (see Exhibits 8 and 9). Average height, weight and head circumference were found to be significantly different from the 50th percentile of normals, both at baseline and at one year for both sexes. Tricep skinfold thickness and arm circumference for CAPD patients were also found to be significantly below normal at baseline and one year.

Patients were grouped into three age categories and heights and weights were analyzed to determine percent deviation from 50th percen-

EXHIBIT 8

MEAN PERCENT DEFICIT FROM NORMAL
50TH PERCENTILE VALUES

Anthropometric Measurement	N	MALE Mean % deficit from normal	N	FEMALE Mean % deficit from normal
Height				
Initial	78	11%	66	10%
1 year	81	14%	65	12%
Weight				
Initial	85	17%	83	21%
1 year	89	22%	80	26%
Head Circumference				
Initial	9	5%	5	5%
1 year	6	10%	2	15%
Arm Circumference				
Initial	27	11%	23	11%
1 year	27	14%	24	9%
Tricep Thickness				
Initial	33	7%	24	35%
1 year	34	22%	26	28%

148

EXHIBIT 9

MEAN PERCENT DEFICIT IN ANTHROPOMETRIC MEASUREMENTS
FROM NORMAL 50TH PERCENTILE VALUES

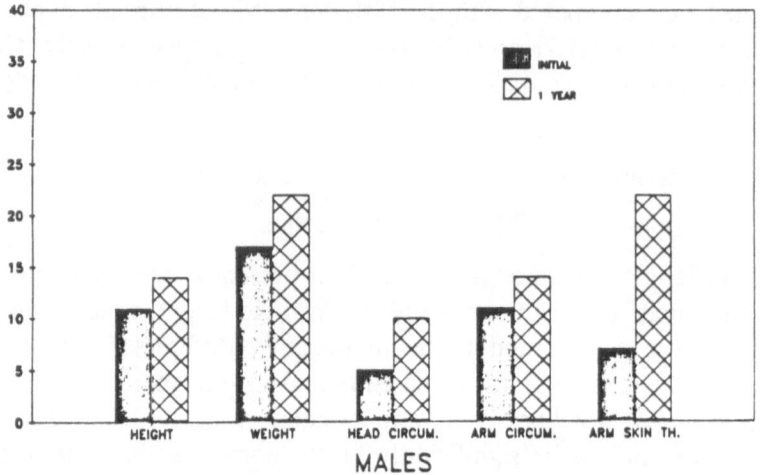

MALES

MEAN PERCENT DEFICIT IN ANTHROPOMETRIC MEASUREMENTS
FROM NORMAL 50TH PERCENTILE VALUES

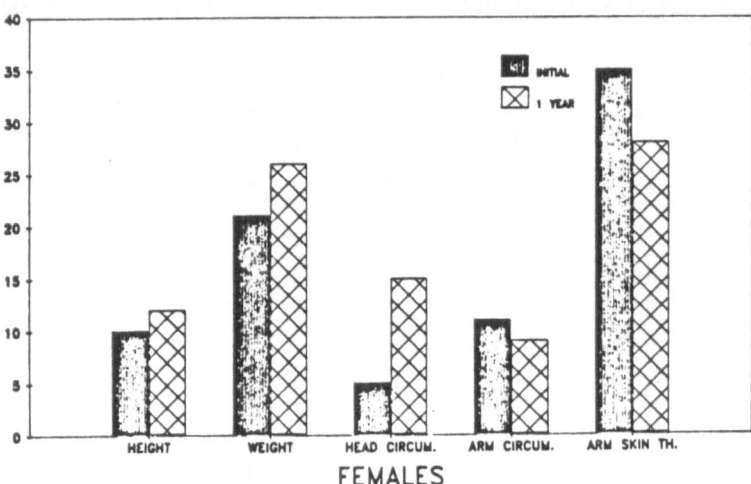

FEMALES

tile values. Exhibits 10 and 11 present mean percent deficits at baseline and one year for heights and weights, grouped by age and sex. Significant growth deficits continued to be observed for the youngest patients in both sexes after one year on CAPD/CCPD; and, age and age by sex interactions were observed in analyses of weight changes.

Median differences in height, weight, head and midarm circumference and tricep skinfold thickness following 1 year of CAPD therapy are given in Exhibit 12. Summary data are presented by age grouping, based

EXHIBIT 10

MEAN PERCENT DEFICIT IN HEIGHT
FROM NORMAL 50TH PERCENTILE VALUES

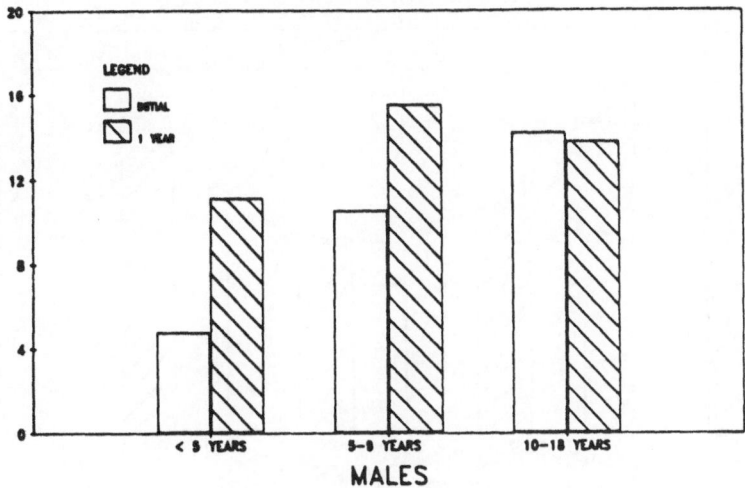

MALES

MEAN PERCENT DEFICIT IN HEIGHT
FROM NORMAL 50TH PERCENTILE VALUES

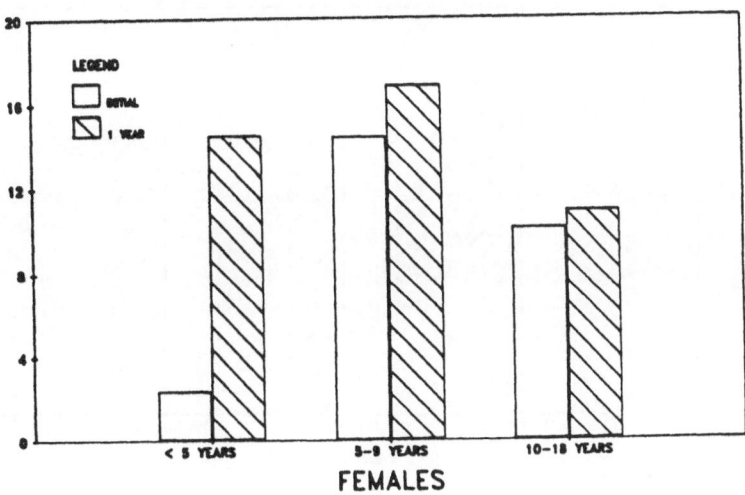

FEMALES

on the age of CAPD/CCPD initiation. The median growth and weight gain of children beginning CAPD/CCPD under 1 year of age is 12 cm and 3 kg, respectively. Median height, following 1 year of therapy for 15–20 year olds, is 154 cm, and median weight is 49 kg. Such results suggest that while children continue to grow on CAPD/CCPD, they are not able to regain lost ground.

150

EXHIBIT 11

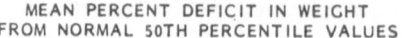

MEAN PERCENT DEFICIT IN WEIGHT
FROM NORMAL 50TH PERCENTILE VALUES

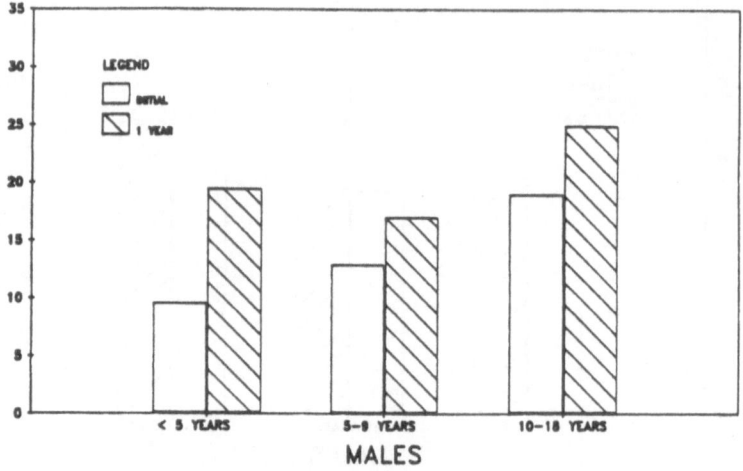

MALES

MEAN PERCENT DEFICIT IN WEIGHT
FROM NORMAL 50TH PERCENTILE VALUES

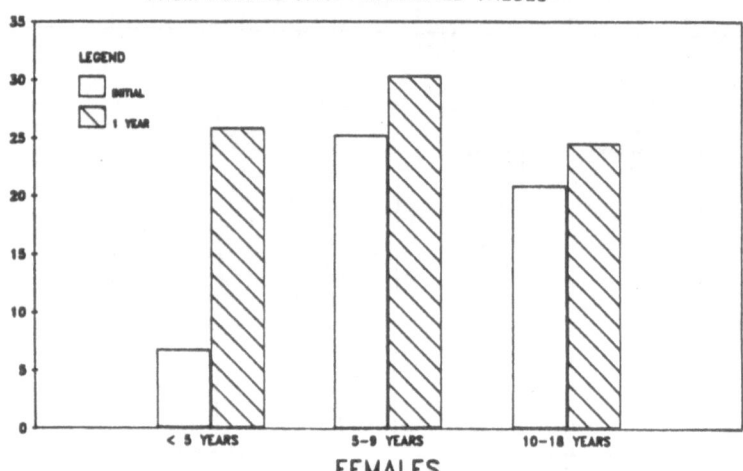

FEMALES

School Attendance

Clinics were asked to assess the school attendance for their patients, and data were received for 174 patients. Results are presented in Exhibit 13, according to the age of the child at the time of assessment. Note that more than three quarters of the children between the ages of 4 and 19 were attending school on a full time basis; full time attendance for children under 5 implies full time nursery school. Notably only 3% of

EXHIBIT 12

ANTHROPOMETRIC ASSESSMENT BY AGE OF
CAPD/CCPD INITIATION

Anthropometric Measurement	Age at CAPD/CCPD Initiation				
	< 1	1-4	5-9	10-14	15-20
HEIGHT					
N	13	17	33	44	35
Median Initial (cm)	56	83	110	137	154
Median 1 year change (cm)	12	4	4	3	0
WEIGHT					
N	12	18	39	55	47
Median Initial (kg)	4	13	20	31	49
Median 1 year change (kg)	3	1	2	2	1
HEAD CIRCUMFERENCE					
N	12	3	0	0	0
Median Initial (cm)	36	46	-	-	-
Median 1 year change (cm)	4	1	-	-	-
ARM CIRCUMFERENCE					
N	5	6	14	15	14
Median Initial (cm)	14	14	17	18	24
Median 1 year change (cm)	0	1	1	1	1
TRICEP CIRCUMFERENCE					
N	7	9	15	15	15
Median Initial (cm)	8	7	7	9	11
Median 1 year change (cm)	0	2	-1	0	0

children between the ages of 9 and 15 were incapable of receiving any kind of schooling; and, all children of school age at the time of assessment were capable of receiving some type of schooling.

Therapy Following CAPD/CCPD Termination

One hundred thirty-seven of the 204 for whom reports were available (67%) had received a transplant and 36 of the 204 (18%) had changed to in-center hemodialysis following termination of CAPD/CCPD (see Exhibit 14). Transfer to home dialysis or in-center IPD occurred in 2% of the reporting sample. Eight patients (4%) transferred to medical

EXHIBIT 13

SCHOOL ATTENDANCE STATUS
BY AGE OF ASSESSMENT

School Attendance Status	Total		Age Group				
	N	%	≤ 4 (n=21)	5-9 (n=34)	10-14 (n=63)	15-18 (n=36)	≥ 19 (n=20)
Full time	116	67	19	82	81	75	29
Regular part time	13	8	0	15	8	5	0
Irregular part time	6	3	0	3	5	3	7
Tutored at home	2	1	0	0	3	0	0
Not attending school: capable	10	6	0	0	0	14	14
Not attending school: incapable	2	1	0	0	3	0	0
Not of school age	25	14	81	0	0	3	50
TOTAL	174	100	100	100	100	100	100

EXHIBIT 14

STATUS FOLLOWING CAPD/CCPD TERMINATION

Status	Number	Percent
Transplantation	137	67
In-center Hemodialysis	36	18
Death	14	7
Medical Management	8	4
Home Hemodialysis	3	1
In-center IPD	2	1
Not Stated	4	2
TOTAL	204	100

management, six of whom experienced a return in kidney function. Terminal cancer was the cause of transfer off CAPD/CCPD to medical management for the remaining two patients. Reasons for discontinuing CAPD/CCPD therapy were requested. Exhibit 15 summarizes clinic reports of reasons which contributed to the termination of CAPD/CCPD. Note that multiple reasons for discontinuation of CAPD/CCPD were permitted for any patient. As would be expected,

EXHIBIT 15

REASONS CONTRIBUTING TO TERMINATION OF CAPD/CCPD
(NOT MUTUALLY EXCLUSIVE)

Reason	Number (n=204)	Percent
Availability of a kidney for transplant	137	67%
Other	67	33%
Reasons for non-transplant patients	n=67	
Excessive peritonitis	29	43
Exit site/tunnel infection	18	27
Patient/Family choice; inability to cope	15	22
Hospitalization for CAPD-related complications	14	21
Death	14	21
Catheter leaks and malfunctions	9	13
Peritoneal dialysis unable to maintain fluid balance	8	12
Catheter failure	7	10
Desire for change; i.e., medical staff take responsibility	7	10
Return of kidney function	6	9
Peritoneal dialysis unable to maintain solute balance	4	6
Hospitalization for other than CAPD-related complications	1	1
Hernia	1	1
Visual/manual impairment	1	1
Socioeconomic reasons	0	0
Other medical reasons	7	10
Other	7	10

transplantation was the most frequently given reason for leaving CAPD/CCPD (67% of patients). Of the 67 patients not receiving a transplant, 29 (43%) were reported to have had excessive peritonitis which contributed to the decision to terminate peritoneal dialysis, while 18 (27%) listed exit site/tunnel infections as a factor in the decision. Peritonitis and exit site/tunnel infections were simultaneously given for 14 patients (21%), while catheter complications (i.e. leak, malfunction, or failure) in conjunction with excessive peritonitis and/or exit site/tunnel infections accounted for 7 terminations of CAPD/CCPD (10%).

Following the identification of all causes contributing to the termination of peritoneal dialysis, the primary reason for such decision was requested. Results are summarized in Exhibit 16. Here again, transplan-

154

EXHIBIT 16

PRIMARY REASON FOR TERMINATING CAPD/CCPD
(MUTUALLY EXCLUSIVE)

Reason	Number	Percent (n=204)
Availability of a kidney for transplant	137	67%
Other	67	33%
Reasons for non-transplant	n=67	
Death	14	21
Excessive peritonitis	10	15
Patient/Family choice; inability to cope	7	10
Return of kidney function	6	9
Exit site/tunnel infection	4	6
Peritoneal dialysis unable to maintain fluid balance	3	4
Catheter failure	3	4
Peritoneal dialysis unable to maintain solute balance	3	4
Catheter leaks and malfunctions	2	3
Hospitalization for CAPD-related complications	2	3
Hospitalization for other than CAPD-related complications	2	3
Desire for change; i.e., medical staff take responsibility	0	0
Visual/manual impairment	0	0
Hernia	0	0
Socioeconomic reasons	0	0
Other medical reasons	6	9
Other	3	4
Terminated CAPD/CCPD primary reason - not stated	2	3

tation was found to be the primary reason for terminating CAPD/CCPD in the majority of all cases. For nontransplanted cases, death was listed as the primary reason for termination of CAPD/CCPD (21%). Excessive peritonitis, exit site/tunnel infections and catheter complications accounted for 10 (15%), 4 (6%), and 5 (7%) of patients, respectively. Of the seven patients whose primary reason was coded as 'patient/family choice; inability to cope,' 5 had claimed a CAPD/CCPD related complication as a contributing reason.

Discussion

This report contains data on 320 pediatric patients who began CAPD/CCPD prior to 20 years of age. Unfortunately, the study population represents only 66% of the 485 registered pediatric patients eligible for study. Preliminary analyses of the characteristics of the 165 patients for whom data were not submitted reveals a small but detectable bias in favor of younger patients within the study group (Exhibit 1). Among the 320 questionnaires returned, many lacked data on specific study questions, especially those relating to growth and development. Thus, interpretation of data analyses from this study is limited.

The most common primary renal disease in this patient population was found to be aplastic/hypoplastic/dysplastic kidneys. This represents a departure from most pediatric series and may reflect the somewhat younger age of the present study population [3,4]. The importance of renal transplantation, as the preferred renal replacement therapy for children [5] is clearly evident from this study. Within 12 months of initiating CAPD/CCPD, 21% of the study group had been transplanted, 17% were on a cadaveric transplant waiting list and had low antibody titers and 3% were scheduled for live donor transplantation. Only 18% had no immediate plans for transplantation and another 8% were on the cadaver waiting list but had high antibody titers. This strong preference for transplantation for pediatric patients is also reflected by the fact that 2/3 of the patients who terminated CAPD/ CCPD did so to obtain a renal allograft.

Data on growth and sexual maturation were provided for approximately one half of the 320 questionnaires received by the Data Coordinating Center. This poor showing suggests that many physicians may not be documenting the growth of their pediatric patients. Despite these limitations, this study still represents the largest known collection of pediatric patients treated with CAPD/CCPD for ≥ 1 year for whom anthropometric and maturation data have been reported. The median age of pubertal onset (Stage ≥ 2) for normal boys is estimated to be about 11 years [6]. Our study found more than half (55%) of boys ages 11–12 had not reached puberty. Mean age of pubertal onset in normal girls is estimated to be 10.5 years, [7] while median age for girls in stage 2 in this sample was reported to be 12.2 years. Similarly, median age of menarche in normal girls was earlier (12.8 years) [7] compared to the median age of menarche in this ESRD sample (15 years). These data consistently suggest a delay in pubertal onset for CAPD patients when compared to normals, a finding which has been reported in children treated with hemodialysis and transplantation [8,9].

156

Of particular interest is the dramatic deficit in height from normal 50th percentile values which occurred during the first year of CAPD/CCPD among children less than 5 years of age. Poor growth is a hallmark of renal failure in infants and very young children [10]. Clearly initiation of CAPD/ CCPD does not forestall this consequence of ESRD in young children, a finding which has been noted in other smaller series of pediatric CAPD/CCPD patients [11,12]. The role of nutritional supplementation via tube feedings proposed by some to improve growth in these patients was not addressed by the present study [13].

References

1. National Center for Health Statistics. Growth curves for children. Hamill PVV, ed. National Center in Health Statistics. 1977. Vital and Health Statistics Series 11. Data from the National Health Survey no. 165. [DHEW publication no (PHS) 78-1650].
2. Frisancho AR. New norms of upper limb fat and muscle areas for assessment of nutritional status. Am J Clin Nutr 1981; 34:2540-2545.
3. Potter DR, Holliday MA, Piel CF, et al. Treatment of end-stage renal disease in children: a 15-year experience. Kidney Int 1980 Jul; 18(1):103.
4. Broyer M. Incidence and etiology of ESRD in children. In: Fine RN and Gruskin AB, eds. End Stage Renal Disease in Children. Philadelphia: W.B. Saunders, 1984:14-16.
5. Fine RN. Renal transplantation in children. J Pediatr 1982; 100:754.
6. Marshall WA, Tanner JM. Variations in patterns of pubertal changes in boys. Arch Dis Child 1970; 45:13.
7. Marshall WA, Tanner JM. Variations in patterns of pubertal changes in girls. Arch Dis Child 1969; 44:291.
8. Kleinknecht C, Broyer M, Gagnadoux M, et al. Growth in children treated with long term dialysis: A study of 76 patients. In: Hamberger J, Crosnier J, Grunfeld J, Maxwell MH, eds. Advances in Nephrology. Volume 99. Chicago: Chicago Year Book Medical Publishers, 1980:133.
9. Ferraris J, Saenger P, Levine L, et al. Delayed puberty in males with chronic renal failure. Kidney Int 1980 Sep; 18:344.
10. Alexander SR. Treatment of infants with ESRD. In: Fine RN and Gruskin AB, eds. End-Stage Renal Disease in Children. Philadelphia: W.B. Saunders, 1984:17-29.
11. Broyer M, Rizzoni G, Douckernoollse R, et al. CAPD in children: data from the European Dialysis and Transplant Association (EDTA) Registry. In: Fine RN, Scharer K, and Mehls O, eds. CAPD in Children. New York: Cerlin, Springer-Verlag, 1985:36-37.
12. Potter DE, San Luis E, Wipfler JE, et al. Comparison of continuous ambulatory peritoneal dialysis and hemodialysis in children. Kidney Int 1986; 30:S11-S14.
13. Wassner SJ, Abitbol C, Alexander SR, et al. Nutritional requirements for infants with renal failure. Am J Kidney Dis 1986 Apr; 7:300.

E. Complications of Peritoneal Catheters*

Introduction

In 1973, Tenckhoff demonstrated the feasibility of peritoneal dialysis as a long term treatment for chronic renal failure, and his modification of the silicone-rubber peritoneal catheter for repeated access to the peritoneum was an important factor in the success of this modality of treatment. However, complications associated with the use of these catheters were recognized early in the course of their use. The most serious complications included: catheter exit-site infection, catheter cuff erosion, tunnel abscess, pericatheter leak, and obstruction to flow. To overcome such problems, a number of changes in peritoneal catheter design have been seen.

Most of the design modifications that have been proposed address specific complications observed in earlier designs. To overcome the problem of catheter cuff erosion, a single cuff straight catheter with the cuff implanted in the preperitoneal position was developed; another approach has been the use of a subcutaneous cuff with a fabric flange. In some instances different material (expanded polytetrafluoroethylene) has been used instead of the customary polyester cuff.

Other modifications have dealt with the problem of obstruction to flow. Several designs claim to overcome the problems of obstruction by omentum and migration within the peritoneal cavity. These include: the column-disc catheter designed by Ash, the Toronto Western Hospital catheter, with its intra-abdominal discs — as well as a number of other catheters which incorporate balloons in the distal limb to deflect

---

* The material contained in this report will be published as follows:
   Lindblad AS, Hamilton RW, Novak JW. A retrospective analysis of catheter configuration and cuff type. A National CAPD Registry Report. In press, *Peritoneal Dial Bull.*

adherent bowel. Although each catheter has had its advocates, comparative clinical trials have been few, limited in scope, and seldom have employed randomized controls.

Subjects and Methods

The purpose of this study was to determine the natural history of implanted peritoneal catheters and to estimate survival distributions for different types of catheters. Data relating to the frequency and character of catheter complications as well as reasons for catheter removal were solicited from a random sample of 2,000 registered patients.

Only Class 1 patients who were ≥ 20 years of age at CAPD/CCPD initiation were considered eligible for this study. Patients must have begun CAPD/CCPD after 1981 and prior to September 1, 1985 — thereby allowing for at least one year of follow-up. Only patients from currently active centers were considered. Information was abstracted from hospital and clinic records by center personnel on study specific forms; and data submitted to the Data Coordinating Center were processed and additionally checked for errors.

Results

Study forms were returned for 1,582 (79%) of the 2,000 patients sampled. Of the forms received, 77 contained no information. As a

EXHIBIT 1

COMPARISON OF SELECTED CHARACTERISTICS FOR
PATIENTS FOR WHOM DATA FORMS WERE RECEIVED
WITH THOSE FOR WHOM DATA WERE NOT RECEIVED

| | Data Form | |
| | Received | Not Received |
Characteristic	(n = 1,505)	(n = 495)
% Male	55	54
% White	77	77
% Prior ESRD Therapy	55	60
% Age		
20 - 29 years	10	11
30 - 39 years	16	14
40 - 49 years	17	17
50 - 59 years	23	25
60 - 69 years	22	23
$\geq$ 70 years	12	11
Median Age	53 years	53 years

result, the analysis which follows is based on 75% of the sampled population. Exhibit 1 compares selected characteristics of the 1,505 patients for whom catheter information was received with the 495 patients for whom study data was not provided. The two populations are nearly identical, suggesting that data from this study is probably representative of the general adult registry population.

Exhibit 2 summarizes first catheter and cuff types for the study patients. Twenty-seven percent of those patients (404/1,505) reported the

EXHIBIT 2

NUMBER OF PATIENTS BY FIRST CATHETER AND FIRST CUFF TYPE

First Catheter Type	Total N	(%)	Double Cuff	Single Cuff Deep Fascia	Single Cuff Subcutaneous	Other	Unknown
Standard, straight	957	(64)	753	116	66	0	22
Standard, curled	330	(22)	218	73	21	14	4
Toronto Western, straight	94	(6)	78	9	6	0	1
Column-disc (Ash)	49	(3)	45	3	0	0	1
Gore-Tex	28	(2)	1	6	7	0	14
Other	2	(.1)	1	0	0	1	0
Unknown	45	(3)	32	1	0	0	12
TOTAL	1505	(100)	1128 (75)	208 (14)	100 (7)	15 (1)	54 (4)

EXHIBIT 3

NUMBER OF PATIENTS BY SECOND CATHETER AND SECOND CUFF TYPE

Second Catheter Type	Total N	(%)	Double Cuff	Single Cuff Deep Fascia	Single Cuff Subcutaneous	Other	Unknown
Standard, straight	234	(58)	176	38	9	0	11
Standard, curled	122	(30)	88	23	5	3	3
Toronto Western, straight	15	(4)	13	2	0	0	0
Column-disc (Ash)	19	(5)	15	0	0	0	4
Gore-Tex	7	(2)	1	0	2	0	4
Other	2	(<1)	1	0	0	0	1
Unknown	5	(1)	4	0	0	0	1
TOTAL	404	(100)	298 (74)	63 (16)	16 (4)	3 (1)	24 (6)

use of a second catheter (Exhibit 3), and 22 percent (88/404) of those who had a second catheter reported the use of a third catheter (Exhibit 4). As information was sparse on the Toronto Western swan neck and Missouri swan neck catheters, these types were included in the 'other' category. Eighty-five patients who had separately reported a catheter replacement to the Registry during routine reporting did not provide second catheter type information and 46 patients reporting at least two replacements did not provide third catheter information.

A standard straight double cuff catheter is the most frequently chosen type of catheter/cuff, irrespective of the number of catheters that were previously implanted. Note that they account for 50% (753/1505) of first catheters, 44% (176/404) of second catheters and 44% (39/88) of third catheters (see Exhibits 2, 3 and 4). Standard curled double cuff catheters were used as first catheters in 15% of patients and as second and third catheters in 21% and 16% of patients with replacements, respectively. Less frequently used were Toronto-Western straight, Column-Disc (Ash) and Gore-Tex catheters, which when combined were used in 11% of patients as first catheters, 10% as second catheters and 15% as third catheters. Three reports of patients using single cuff Column-Disc (Ash) catheters and three reports of patients with a double-cuff Gore-Tex catheter were received. As Column-Disc catheters do not routinely come with a single cuff design and Gore-Tex catheters are not supplied with a double-cuff, these 6 responses are of questionable accuracy.

Selected patient characteristics according to catheter and cuff types are detailed in Exhibit 5. In general, the patient variables studied appear

EXHIBIT 4

NUMBER OF PATIENTS BY THIRD CATHETER AND THIRD CUFF TYPE

| Third Catheter Type | Total | | Double Cuff | Third Cuff Type | | | |
	N	(%)		Single Cuff Deep Fascia	Single Cuff Subcutaneous	Other	Unknown
Standard, straight	50	(57)	39	8	1	0	2
Standard, curled	22	(25)	14	5	1	1	1
Toronto Western, straight	2	(2)	0	2	0	0	0
Column-disc (Ash)	6	(7)	5	0	0	0	1
Gore-Tex	5	(6)	1	0	0	0	4
Other	3	(3)	2	0	0	0	1
TOTAL	88	(100)	61 (69)	15 (17)	2 (2)	1 (1)	9 (10)

EXHIBIT 5

SELECTED CHARACTERISTICS
BY FIRST CATHETER TYPE AND FIRST CUFF TYPE

	N	% Male	% White	% Prior ESRD	% Diabetic	Median Age
Catheter Type:						
Standard, straight	957	55	75	56	24	53
Standard, curled	330	53	81	51	30	51
Toronto Western (straight)	94	61	83	53	23	56
Column-disc (ASH)	49	54	79	50	38	52
Gore-Tex	28	68	82	54	18	53
Unknown	45	55	79	76	28	49
Cuff Type:						
Double	1128	55	78	54	25	53
Single (Deep fascia)	208	60	76	58	28	51
Single (Subcutaneous)	100	45	67	56	19	52
Unknown	54	54	77	60	33	53

to be evenly distributed among the catheter and cuff types. Only Gore-Tex catheter patients, who were less frequently observed to be diabetic, and 'unknown' catheter types, who more frequently received prior ESRD therapy, were statistically maldistributed.

Catheter Survival

Survival probabilities according to catheter and cuff type were calculated using the methods of Kaplan Meier [1] and are presented in Exhibit 6. Patients whose only reason for catheter removal was coded as death, transfer to another modality, or transplantation or whose catheters remained in place at last contact, were censored. Catheter survival times for these patients contribute information up to the point of last contact.

. A Cox proportional hazards model [2] was used to assess catheter and cuff differences with respect to catheter survival adjusted for prognostic variables. The complete model included age, sex, diabetic glomerulosclerosis diagnosis, prior ESRD therapy status, race, catheter configuration,

162

EXHIBIT 6

PROBABILITY OF CATHETER SURVIVAL (%) FOR SELECTED TIME POINTS
BY CATHETER TYPE (95% CONFIDENCE INTERVAL)

First Catheter and Cuff Type	6 Prob.	6 95% CI	12 Prob.	12 95% CI	18 Prob.	18 95% CI	24 Prob.	24 95% CI	36 Prob.	36 95% CI
STANDARD, STRAIGHT										
Double cuff	83	(80,86)	70	(66,74)	60	(55,65)	51	(45,56)	33	(27,40)
Single cuff (deep)	73	(63,81)	60	(49,70)	44	(33,56)	33	(22,47)	22	(12,35)
Single cuff (SubQ)	79	(67,87)	69	(55,80)	55	(40,69)	55	(40,69)	36	(19,56)
STANDARD, CURLED										
Double cuff	85	(79,90)	69	(61,76)	51	(42,60)	43	(33,54)	34	(21,49)
Single cuff (deep)	81	(69,88)	70	(57,80)	64	(50,76)	49	(32,65)	6	(2,19)
Single cuff (SubQ)	78	(54,90)	57	(33,77)	*		*		*	
TORONTO WESTERN, STRAIGHT	80	(70,88)	69	(58,79)	52	(39,64)	35	(23,49)	22	(11,38)
COLUMN-DISC (ASH)	81	(67,90)	71	(53,84)	59	(40,76)	47	(32,73)	*	
GORE-TEX	85	(67,94)	57	(37,74)	41	(23,62)	*	*	*	

Months on CAPD

*Probability estimates with confidence interval widths exceeding 45 are not shown.

cuff type and catheter by cuff interactions. Only the standard straight, standard curled, Column-Disc (Ash), Gore-Tex and Toronto Western straight catheters were assessed as sample sizes in all other catheter types were too small to permit analysis. Prior treatment for end-stage renal disease was found to be associated with shorter catheter survival; no other covariate appears to be significantly related to catheter survival.

No overall differences in catheter survival among catheter configurations (i.e. straight, curled, column-disc, Gore-Tex, Toronto Western) were identified in the surveyed patients. Pairwise comparisons, however, suggest improved survival for the standard double cuff catheter versus the Toronto Western catheter. A significant difference in length of catheter survival with respect to cuff type was observed, e.g. catheters using a single cuff located in the deep fascia have a shorter survival than double cuff catheters (relative risk = 1.4). These deep single cuff catheters are also observed to have shorter survival times than single cuff catheters where the cuff is located in the subcutaneous tissue (relative risk 1.4). No difference with respect to catheter survival was observed between catheters with a double cuff versus catheters with subcutaneously placed single cuffs and no catheter configuration by cuff

EXHIBIT 7

PROBABILITY OF CATHETER SURVIVAL
BY CUFF TYPE

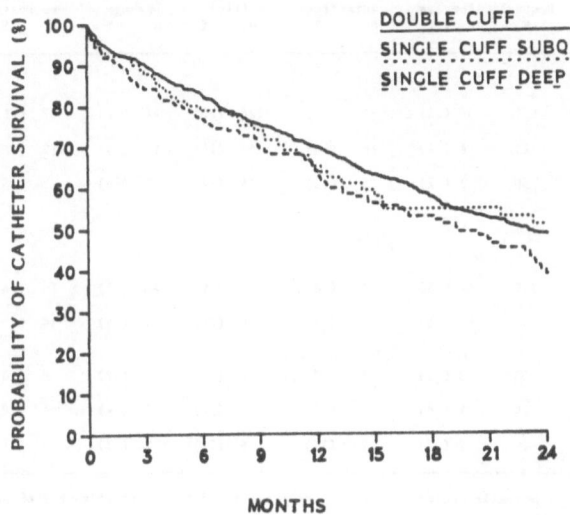

type interaction was observed. Cumulative survival probabilities by cuff type are graphically illustrated in Exhibit 7.

Reasons for Catheter Removal

Exhibit 8 depicts the proportion of patients whose first catheter was removed for specified reasons by cuff type and catheter configuration. Since multiple reasons may have been given for a catheter's removal, the reasons listed are not mutually exclusive. Transfers included transfer to hemodialysis, transplants, or death. All forms with 'other' complication coded as 'yes' were hand reviewed for reclassification when appropriate. It is important to note that testing differences between three cuff types and five catheter configurations among seven reasons for removal results in 91 tests. By chance alone one would expect a statistically significant difference for one out of every 20 tests at the .05 level. Nonetheless, as this is an exploratory analysis, differences observed will be noted in the text which follows.

Of the seven possible reasons for removal only two, exit site infection and peritonitis appeared to be disproportionately distributed among the cuff types. Exit site infections were reported in proportionately more patients using a single subcutaneously placed cuff (13%) than for

EXHIBIT 8

COMPLICATIONS RESULTING IN CATHETER REMOVAL
BY CATHETER CONFIGURATION AND CUFF TYPE

First Catheter and Cuff Type	Total Pts. N	Total Removals N	Tunnel Abscess		Exit Site Infection		Reason for Removal* Perito- nitis		Leakage		Failure to Drain		Transfer		Other	
			N	%	N	%	N	%	N	%	N	%	N	%	N	%
CUFF TYPE																
Double	1128	627	50	(4)	76	(7)	228	(20)	27	(2)	67	(6)	259	(23)	82	(7
Single (deep)	208	125	8	(4)	16	(8)	50	(24)	11	(5)	12	(6)	46	(22)	23	(11
Single (subQ)	100	50	2	(2)	13	(13)	14	(14)	5	(5)	3	(3)	21	(21)	7	(7
CATHETER TYPE																
Standard, straight	957	519	44	(5)	75	(8)	184	(19)	26	(3)	60	(6)	200	(21)	74	(8
Standard, curled	330	198	16	(5)	22	(7)	68	(21)	15	(5)	18	(5)	80	(24)	28	(8
Toronto Western, straight	94	60	3	(3)	7	(7)	28	(30)	2	(2)	0	(0)	36	(38)	6	(6
Column-Disc (ASH)	49	24	1	(4)	2	(4)	12	(24)	2	(4)	4	(8)	8	(16)	2	(4
Gore-Tex	28	20	2	(7)	9	(32)	6	(21)	2	(7)	2	(7)	8	(29)	5	(18

*Reasons for removal are not mutually exclusive. Percentages are based on the total number of patients with each catheter type.

patients using a double cuff (7%). However peritonitis, as a contributing cause for catheter removal, was claimed in proportionately fewer patients using a subcutaneously placed single cuff (14%) than in patients using a single cuff placed in the deep fascia (24%).

Among the five catheter configurations, patients using the Toronto-Western catheter were more likely to claim peritonitis and transfer as a reason for catheter removal than patients using a standard type catheter. However, no patients using a Toronto Western catheter claimed failure to drain as a reason contributing to catheter removal while a range of 5%–8% was claimed for the remaining four catheters. Exit site infection was a common complication precipitating catheter removal among patients using the Gore-Tex catheter (32%) while it accounted for no more than 8% of patients using other catheter types.

Second Catheter Survival

Second catheter survival was compared with first catheter survival in a survival analysis; no association between the length of first catheter survival and the probability of second catheter survival was found in those patients who received a second catheter. First catheter survival irrespective of catheter type was longer than second catheter survival (median 22 months, versus 15 months, respectively). These observations imply that although the length of first catheter survival is not predictive of second catheter life, in general, one expects a substantial decrease in the life of second catheter. This result suggests the group of patients, who for complications or other reasons have their first catheter removed, may be predisposed to failure of the second catheter.

Discussion

The single straight catheter with double cuffs is the most widely used peritoneal access system. There are wide beliefs that the deep cuff is important in preventing leaks and that a cuff in the subcutaneous tissue, usually about 2 cm below the skin, stabilizes the catheter near the exit site and reduces exit-site trauma. The role of the cuffs in preventing the movement of bacteria through the tunnel has recently been challenged; early colonization of catheter surfaces along the entire length of the catheter have been noted in catheters removed from patients with or without a history of infection [3]. The formation of a biofilm on catheters is now held to be common and the role of the biofilm in precipitating infections, is unclear.

Single subcutaneous cuffs were not invariably associated with higher leak rates than systems containing the deep cuff. However, our survey lacks information relative to variables that may have an impact on leak rate. Lateral placement of the deep cuff in the fascia, in rectus muscle or in the body of the rectus muscle may yield lower leak rates than mid-line placements [4]. The depth of placement of a single subcutaneous cuff can be important particularly if the placement is in deep to mid-line fascia or superficial rectus fascia.

Single deep cuffs with presumably more mobility at the exit site were not found to be associated with consistently higher rates of exit site infection or tunnel abscesses. In fact, patients with subcutaneously placed cuffs report proportionately more exit site infections than patients with either single cuffs placed in the deep fascia or double cuffs. This latter observation is supported by data from a recent publication of a single center study which found a higher incidence of exit site complications as a reason for catheter removal in patients using the subcutaneously placed cuff versus those patients using the double cuff [5]. Recent evidence suggests that the direction of the exit hole may impact on the incidence of exit-site infection and could be a variable for those systems containing the subcutaneous cuff.[6] In addition, some patients are more successful at immobilizing their external catheter

166

segments during activities and thereby reducing trauma to the exit site.

Prior ESRD therapy was found to be significantly associated with a decrease in catheter survival. Although no reason for this result is apparent, future studies on catheter survival should consider inclusion of this variable in analysis.

The results do not clearly show major differences in catheter survival related to the choice of catheter configuration; however, the suggestion of improved catheter survival in patients using a standard catheter versus patients using a Toronto-Western catheter is supported by others [5]. The better catheter survival with the double cuff catheter and single subcutaneously placed catheter versus the single cuff catheter placed in the deep fascia is not readily explained. Patient selection factors across all centers have an unknown impact on catheter survival. Additionally, surgical technique, postoperative care, and catheter break in techniques are likely to be more uniform in a single center study as opposed to a broad scale multi-institutional study. The results reported should be viewed with these caveats in mind. Further study to confirm these observations, ideally in a randomized setting, is needed before extrapolating to broad scale practice.

References

1. Kaplan E and Meier P. Nonparametric estimation from incomplete observations. J Am Stat Soc 1958; 53:457–458.
2. Cox DR. Regression models and life tables. J Stat Soc B 1972; 34:200.
3. Dasgupta MK, Ulan RA, Bettcher KB, Burns V, Lam K, Dosseter JB, Costerton JW. Effect of exit site infection and peritonitis on the distribution of biofilm encased adherent bacterial microcolonies on Tenckhoff catheters in patients undergoing CAPD. In: Khanna R, Nolph KD, Prowant BF, Twardowski ZJ, and Oreopoulos DG, eds. Advances in CAPD. Proceedings of the 6th Annual CAPD Conference. Toronto: University of Toronto Press, 1986:102–109.
4. Helfrich GB, Pechan BW and Alijani MR. Reduced catheter complications with lateral placement. Peritoneal Dial Bull 1983 Oct-Dec; 3:(4) S2–S4.
5. Flanigan MJ, Ngheim DD, Schulak JA, Ullrich GE, Freeman RM. The use and complications of three peritoneal dialysis catheter designs: A retro spective analysis. Trans Am Soc Artif Intern Organs 1987 Jan-Mar; 33(1):33–38.
6. Twardowski ZJ, Nolph KD, Khanna R, Prowant BF, Ryan LP and Nichols WK. The need for a 'swan neck' permanently bent, accurate peritoneal dialysis catheter. Peritoneal Dial Bull 1985 Oct-Dec; 5(4):219–225.

F. The Effects of CAPD on Hypertension Control*

Introduction

Hypertension (elevated systolic and diastolic blood pressure) is common in patients with chronic renal disease and is estimated to affect about 80% of patients entering dialysis. Confirmation of that estimate in a sufficiently large sample of entering ESRD patients is not available for any therapeutic modality, nor are responses to antihypertensive therapy known. In the general population, several classic studies [1–3] have indicated that high blood pressure is a leading risk factor predisposing to stroke, heart failure, and kidney failure, and that blood pressure control is generally a worthy therapeutic objective. Indeed, patients with diastolic pressures in excess of 105 mm Hg who sustain a reduction of blood pressure by any means can usually expect prolonged useful life from reduced occurrences of stroke, congestive heart failure and renal failure.

Definitive evidence that a reduction to 'normal blood pressure' will offer the same benefit in a dialysis population is not available. Although hypertension in the patient who comes to dialysis is common, the prevalence of this condition in adequate samples of patients entering dialysis has not been fully characterized. While blood pressure response to attainment of desirable 'dry weight' is excellent in many dialyzed patients, others require medication to maintain pressure control and some fail to have their blood pressure controlled due to various causes including salt and water non-compliance, hyper-hormonal states and/or inadequate medication.

* The material contained in this report will be published as follows:
Lindblad AS, Hamilton RW, Novak JW. A retrospective analysis of catheter configuration and cuff type. A National CAPD Registry Report. In press, *Peritoneal Dial Bull*.

This special study of the National CAPD Registry was designed to estimate the percent of Registry patients who have a history of hypertension, their status at the initiation of CAPD/CCPD and the effect of CAPD/CCPD on hypertension by assessing blood pressures and medication usage at one month and one year after CAPD/CCPD initiation.

Subjects and Methods

A random sample of 400 patients entered onto the CAPD Registry was selected. Patients were required to have been at least 20 years of age and new to CAPD/CCPD at the time of registration. All subjects must have begun CAPD/CCPD after 1981 and prior to September 1985, and were to have been under the care of a currently active Registry center. Prior hypertension history was obtained and blood pressure, weight and hypertensive medication assessments were requested at baseline (within two weeks prior to CAPD initiation), 1 month, 1 year and at last contact while on CAPD/CCPD. Use of diuretics, beta blockers, vasodilators, central sympatholytics and converting enzyme inhibitors were separately assessed.

Results

Responses were obtained for 209 (52%) of the sampled patients despite multiple written and telephone contacts to non-responding institutions. Because the potential for important non-response biases exist, all conclusions should be tempered by this consideration. Although this was the smallest study in terms of number of patients, its response rate was the lowest in this series of Registry studies. This suggests that the blood pressure/medication profiles requested were not readily available to a substantial number of the clinics. The sample sizes for the analyses vary depending upon response rate and withdrawal from CAPD/CCPD therapy.

Exhibit 1 details some presenting characteristics, by response status, of the study patients. Study patients demographics are comparable to Registry patients on the whole, and, patients age, sex, prior therapy and diabetes status are generally comparable between study participants and for those whom special study data were not received—although a higher proportion of participants were white.

Hypertension history for the study patients is summarized in Exhibit 2. Seventy-seven percent of the participating patients are regarded as

EXHIBIT 1

BACKGROUND CHARACTERISTICS OF SELECTED SAMPLE

	Participants n = 209	Non-Participants n = 191
Sex - % Male	58	51
Race - % White	81	71
Prior ESRD Therapy %	52	56
Diabetes - % diabetic glomerulosclerosis	22	25
Median Age (years)	52	52

EXHIBIT 2

HYPERTENSION HISTORY

		Proportion	Percent
Is patient hypertensive - Yes		160/209	76.6%
Has patient ever taken Anti-hypertensives	Unknown	12/209	5.7
	No	51/209	24.4
	Yes	146/209	69.9
Medication History			
Diuretics		70/146	47.9
Central sympatholytics		64/146	43.8
Beta blockers		71/146	48.6
Vasodilators		53/146	36.3
Converting enzyme inhibitors		9/146	6.2
Duration of Pre-CAPD therapy	None	7/146	4.8
	$\leq$ 1 year	17/146	11.6
	1-4 years	43/146	29.5
	5-9 years	16/146	11.0
	10-14 years	9/146	6.2
	$\leq$ 15 years	5/146	3.4
	Unknown	49/146	33.6
Time since hypertension diagnosis	Mean	7.7 years	
	Median	4.8 years	
Duration of anti-hypertensive therapy	Mean	5.6 years	
	Median	3.3 years	

having a history of hypertension at baseline, with the 95% confidence interval ranging from 71% to 82%. Over 90% of the hypertensives are known to have received antihypertensive medications at some time. Beta blockers, diuretics, central sympatholytics and vasodilators were used by 36% to 49% of the hypertensive patients. Median time since diagnosis of hypertension is 4.8 years, and the median hypertensive patient has a medication history of 3.3 years. Only 7 patients with a medication history were reported not to have been receiving medication immediately

170

EXHIBIT 3

MEAN BLOOD PRESSURE AND
WEIGHT CHARACTERISTICS

	Baseline	1 month	1 year	Last contact
Blood pressures:				
Systolic	147.6	137.3	140.3	136.5
Diastolic	83.9	79.9	82.9	80.3
N	151	167	122	148
Weight:				
Kg	66.8	66.9	68.9	68.1
N	139	160	120	144

prior to entry onto CAPD, but for all patients, this duration was frequently not known.

Mean blood pressure and weight values for the cohort are detailed in Exhibit 3. At baseline, mean blood pressure was 148/84 mm Hg, with substantial patient to patient variability as indicated by a standard deviation of 27 mm Hg for systolic and 15 mm Hg for diastolic pressure. These variances were statistically constant at all the other time points. Mean baseline pressures for 1A (no prior ESRD therapy) and 1B patients were equivalent, the two groups differing by less than 1 mm Hg for both measures. Note that the median time to last contact is 18

EXHIBIT 4

CHANGE IN BLOOD PRESSURE FROM BASELINE

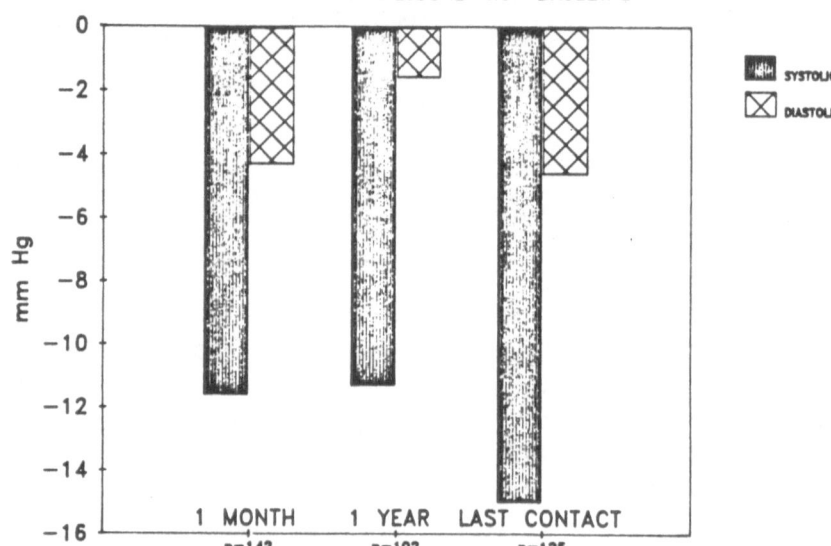

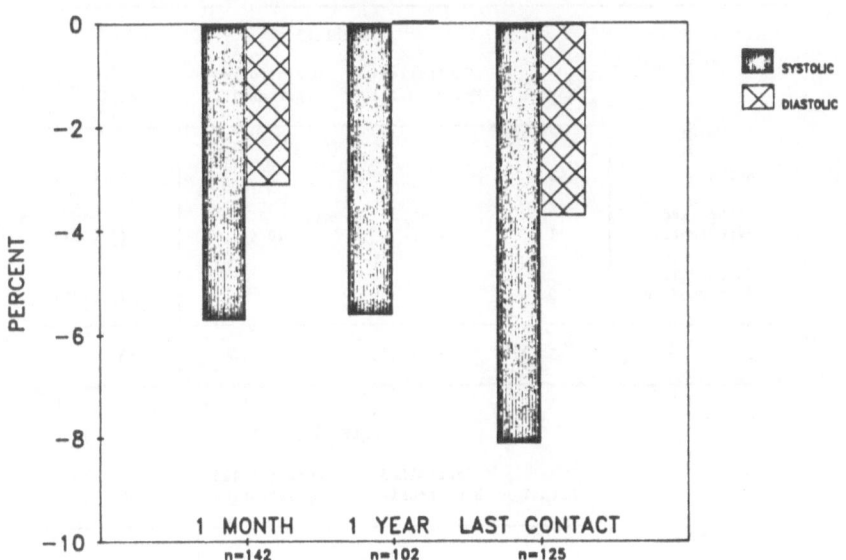

EXHIBIT 5

PERCENT CHANGE IN BLOOD PRESSURE FROM BASELINE

months. The decreases in blood pressure, which are summarized in Exhibit 3, are more rigorously characterized in Exhibits 4 and 5, where absolute and percent decreases from baseline are graphically presented. Significant decreases from baseline are observed for all systolic measurements and for diastolic measures at one month and at last contact. Systolic pressure decreases exceed 11 mm Hg and range from 5.6% to 8.1% of baseline levels as a percent of baseline. Systolic pressure decreases are significantly greater than diastolic pressure decreases for all time periods. For 96 patients with weight recorded both at baseline and 1 year, a significant mean weight gain of 2 kilograms (.9 to 3.1, 95% CI) was observed. Decreases in blood pressure were similar, irrespective of prior ESRD therapy status (Class 1A or 1B).

To accurately assess the impact of CAPD on patients' hypertension, one must simultaneously consider blood pressure levels and medication approaches. Accordingly, patients were categorized as 1) uncontrolled hypertensive—diastolic > 90 despite receiving anti-hypertensive medications, 2) controlled hypertensive—diastolic pressure ≤ 90, receiving medication, and 3) normal—all non-medicated patients. Thus, a few untreated patients with elevated blood pressure are included as normal in Exhibits 6 and 7. Cross tabulation of baseline versus 1 month and baseline versus 1 year status is presented in Exhibit 6. Note that at both time periods, a significant increase in the frequency of normal patients and a concomitant decrease in uncontrolled hypertensives was observed.

EXHIBIT 6

BLOOD PRESSURE AND MEDICATION CATEGORIZATIONS

	BASELINE			
	Normal	Controlled Hypertensive	Uncontrolled Hypertensive	Total
1 MONTH:				
Normal	42	11	2	55 (41%)
Controlled Hypertensive	1	44	18	63 (47%)
Uncontrolled Hypertensive	0	9	7	16 (12%)
Total	43 (32%)	64 (48%)	27 (20%)	134

	BASELINE			
	Normal	Controlled Hypertensive	Uncontrolled Hypertensive	Total
1 YEAR:				
Normal	29	14	6	49 (51%)
Controlled Hypertensive	0	20	10	30 (31%)
Uncontrolled Hypertensive	0	12	5	17 (18%)
Total	29 (30%)	46 (48%)	21 (22%)	96

For example, the proportion of normals is increased from 30% at baseline to 51% at one year.

Exhibit 7 graphically displays the conditional outcome probabilities for the two time periods. Note that less than 26% of uncontrolled hypertensives at baseline remain in that category at either follow-up period. Mean diastolic blood pressure for the 17 uncontrolled patients at 1 year is 104 mm Hg. Further, 7% of uncontrolled hypertensives are converted to normal at one month—which increases to a 29% conversion rate at one year. The controlled hypertensives are converted to normal with similar frequency while those that begin as normal are very likely to remain in that state.

Exhibit 8 presents distributions for the spectrum of classes of drugs used in treating patients at baseline, 1 month and 1 year. Although 32% of patients receiving pharmacologic anti-hypertensives at baseline were receiving diuretics, at one month only 18% and at 1 year only 9% are treated with these agents. Beta blockers, converting enzyme inhibitors and vasodilators are used to equivalent degrees among treated patients

EXHIBIT 7

HYPERTENSION CATEGORIES AT 1 MONTH
BY BASELINE STATUS

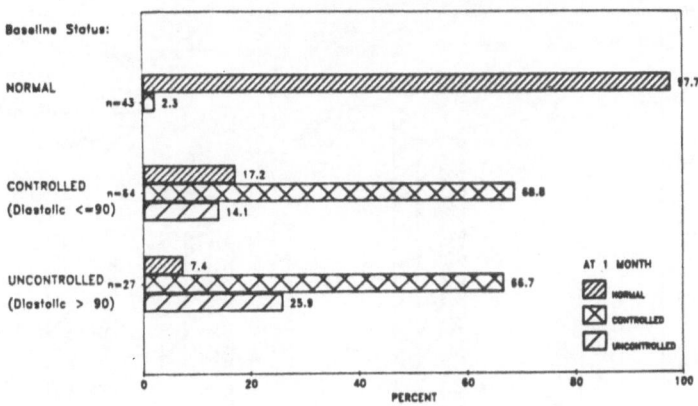

HYPERTENSION CATEGORIES AT 1 YEAR
BY BASELINE STATUS

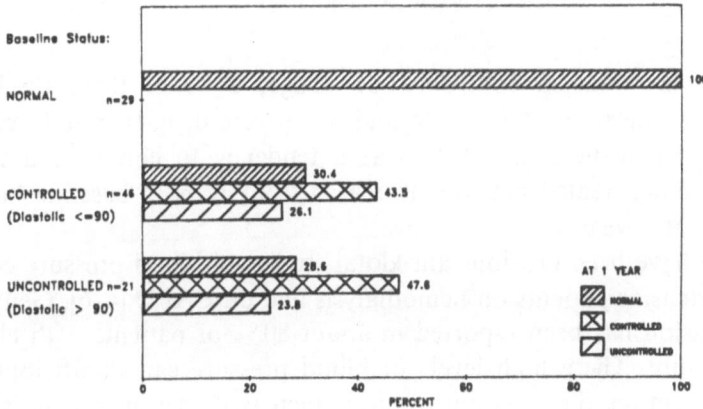

at all time periods studied. Further, there is a suggestion of decreased use of central sympatholytics in patients treated at 1 year.

Discussion

Following the initiation of CAPD therapy in hypertensive patients, early and sustained decreases in systolic and diastolic blood pressure were seen. Patients who began CAPD with normal blood pressure and no anti-hypertensive drugs tended to remain in this status. Most of the patients starting CAPD with blood pressure controlled by antihyperten-

174

EXHIBIT 8

ANTIHYPERTENSIVE MEDICATIONS FOR TREATED PATIENTS

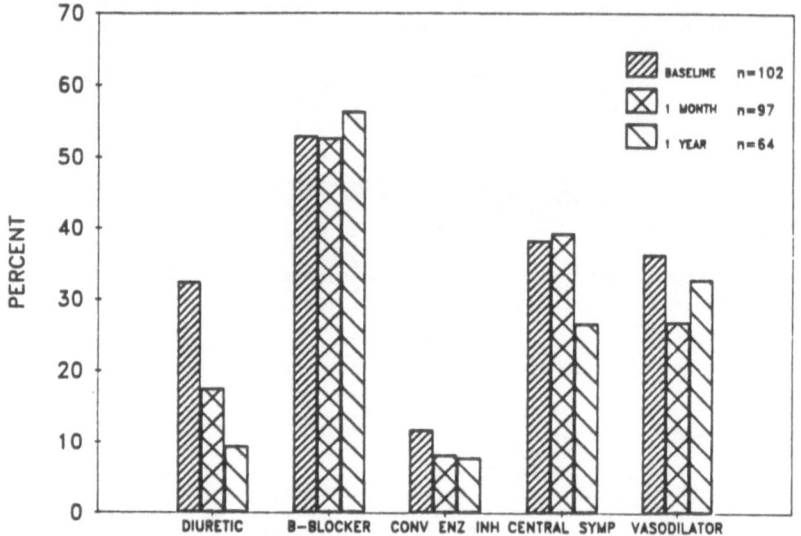

sive agents remained controlled on drugs; 17% of these no longer required medication at 1 month and 30% were drug free at 1 year. Of those using medications, there was a tendency to eliminate diuretics. Usage among treated patients decreased from 32% at baseline but was still 9% at 1 year.

There have been previous anecdotal studies of blood pressure control in hypertensive patients on hemodialysis and on CAPD [4–6]. Generally, hypertension has been reported in about 80% of patients with chronic renal failure. These high levels of blood pressure can be attributed to increases in cardiac output and/or increased peripheral resistance. Cardiac output increases may reflect volume expansion secondary to sodium and water retention or the anemia of chronic renal failure. Increases in peripheral resistance may reflect increased levels of circulating angiotensin II or decreased levels of vasodilators such as prostaglandins, bradykinin, or renal medullary lipids. Also there is recent speculation that volume expansion may be associated with increased blood levels of inhibitors of sodium transport which may increase intracellular sodium and calcium in the cells of vascular walls and enhanced reactivity [7,8]. Although normotension without medication is associated with maintenance of dry weight [4–6,9] in a small group of patients, hypertension may be refractory to volume control and many patients in this category have elevated levels of plasma renin [9–11].

This Registry study showed that 30 % of medicated patients were converted to normal by one year. This is less than the up to 60 % rate reported from isolated series [4] and highlights the continued importance of the hypertension problem. Perhaps the most important finding from this sample of the national population is that 26 % of previously controlled patients were uncontrolled (i.e. diastolic > 90 mm Hg) after one year on CAPD and that 24 % of patients uncontrolled at baseline were still uncontrolled after one year. It remains to be determined whether the uncontrolled patients at one year had problems with increased peripheral resistance in face of good volume control or inadequate volume control related to excessive intakes of sodium and water and/or poor ultrafiltration.

References

1. The Multiple Risk Factor Intervention Trial (MRFIT). JAMA 1976; 235:825.
2. The Veteran's Administration Cooperative Study Group on Antihypertensive Agents. Effects on treatment or mortality in hypertension. I. Results in patients with diastolic blood pressures averaging 115 to 120 mm Hg. JAMA 1967; 202:1028–1034.
3. The Veteran's Administration Cooperative Study Group on Antihypertensive Agents. Effects on treatment or mortality in hypertension. II.- Results in patients with diastolic blood pressures averaging 90 to 114 mm Hg. JAMA 1978; 213:1143–1152.
4. Young MA, Nolph KD, Dutton S and Prowant B. Antihypertensive drug requirements in continuous ambulatory peritoneal dialysis. Peritoneal Dial Bull 1984 Apr-Jun; 4(2):85–88.
5. Lazarus JM, Hampers CL and Merrill JP. Hypertension in chronic renal failure. Arch Intern Med 1974; 133:1059.
6. Russel RP and Whelton PK. Hypertension in chronic renal failure. Am J Nephrol 1983 Mar-Jun; 3(2–3):185.
7. Huot SJ, Pamnani MB, Clough DL and Haddy FJ. The role of sodium intake, the Na-K pump and a ouabain like humoral agent in the genesis of reduced renal mass hypertension. Am J Nephrol 1983 Mar-Jun; 3(2–3):92–99.
8. de Wardener HE and MacGregor GA. The role of a circulating inhibitor of Na-K ATPase in essential hypertension. Am J Nephrol 1983 Mar-Jun; 3(2–3):88–91.
9. Vertes V, Cangian JL, Berman LB and Gould A. Hypertension in end-stage renal disease. N Engl J Med 1969; 280:978.
10. Weidman P, Maxwell MH and Lupu AN. Plasma renin activity and blood pressure in terminal renal failure. N Engl J Med 1971; 285:757.
11. Weidman P and Maxwell M. The renin angiotensin-aldosterone system in terminal renal failure. Kidney Int 1976; 8:S219.

Special Reports—1986

Introduction to Special Reports A–C:

Factors Associated with Morbidity and Mortality among Patients on CAPD

The registry report issued in January 1985 contained a special report on prognostic factors associated with the first episode of peritonitis. The factors considered in the analysis were the patients' age, sex, race, living arrangement (with or without family), history of diabetes, and prior therapy for ESRD. A two stage statistical analysis was used, the first to identify which of these factors were individually associated with the risk of peritonitis. The second stage assessed the relative importance of the factors identified in stage one.

The result of the analysis of peritonitis risk is summarized in the following table. It was found that non-diabetic patients who were 20–59 years of age, white, lived without family, and had no prior ESRD therapy, were at relatively low risk. A patient with these characteristics was designated as a 'baseline patient' and the magnitudes of the additional risks were determined for patients who differed with respect to one or more traits.

The same methodology was used in the three reports that follow, pertaining to:
— First Hospitalization for CAPD—Related Complications.
— Transfer off CAPD.
— Death while on CAPD.

TABLE 1.   Examples of Additional Risks (%) of Developing First Peritonitis for Patients with Various Characteristics as Compared with a "Baseline Patient"

| | TRAIT | | | | | % |
	DIABETIC STATUS	AGE	RACE	LIVING ARRANGEMENT	PRIOR ESRD THERAPY	ADDITIONAL RISK
"BASELINE PATIENT"	Non-Diabetic	20-59	White	Without Family	No Prior Therapy	0.0 *
(1)				With Family		-5.2
(2)			Black			14.5
(3)		<20				19.5
(4)		≥60				12.2
Patients Differ- (5)					Prior Therapy	9.2
ing from (6)			Black	With Family		49.9
Characteristics (7)		≥60	Black			28.4
of "Baseline (8)		≥60		With Family		6.4
Patient" with (9)		≥60	Black	With Family		68.2
respect to (10)		≥60	Black	With Family	Prior Therapy	83.7
traits listed (11)	Diabetic					13.6
on each line (12)	Diabetic	≥60				27.5
(13)	Diabetic	≥60	Black			45.9
(14)	Diabetic		Black	With Family		70.4
(15)	Diabetic	≥60	Black	With Family		91.2
(16)	Diabetic	≥60	Black	With Family	Prior Therapy	108.8

*By definition of a "baseline patient"

A. Factors Associated with First Hospitalization for CAPD-Related Complications*

Introduction

Patients receiving CAPD may develop peritonitis or exit site or tunnel infections, or have catheter malfunctions which are sufficiently severe or persistent to require hospitalization. Such hospitalizations add to the overall cost of CAPD and could adversely affect its acceptability.

The National CAPD Registry reports that 35% of patients receiving CAPD for ESRD were hospitalized for CAPD-related complications within six months of beginning treatment; 53% within 12 months [1]. Since it is unlikely that all patients have an equal probability of being hospitalized, the purpose of this study is to examine the relationship between the first hospitalization for CAPD-related complications and a number of patient characteristics for which information is available in the Registry. Specifically, the role of patients' age, sex, race, living arrangement (with or without family), diabetic glomerulosclerosis, and prior therapy for ESRD are examined to determine whether they are associated with hospitalization. The relationship between these variables and duration of hospitalization for CAPD-related complications will not be addressed in this analysis; neither will the relationship of these variables to other causes of hospitalization (e.g., coronary disease).

Subjects and Methods

Fifty-nine hundred, eighty-four (5,984) of the 8,829 CAPD patients with follow-up information in the National CAPD Registry comprise the

* The material contained in this report has been published as follows:
  Nolph KD, Cutler SJ, Steinberg SM, Novak JW, Hirschman GH. Factors associated with morbidity and mortality among patients on CAPD. *Trans Am Soc Artif Intern Organs* 33:57–65, 1987.

study group. All patients were followed by the Registry from the time they began CAPD—either as first ESRD therapy, or after transfer off another treatment modality, or after failure of transplant graft. The 2,845 Registry patients not included in this study started CAPD therapy prior to registration. The lack of information regarding these patients' early hospitalization experience while on CAPD required their exclusion from the present study. Demographic information (age, race, sex, living arrangement), the nature of the patients' primary renal disease, and whether there was prior ESRD therapy were available for all patients included in the study.

In order to determine the relationship between time to first CAPD-related hospitalization and the other variables studied, a two-stage analysis was employed. In the first stage, the Mantel-Haenszel [2] procedure was used to determine the presence of association between each variable and time to first CAPD-related hospitalization. For each of the six variables, the patients were classified into two subgroups and the Mantel-Haenszel technique was used to estimate the risk of the first CAPD-related hospitalization in each subgroup relative to the other. This method was first applied to the total study population to find the overall risk associated with each factor. The same method was then applied within subgroups, in order to identify possible interactions between the variables being studied. This approach may best be explained through an example. The relative risk of first CAPD-related hospitalization was first assessed for each variable (e.g., diabetics versus nondiabetics), and then separately within various subgroups (e.g., with respect to age). If results obtained varied considerably among the subgroups, an interaction between the variable divided into subgroups and the one under study was suggested.

Estimates of the relative risks were next converted into risk scores by multiplying the common logarithms of the relative risks by 100. The resulting risk scores are such that if two subgroups (e.g., male and female) had identical risks of first CAPD-related hospitalization by a certain time, the risk score will be zero (0). In such a case, we might reasonably conclude that sex had no impact on outcome. A risk score of 8 to 12 corresponds to an excess risk of first CAPD-related hospitalizations (for example, for diabetics as compared to non-diabetics) of 20 to 30 percent during a defined follow-up period. Scores of 8 to 12 may be clinically meaningful, but may be unrecognized in an individual clinic. Variables characterized by risk scores larger than 12 are likely to be noticed in a moderate size nephrology practice and, therefore, considered of importance. Risk scores as small as 4 or 5 may indicate a 'statistically' significant difference in a large patient population; however, since these scores are indicative of excess risks of only 10 to 12 percent, they need to be interpreted more conservatively.

In the second stage of the analysis, the individual factors and the potentially important interactions are evaluated simultaneously—through the use of a multivariate mathematical model. Specifically, the Proportional Hazards Method of Cox[3] was used to evaluate the impact of each selected factor on time to first CAPD-related hospitalization, while adjusting for the influence of the other variables included in the model. With this technique, changes in risk attributable to each factor are calculated while taking account of other pertinent characteristics. The resulting parameter estimate for each factor represents its individual prognostic importance. For example, the risk associated with living with family versus living without family on first CAPD-related hospitalization may be examined by mathematically holding effects of sex, age, race, disease, and treatment history fixed at some level. The results of such an analysis provide a clearer picture of the influence of each of the variables studied on time to first CAPD-related hospitalization.

In summary, the results of applying the Cox model makes possible a description of the risk of first CAPD-related hospitalization for patients with a variety of characteristics as compared to a 'baseline' patient group. To implement the model, it is customary to select as a baseline, a set of characteristics associated with a presumed low risk patient. In this analysis, the baseline group was defined to possess the following traits: white, 20–59 years of age, male, non-diabetic, with no prior ESRD therapy. The risk for all other patient groups is expressed as 'percent additional risk' relative to the baseline group. The additional risks refer to probabilities averaged over successive small intervals of time, but do not provide a precise measure of the cumulative difference in probability over an extended period of observation.

Results

(a) Stage One Analysis

Table 1 displays summary information on the risk scores associated with each of the factors individually studied. Being under 20 years of age as compared with being between 20 and 59 years of age, with a risk score of 13.3, is the individual factor most closely associated with early first hospitalization for CAPD-related complications. Primary renal disease, living arrangement, sex, and race were each of moderately low importance with risk scores between 3.7 and 5.1. Age over 60 and previous

184

TABLE 1.   Risk Scores of Subgroup A / Subgroup B for Each of Six Factors
that May be Related to First Hospitalizations for
CAPD-Related Complications

FACTOR RELATIVE RISK		RISK SCORE	TOTAL NUMBER OF PATIENTS*
Previous ESRD Therapy		0.9	3747
No Previous ESRD Therapy			2237
Race:	Black	3.7	996
	White		4610
Sex:	Female	3.8	2655
	Male		3329
Living Arrangement:	Without Family	4.7	1050
	With Family		4934
Renal Disease:	Diabetic**	5.1	1345
	Non-Diabetic		4639
Age:	Under 20	13.3	321
	20-59		3673
Age:	60 & over	1.3	1949
	20-59		3673

*Number of patients in Subgroup A / Number of patients in Subgroup B

**Primary renal disease is Diabetic Glomerulosclerosis.

ESRD therapy were each very poorly associated with time to first hospitalization for CAPD-related complications.

The impact of each factor within the various patient subgroups is provided in Table 2, in order to identify possible interaction terms to be included in the Cox model. Note that even though age over 60 and previous ESRD therapy were of little importance individually, they are included in examination of subgroups to determine whether there are effects in selected subgroups. Because of the limited number of young patients, the variation in risk among subgroups of patients under age 20 was not analyzed. Interactions are identified by letters (a) through (d) in Table 2.

The effect of race (black versus white) within individual subgroups is presented in column 1 of Table 2. Blacks without previous ESRD treatment are at lower hospitalization risk than whites without previous ESRD treatment (risk score of -1.5), whereas the reverse is true among those with previous ESRD therapy (risk score 6.1). This interaction between race and previous therapy will be examined in a Cox model.

The effect of prior therapy is relatively consistent and low among subgroups, with exception of its somewhat greater effect in diabetics

TABLE 2.   Risk Scores for Various Characteristics when Examined within Individual Subgroups

SUBGROUP	BLACK WHITE (1)	PRIOR THERAPY NO PRIOR THERAPY (2)	OVER 60 20-59 (3)	DIABETIC* NON-DIABETIC (4)	FEMALE MALE (5)	NO FAMILY FAMILY (6)
White		-0.3** a	1.4	4.7	4.0	4.0
Black		7.5	0.1	3.5	2.8	4.5
No Previous ESRD Tx	-1.5** a		2.8	3.1 b	2.6	4.2
Previous ESRD Tx	6.1		0.4	7.3	4.6	5.0
Under 20 Years of age	2.3	4.0		***	-4.0** c	***
20-59 Years	4.5	1.9		6.6	3.7	6.0
60 Years and Older	3.2	-0.6**		5.4	5.6	3.7
Non-Diabetic	4.1	0.5 b	2.2		3.9	5.3
Diabetic	2.6	4.3	1.0		3.5	4.2
Male	3.9	0.0	0.7	5.2		6.9 d
Female	2.8	2.0	2.7	4.9		2.0
Lives With Family	3.3	0.9	1.7	5.5	4.5	
Lives Without Family	3.7	1.6	-0.6**	4.8	-0.2** d	

*Renal Disease is diabetic glomerulosclerosis.

**The group in the numerator is at lower risk than the group in the denominator.

***Insufficient patients for calculation to be reliable.

than in non-diabetics. This interaction will also be included in the model. There are no identifiable interactions involving age over 60 that should be included in the Cox model. The risk of CAPD-related hospitalization is lower in females under 20 than in males under 20 (risk score of -4.0), but the reverse is true above age 20 (risk score of 3.7). Finally, there is a noticeably greater risk for males living apart from their family than for females living apart from their family.

In summary, all individual factors considered in the analysis should be included in the Cox model. In addition, those interactions mentioned will be incorporated and tested as well.

(b) Stage Two Analysis

Terms for seven individual variables (diabetic status, age < 20, age > 60, sex, prior ESRD therapy, race, and living arrangement) and four interactions (prior ESRD therapy × race, prior ESRD therapy × diabetic status, living arrangement × sex, and age < 20 × sex) were included in an initial proportional hazards model. The model fitting indicated that the interactions were each statistically non-significant in the presence of all the individual variables included, and could be

TABLE 3.   Parameter Estimates and Standard Errors of Jointly
Considered Prognostic Variables, Obtained Through the
Use of the Final Cox Proportional Hazards Model

VARIABLE	PARAMETER ESTIMATE	STANDARD ERROR	P-VALUE *
Diabetic **	.127	.048	.008
Age, < 20	.459	.079	< .0001
Age, ≥ 60	.097	.042	.021
Prior ESRD Therapy	.129	.041	.002
Race (Effect of Black Race)	.128	.049	.010
Sex (Effect of Female)	.128	.039	.001

*If the p-value is < .05, the parameter estimate is unlikely to
differ from zero because of chance.

**Primary renal disease is diabetic glomerulosclerosis.

eliminated. A second model was fitted with only the seven individual
variables, and all but living arrangement (p = .994) were found to be
statistically significant. A final model was constructed with the six

TABLE 4.   Examples of Additional Risks of First Hospitalization for CAPD-Related
Complications for Patients with Various Characteristics as Compared
with a "Baseline Patient"

		TRAIT					
		DIABETIC STATUS	AGE	RACE	SEX	PRIOR ESRD THERAPY	% ADDITIONAL RISK
"Baseline Patient"		Non-diabetic	20-59	White	Male	No	0.0 *
	(1)	Diabetic					13.5
	(2)		< 20				58.2
	(3)		≥ 60				10.2
	(4)			Black			13.7
Patients Differing	(5)				Female		13.7
from Characteristics	(6)					Yes	13.8
of "Baseline Patient"	(7)	Diabetic		Black			29.0
with respect to	(8)	Diabetic				Yes	29.2
traits listed on	(9)	Diabetic		Black	Female		46.7
each line	(10)	Diabetic		Black		Yes	46.8
	(11)	Diabetic		Black	Female	Yes	66.9
	(12)	Diabetic	< 20				79.7
	(13)		< 20	Black			79.9
	(14)	Diabetic	< 20	Black			104.2
	(15)		< 20	Black	Female		104.4
	(16)	Diabetic	< 20			Yes	104.4
	(17)	Diabetic	< 20	Black	Female		132.1
	(18)	Diabetic	< 20	Black		Yes	132.3
	(19)		< 20	Black	Female	Yes	132.6
	(20)	Diabetic	< 20	Black	Female	Yes	164.1

*By definition of a "baseline patient."

remaining individual variables, and the parameter values obtained are presented in Table 3. Each term of the model has a statistically significant effect on time to first CAPD-related hospitalization, while accounting for the influence of the other characteristics. All terms increase the risk of first hospitalization for CAPD-related complications.

The parameter values in Table 3 are used to estimate the additional risk of being hospitalized for CAPD-related complications for patients with various combinations of characteristics. Additional risk is calculated as a percentage compared to the risk for a 'baseline patient.' The arithmetic procedure for using the parameters in Table 3 to produce the risk estimates in Table 4 has appeared previously [1]. In all cases, traits that differ from those of the 'baseline patient' result in an increased risk of first CAPD- related hospitalization. Being under 20 leads to greatly increased risk, and the more traits that differ, the greater the increase in risk.

Discussion

Information regarding types of patients that are susceptible to early hospitalization can identify high-risk patients and direct more careful attention to those patients likely to require earlier hospitalization.

The exploratory, univariate analysis indicated that only age < 20 was a largely important factor. Race, sex, and living arrangement were also potentially important. A number of minor interactions were identified that were included in the multivariate analysis. The multivariate analysis indicated that living arrangement and all of the interactions were not important, but that all other individual factors were important.

Patients who are under 20 and have more than two other risk factors might be considered for additional training or other approaches to prevent the types of infections and complications that can lead to hospitalization.

The Registry is limited to patients placed on CAPD and, therefore, information is not available on the characteristics of patients that require hospitalization related to other treatment modalities. Patients identified as being at high risk for CAPD-related hospitalization have an unknown, not necessarily better or worse, risk for hospitalization if treated with another therapy.

There are no randomized prospective comparisons of the hospital days per year anticipated with other therapies (total days or days for dialysis complications). Thus, differences in hospital days may be due to

188

differences in case-mix as well as problems with therapy. Multiple recent reports list total hospital days per year for patients on CAPD, center hemodialysis, and home hemodialysis [1,4–7]. Total hospital days per year in non-diabetics between the ages of 20 and 60 years are presented in some of these reports. Only the analyses of CAPD experiences categorize hospital days into total days and days for dialysis complications. Mean values for home hemodialysis total days per year range from 9 to 15. Mean values for center hemodialysis total days per year range from 3 to 25; days per year for dialysis complications on CAPD range from 1 to 10.

It is obvious that hospitalization days per year with any chronic dialysis therapy can be influenced not only by risk factors which we have identified for the CAPD population, but also by other risk factors which may not be followed by our Registry and/or which may be unique to specific forms of therapy. Also, we do not have information available on the criteria used in selecting patients for CAPD and the variation in criteria among treatment centers. As a result the data analyzed only reflect the information provided to the Registry. For all of these reasons the analysis can not be used to guide selection of patients for CAPD or other forms of therapy. However, the findings can prove useful in identifying patients at increased risk for hospitalization, within the CAPD Registry experience, and in developing more extensive monitoring and training programs for such patients.

Refernces

1. Report of the National CAPD Registry of the National Institutes of Health. Characteristics of participants and selected outcome measures for the period January 1, 1981 through August 31, 1984. NIADDK, 1985.
2. Mantel N. Evaluation of survival data and two new rank order statistics arising in its consideration. Cancer Chemother Rep 1966; 50:163–170. 3. Cox DR. Regression models and life tables (with discussion). J Royal Stat Soc (B) 1972; 35:187–220.
3. Nolph KD, Pyle WK, Hiatt M. Mortality and morbidity in continuous ambulatory peritoneal dialysis: Full and selected Registry populations. ASAIO 1983 Oct-Dec; 6(4):220–226.
4. Mion CM, Mourad G, Canaud B, et al. Maintenance dialysis: A survey of 17 years' experience in Langueddoc-Roussillon with a comparison of methods in a 'standard population'. ASAIO 1983 Oct-Dec; 6(4):205–213.
5. Khanna R, Wu G, Vas S, Oreopoulos DG. Mortality and morbidity on continuous ambulatory peritoneal dialysis. ASAIO 1983 Oct-Dec; 6(4):197–204.
6. Blagg CR, Wahl PW, Lamers JY. Treatment of chronic renal failure at the Northwest Kidney Center, Seattle, from 1960–1982. ASAIO 1983 Oct-Dec; 6(4):170–175.

B. Factors Associated with Transfer off CAPD*

Introduction

The National CAPD Registry reported that, within one year of starting CAPD, 20 % of patients will have transferred from CAPD (by life table analysis; considering patients who died or received a kidney transplant as withdrawn from follow-up) [1]. By the end of the second year, 34 % of patients will have transferred from CAPD. Most of those who transfer (86%) go to hemodialysis. Smaller percentages elect intermittent peritoneal dialysis, have some return of kidney function, or choose medical management without dialysis. The main reasons reported to the Registry for such transfers are medical reasons (such as visual impairment), excessive peritonitis, failure of the procedure to meet fluid/biochemical standards and patient/family choice.

In order to identify patients with a high probability of transfer off CAPD, this analysis examines the relationship between transfer off CAPD and patient characteristics for which information is available in the Registry. Specifically, the role of age, sex, race, living arrangement (with or without family), diabetic glomerulosclerosis and prior ESRD therapy are examined to determine whether they are associated with the transfer off CAPD to hemodialysis, IPD or no therapy. This analysis will not examine factors associated with the receipt of a kidney transplant, since such transplants are likely to be influenced as much by the availability of a suitable kidney as by the recipient's characteristics at the initiation of maintenance therapy.

* The material contained in this report has been published as follows:
Nolph KD, Cutler SJ, Steinberg SM, Novak JW, Hirschman GH. Factors associated with morbidity and mortality among patients on CAPD. *Trans Am Soc Artif Intern Organs* 33:57–65, 1987.

Increased understanding of factors which predispose to transfer from CAPD may be useful in selecting patients for CAPD and/or in considering ways to reduce transfer.

Subjects and Methods

Fifty-nine hundred, eighty-four (5,984) of the 8,829 CAPD patients with follow-up information in the National CAPD Registry comprise the study group. All study patients were followed by the Registry from the time they began CAPD—either as first ESRD therapy, or after transfer off another treatment modality, or after failure of transplant graft. The 2,845 Registry patients not included in this study started CAPD therapy prior to registration. These patients were on CAPD when their treatment centers joined the registry program. The lack of information regarding these patients' early experience on (and off) CAPD required their exclusion from the present study.

In order to determine the relationship between probability of transfer and the other variables studied, a two-stage analysis was employed. In the first stage, the Mantel-Haenszel [2] procedure was used to determine the presence of association between each variable and the probability of transfer. For each of the six variables, present at initiation of CAPD, the patients were classified into two subgroups and the Mantel-Haenszel technique was used to estimate the relative risk of transfer for one subgroup relative to the other. This method was first applied to the total study population to find the overall risk associated with each factor. The same method was then applied within subgroups, in order to identify possible interactions between the variables being studied.

This approach may best be explained through an example. The relative risk of transfer was first assessed for each variable (e.g., all diabetics versus all nondiabetics). Comparison of diabetics and nondiabetics was then made within sub-groups pertaining to other characteristics, e.g. age. If results obtained varied considerably among subgroups, an interaction between the variable divided into subgroups (e.g., age) and the one under study (e.g., diabetic status) was indicated.

Estimates of the relative risks were next converted into risk scores by multiplying the common logarithms of the relative risks by 100. The resulting risk scores are such that if two subgroups (e.g., male and female) had identical risks of transferring off CAPD by a certain time, the risk score will be zero (0). In such a case, we might reasonably conclude that sex had no impact on outcome. A risk score of 8 to 12 corresponds to an excess of transfers (for example, for those living without family as opposed to those living with their family) on the order of 20 to 30 percent during a defined follow-up period. Scores of 8 to 12 may be clinically meaningful, but may be unrecognized in an individual clinic. Variables characterized by risk scores larger than 12 are likely to be noticed in a moderate size nephrology practice and, therefore, considered of importance. Risk scores as small as 4 or 5 may indicate a 'statistically' significant difference in a large patient population; however, since these scores are indicative of excess risks of only 10 to 12 percent, they need to be interpreted more conservatively. A potential interaction will be identified when the risk scores differ between subgroups by at least 4 units.

In the second stage of the analysis, the individual factors and the potentially important interactions were evaluated simultaneously—through the use of a multivariate mathematical model. Specifically, the Proportional Hazards Method of Cox [3] was used to evaluate the impact of each selected factor on time to transfer, while adjusting for the influence of the other variables included in the model. Models are constructed with progressively fewer variables until the final model consists of statistically significant parameters. With this technique, changes in risk attributable to each factor are calculated while taking account of other pertinent characteristics. The resulting risk estimate for each factor represents its individual prognostic importance. For example, the risk associated with living with family versus living without family on the probability of transfer off CAPD may be examined by mathematically holding the effects of sex, age, race, diabetes, and treatment history fixed at some level. The results of such an analysis provide a clearer picture of the influence of each of the variables studied on transfer probability.

The results of applying the Cox model makes possible a description of the risk of transfer for patients with different characteristics as compared to a 'baseline' patient group. To implement the model, it is customary to select as a baseline, a set of characteristics associated with a presumed low risk patient. The risk for all other patient groups is expressed as 'percent additional risk' relative to the baseline group. The additional risks refer to probabilities averaged over successive small intervals of time, but do not provide a precise measure of the cumulative difference in probability over an extended period of observation.

Results

(a) Stage One Analyses

Table 1 summarizes information on risk scores associated with each of the factors studied. None of the factors as they are examined individually indicate substantial and clear association with transfer. Patients living without family (compared to those with family) have the highest risk of transfer with a score of 8.8 (roughly 22% increased risk) followed by blacks (compared to whites) with a score of 5.7 and diabetics (compared to non- diabetics) with a score of 5.5. Age, sex, and history of previous ESRD therapy do not appear to influence the probability of transferring off CAPD when examined using this approach.

In order to identify possible interaction terms to be included in the Cox models, the impact of each factor on time to transfer within various patient subgroups is assessed in Table 2. The possible variation of risk among subgroups is examined for all variables, even if the overall risk for a variable is small. The variation in risk among subgroups of patients under age 20 was not analyzed, however, because of the limited

TABLE 1. Risk Scores of Subgroup A for Each of Six Factors that May be Associated with Transfer Off CAPD (Subgroup B)

FACTOR COMPARISON		RISK SCORE	TOTAL NUMBER OF PATIENTS*
Previous ESRD Therapy			3747
No Previous ESRD Therapy		-0.3	2237
Race:	Black		996
	White	5.7	4610
Sex:	Female		2655
	Male	1.1	3329
Living Arrangement:	Without Family		1050
	With Family	8.8	4934
Renal Disease:	Diabetic**		1345
	Non-Diabetic	5.5	4639
Age:	Under 20		321
	20-59	2.4	3673
Age:	60 & over		1949
	20-59	-0.4	3673

* Number of patients in Subgroup A
Number of patients in Subgroup B

** Primary renal disease is Diabetic Glomerulosclerosis

TABLE 2.   Risk Scores for Various Characteristics When Examining within Individual Subgroups

SUBGROUP	BLACK WHITE (1)	PRIOR THERAPY NO PRIOR THERAPY (2)	OVER 60 20-59 (3)	DIABETIC* NON-DIABETIC (4)	FEMALE MALE (5)	NO FAMILY FAMILY (6)
White		-1.1**	0.5 g	6.4 a	1.7	8.8
Black		2.3	-3.8**	1.6	-1.5**	5.4
No Previous ESRD TX	3.5		2.3 c	1.0 d	0.3	10.6
Previous ESRD TX	6.8		-2.0**	9.2	1.6	7.8
Under 20 Years Old	0.8	9.9 b		***	-5.6**	***
20-59 Years Old	7.3 f	0.4 c		5.6	0.5 i	9.9
Over 60 Years Old	2.9 g	-3.8**		5.9	3.5	6.5
Non-Diabetic	6.9 a	-1.7**	0.2		0.8	11.1 e
Diabetic	1.7	6.3 d	0.3		2.2	-0.7**
Male	7.3	-1.0**	1.6**	5.0		11.1 h
Female	4.0	0.4	1.5	6.1		6.2
Lives With Family	5.8	0.0	0.2	7.7 e	1.6 h	
Lives Without Family	3.1	-1.8**	2.8**	-4.3**	-2.8**	

*Renal Disease is diabetic glomerulosclerosis.

**The group in the numerator is at lower risk than the group in the denominator.

***Insufficient patients for calculation to be reliable.

number of young patients. Interactions are identified by letters (a) through (i) in Table 2.

The effect of race (black versus white) within individual subgroups is presented in column 1 of Table 2. Generally the scores are indicative of moderately small risks, ranging between 0.8 and 7.3. Six subgroups exhibited scores of at least 4.0, indicating moderate importance. An interaction is exhibited in the variation in risk between diabetics and nondiabetics (a). Other interactions involve age, and are denoted by (f) and (g).

In 5 of the 11 sub-groups examined in column 2 (prior therapy vs. no prior therapy), patients with a history of prior therapy for ESRD had a lower risk (negative risk scores). In contrast, risk scores of 9.9 and 6.3 were obtained in two other subgroups. The variability in the direction of the effect of prior therapy, suggests that some interactions associated with this variable are worth considering in the model, specifically interactions between age and prior therapy, (b) and (c), and diabetes and prior therapy (d).

Effects of age ≥ 60 are all small in magnitude. Nonetheless, there are 2 interactions, involving race (g), and prior therapy (c) (noted previously in columns 1 and 2) that are to be considered in the Cox analysis.

The impact of diabetes is evident in most subgroups, with the majority of risk scores in the 5.0 to 9.2 range. There is evidence of a noticeable interaction between diabetic status and living arrangement, with a risk score of 7.7 for patients living with family compared to a score of -4.3 for those living without family (e). Sex has a very weak effect, but exhibits variability in direction of effect. Two minor interactions with age (i) and living arrangement (h) are important enough to consider for inclusion in the Cox model. Finally, the effect of living arrangement appears to be moderately strong, and exhibits a marked interaction with diabetic status (e).

In summary, based upon information in Table 2, there is no one single factor that can predict transfer. Also, since there are a large number of effects of opposite direction between subgroups, these differences in direction of risk may indicate small variations about a true, zero effect of the factor under examination. For lack of clear information concerning effects to include or exclude, and the frequency of minor interactions between factors and subgroups, the Cox model will initially include all individual factors plus the identified interactions.

(b) Stage Two Analyses

Terms for all individual variables (prior ESRD therapy, age < 20, age > 60, diabetic status, race, sex, living arrangement) and 9 previously identified interactions (prior therapy $\times$ diabetic status, prior therapy $\times$ age < 20. prior therapy $\times$ age ≥ 60, living arrangement $\times$ diabetic status, race $\times$ diabetic status, race $\times$ age < 20, race $\times$ age ≥ 60, living arrangement $\times$ sex, and sex $\times$ age < 20) were included in the proportional hazards model. None of the interactions were found to be statistically important when the simultaneous impact of the other variables included in the model is accounted for. A second model was constructed, which consisted only of the individual factor effects. This second model indicated that both prior therapy and race were very important statistically, living arrangement was of possible importance, and no other factor was of any consequence. A third model was developed containing the three factors found to be statistically important, with the result that only race and prior therapy were found to be statistically significant (living arrangement resulted in a parameter estimate with a p-value of 0.13). A final model with two factors produced parameter values presented in Table 3.

The table also indicates the percent of additional risk over a baseline characteristic associated with each factor. For this analysis, a baseline patient is white and has not had prior therapy for ESRD before starting on CAPD. If the patient were white, but had prior therapy, there would

TABLE 3. Parameter Estimates and Percent Additional Risks of Jointly Considered Prognostic Variables, Obtained Through the Use of the Final Cox Proportional Hazards Model

VARIABLE	PARAMETER ESTIMATE	STANDARD ERROR	PERCENT ADDITIONAL RISK*	P-Value
Prior ESRD Therapy	.328	.065	38.8	.0000
Race (Effect of Black Race)	.356	.070	42.8	.0000
Both Prior ESRD Therapy & Black			98.2	.0000

*As compared to a white patient without prior ESRD therapy.

be an additional 38.8% chance of transferring off CAPD during the time of this study. If the patient did not have prior therapy, but was black instead of white, there would be an additional 42.8% risk of transferring off during the observation period; and, if the patient was black and had prior therapy, there would be an additional 98.2% risk, a virtual doubling of the probability of transferring off CAPD. These effects are consistent with probabilities for transfer calculated by the life table method: 25% of patients without prior therapy leave CAPD by 19.7 months compared with 13.5 months for those with prior therapy. Also, 25% of whites transfer off CAPD by 16.7 months while 25% of blacks transfer off CAPD by 10.9 months.

Discussion

There are no prospective randomized comparisons of transfer rates from CAPD as compared to center hemodialysis or home hemodialysis. Actuarial cumulative 2–year total drop-outs from hemodialysis and CAPD have been reported for populations considered 'good candidates' for dialysis therapies [4–12]. Usually these restricted populations exclude diabetics, patients less than 20 years of age and patients over 60. Home hemodialysis technique survivals tend to exceed those of CAPD and center hemodialysis; 90% technique survival at 2 years has been reported [8]. Total drop-out survivals, however, are not commonly listed for hemodialysis experiences. Recent reports include 7 actuarial technique survivals for restricted CAPD populations and 2 actuarial technique survivals for center hemodialysis populations [4–12]. Four of six CAPD technique survivals fall below the lowest center hemodialysis technique survival at two years, supporting common impressions that drop-out from CAPD tends to be relatively high compared to hemodialysis experiences. Paradoxically, the best technique survival of these 9 analyses is from CAPD experience [7].

The CAPD Registry cannot determine whether transfer rates from CAPD are higher or lower than from other dialysis therapies. Only CAPD is monitored. We do have the opportunity, however, to detect risk factors for transfer among the outcome measures we follow in the registered CAPD population.

The multivariate analysis herein described considered the simultaneous effects of all factors available to us. Only race and prior ESRD therapy emerged as statistically significant and apparently important risk factors predisposing to transfer. Age, sex, diabetic status and living arrangement were without value in predicting who will transfer, once race and prior therapy are taken into account. This is in contrast to the univariate findings which indicated that living arrangements and diabetic status were of some importance when looked at independently of other variables.

Reasons for earlier transfer off CAPD of blacks and those with prior dialysis therapy are only speculative. One possible explanation is that such transfer results from higher rates of complications or hospitalization. The data from the National CAPD Registry was examined for those who transferred off therapy and this was confirmed in some cases. Blacks who transferred off CAPD had 3.5 episodes of peritonitis per patient year of follow-up compared to a peritonitis rate of 2.3 for whites who transferred. Blacks who transferred off CAPD spent 25.1 days per patient year hospitalized for CAPD related complications compared with 20.0 days for whites who transferred. Blacks who transferred off CAPD had noticeably higher peritonitis rates and longer periods hospitalized for CAPD related complications than did whites who transferred. It also should be noted that each of these rates is considerably higher than the corresponding rates for those who did not transfer. For whites remaining on CAPD there was an average of 1.1 episodes of peritonitis per patient year and an average of 5.3 days of hospitalization for CAPD related complications. For blacks remaining on CAPD the corresponding figures were 1.5 and 6.1.

Those with prior therapy who transferred off CAPD had 2.7 episodes of peritonitis per patient-year while the corresponding figure for those without prior therapy who transferred is 2.4 episodes per patient-year. Those with prior therapy who transferred off CAPD spent an average of 21.0 days per patient-year in the hospital for CAPD-related complications, while those who did not have prior therapy who transferred had a corresponding rate of 22.0 days per patient-year of observation. These values do not differ greatly from each other and cannot provide an explanation for the differences in times to transfer for the two groups of patients. They are, however, considerably higher than rates for patients who did not transfer: 1.1 episodes of peritonitis per patient year and 5.5 days hospitalized per patient year for CAPD-related complications.

The Registry has previously reported the relationships between race and prior therapy in the development of peritonitis [13,14]. This present study goes a step further and indicates that patients with a peritonitis problem transfer off more quickly than patients without peritonitis problems. Also, blacks, who transfer have a greater peritonitis (and hospitalization) risk than whites who transfer, supporting the hypothesis that frequent complications such as peritonitis) may lead to transfer. The explanation for the earlier transfer of patients with prior therapy appears to be independent of the frequency of complications.

Patients who have had previous therapy may be more likely to change for a number of reasons. CAPD may have only intended as a respite for several months to recover from a complication of hemodialysis. Also, those patients who are experienced on another therapy may prefer to return to that therapy once they have been maintained by the CAPD procedure for some time. Since a major feature of CAPD is opportunity for self care, certain types of patients may not be able to handle the responsibility of caring for themselves. Another possibility is that those patients who have previous experience with another modality are able to transfer between modalities because they do not have contraindications to therapeutic alternatives. Also, problem patients on hemodialysis may be transferred to CAPD in hopes of alleviating difficulties; the CAPD experience may be associated with persistence or enhancement of the problems and patients return to the former therapy.

It can be stated after joint consideration of patient traits as discussed in this chapter, that there appears to be no difference in transfer probability dependent on sex, age, diabetic status or living arrangement and that only race and prior therapy affect this outcome. A higher probability of developing complications such as peritonitis probably increases transfer probabilities for blacks. The patient who comes to CAPD from a prior dialysis therapy is more likely to transfer independent of the frequency of complications. Thus, psychosocial, or other factors which led to the decision to transfer to CAPD may not be solved and the patient returns to the prior therapy or tries yet another.

In considering the findings of this analysis, the limitations of the available data must be borne in mind. The Registry is limited to patients placed on CAPD and, therefore, we cannot infer similar or dissimilar prognostic influences for transfer off other modalities. Similarly, information is not available on the criteria used in selecting patients for

CAPD and the variation in criteria among treatment centers. As a result, the data that have been analyzed reflect the identifiable factors that are related to the observed experiences. Even with these limitations, the findings should be useful for identifying patients that are more likely to require change from CAPD to another form of dialysis, and for designing procedures for monitoring patients and anticipating and facilitating transfer in those patients more likely to require change. In addition, these findings may be useful to those interested in identifying questions for further study.

References

1. Nolph KD, Cutler SJ, Steinberg SM, Novak JW. Findings from the NIH National CAPD Registry, January 1985. Trans Am Soc Artif Intern Organs, to appear.
2. Mantel N. Evaluation of survival data and two new rank order statistics arising in its consideration. Cancer Chemother Rep 1966; 50:163–170.
3. Cox DR. Regression models and life tables (with discussion). J Royal Stat Soc (B) 1972; 34:187–220.
4. Capelli JP, Camiscioli TC, Vallorani RD. Comparative analysis of survival on home hemodialysis, in-center hemodialysis and chronic peritoneal dialysis (CAPD-IPD) therapies. Dial & Transplant 1985 Jan; 14(1):38–52.
5. Blagg CR, Wahl PW, Lamers JY. Treatment of chronic renal failure at the Northwest kidney center, Seattle, from 1960–1982. ASAIO 1983 Oct-Dec; 6(4):170–175.
6. Shapiro FL, Umen A. Risk factors in hemodialysis patient survival. ASAIO 1983 Oct-Dec; 6(4):176–184.
7. Khanna R, Wu G, Vas S, Oreopoulos DG. Mortality and morbidity on continuous ambulatory peritoneal dialysis. ASAIO 1983 Oct-Dec; 6(4):197–204.
8. Mion CM, Mourad G, Canaud B, et al. Maintenance dialysis: A survey of 17 years' experience in Langueddoc-Roussillon with a comparison of methods in a 'standard population.' ASAIO 1983 Oct-Dec; 6(4):205–213.
9. Wing AJ, Broyer M, Brunner FP, et al. The contribution of continuous ambulatory peritoneal dialysis in Europe. ASAIO 1983 Oct-Dec; 6(4):214–219.
10. Nolph KD, Pyle WK, Hiatt M. Mortality and morbidity in continuous ambulatory peritoneal dialysis: Full and selected Registry populations. ASAIO 1983 Oct-Dec; 6(4):220–226.
11. Kramer P, Broyer M, Brunner FP, Brynger H, Oules R, Rizzoni G, Selwood NH, Wing AJ, Balas EA. Combined report of regular dialysis and transplantation in Europe, XIV, 1983. Proc of EDTA 1984; 21:2–68.
12. Schriel J, Silins J, Lennox R, MacNaught D, Posen GA, Coll AE. Canadian Renal Failure Register, 1982, Report. Published by the Kidney Foundation of Canada.
13. Nolph KD, Cutler SJ, Steinberg SM, Novak JW. Continuous ambulatory peritoneal dialysis in the United States. A three year study. Kidney Int 1985 Aug; 28(2):198–205.
14. Steinberg SM, Cutler SJ, Novak JW, Nolph KD. Prognostic factors associated with peritonitis among patients on continuous ambulatory peritoneal dialysis. Trans Am Soc Artif Intern Organs, to appear.

C. Factors Associated with Death While on CAPD*

Introduction

Until techniques for transplanting kidneys and for performing chronic dialysis were available, patients with end-stage renal disease (ESRD) faced uremia and death. Currently available therapies do prolong the lives of patients with ESRD, but the life expectancy for these patients is generally shorter than for the population at large.

The National CAPD Registry reports that 14% of those being treated with CAPD die within 1 year and 25% die within 2 years of initiation of CAPD [1]. These figures also include deaths of those who transfer off CAPD and die within 2 weeks after the change. The present study examines the relationship between the time until death in patients treated by CAPD, and patient characteristics for which information is available in the Registry. Specifically we have examined whether patient age, sex, race, living arrangement (with or without family), diabetic glomerulosclerosis and/or prior therapy for ESRD are associated with death while on CAPD. Information on events occurring to patients beyond two weeks after transfer off CAPD is not available to the Registry. Evaluations of patient survivals with any form of therapy are better interpreted once factors associated with a greater risk of death are identified. The findings from this study should not be used to select patients for therapy, however, unless comparable information pertaining to other forms of therapy is considered. Those patients at high risk of death while on CAPD may be at comparable or even higher risk on

* The material contained in this report has been published as follows:
  Nolph KD, Cutler SJ, Steinberg SM, Novak JW, Hirschman GH. Factors associated with morbidity and mortality among patients on CAPD. *Trans Am Soc Artif Intern Organs* 33:57–65, 1987.

other modalities, but that cannot be assessed by the present study. The Registry does not receive information on patient experiences on other treatment modalities.

Subjects and Methods

Fifty-nine hundred, eighty-four (5,984) of the 8,829 CAPD patients with follow-up information in the National CAPD Registry comprise the study group. All study patients were followed by the Registry from the time they began CAPD either as first ESRD therapy, or after transfer off another treatment modality, or after failure of transplant graft. The 2,845 Registry patients not included in this study started CAPD therapy prior to registration. They are survivors from a larger pool of patients put on CAPD without immediate registration and we cannot characterize the various factors leading to death of non-surviving, non-registered cohorts. Demographic information (age, race, sex, living arrangement), the nature of the patients' primary renal disease, and whether there was prior ESRD therapy were available for all patients included in the study.

In order to determine the relationship between time to death while on CAPD and the other variables studied, a two-stage analysis was employed. In the first stage, the Mantel-Haenszel [2] procedure was used to determine the presence of association between each variable and time to death while on CAPD. For each of six characteristics at initiation of CAPD, the patients were classified into two subgroups and the Mantel-Haenszel technique was used to estimate the risk of death in each subgroup relative to the other. This method was first applied to the total study population to find the overall risk associated with each factor. The same method was then applied within subgroups, in order to identify possible interactions between the variables being studied.

This approach may best be explained through an example. The relative risk of dying while on CAPD was first assessed for each variable, (e.g., diabetics vs. non-diabetics) and then separately within various subgroups (e.g., with respect to age). If results obtained varied considerably among the subgroups, an interaction between the variable divided into subgroups and the one under the study was suggested.

Estimates of the relative risks were next converted into risk scores by multiplying the common logarithms of the relative risks by 100. The resulting risk scores are such that if two subgroups (e.g. male and female) had identical risks of dying by a certain time, the risk score will be zero (0). In such a case, we might reasonably conclude that sex had no impact on the probability of dying on CAPD. A risk score of 8 to 12 corresponds to an excess risk of dying (for example, for diabetics as compared to nondiabetics) of 20 to 30 percent during a defined follow-up period. Scores of 8 to 12, implying a 20 to 30 percent excess risk may be clinically meaningful, but may be unrecognized in an individual clinic. Variables characterized by risk scores larger than 12 are likely to be noticed in a moderate size nephrology practice and, therefore, considered of importance. Risk scores as small as 4 or 5 may indicate a 'statistically' significant difference in a large patient population; however, since these scores are indicative of excess risks of only 10 to 12 percent, they need to be interpreted more conservatively.

In the second stage of the analysis, the individual factors and the potentially important interactions are evaluated simultaneously through the use of a multivariate mathematical model. Specifically, the Proportional Hazards Method of Cox [3] was used to evaluate the impact of each selected factor on the probability of dying while on CAPD, while adjusting for the influence of the other variables included in the model. With this technique, changes in risk attributable to each factor are calculated while taking account of other pertinent characteristics. The resulting parameter estimate for each factor represents its individual prognostic importance. For example, the risk associated with living with family vs. living without family may be examined by mathematically holding effects of sex, age, race, disease, and treatment history fixed at some level. The results of such an analysis provide a clearer picture of the influence of each of the variables studied on dying while on CAPD.

In summary, the results of applying the Cox model makes possible a description of the risk of death while on CAPD for patients with a variety of characteristics as compared to a 'baseline' patient group. To implement the model, it is customary to select as a baseline, a set of characteristics associated with a presumed low risk patient. In this analysis, the baseline group was defined to possess the following traits: white, 20–59 years of age, non-diabetic, and with no prior ESRD therapy. The risk for all other patient groups is expressed as 'percent additional risk' relative to the baseline group. The additional risks refer to probabilities averaged over successive small intervals of time, but do not provide a precise measure of the cumulative difference in probability over an extended period of observation.

Results

(a) Stage One Analyses

Summary information on risk scores associated with each factor studied is presented in Table 1. Being diabetic appears to be associated with a large risk of death as indicated by the risk score of 9.7. Those living without family are also shown to be at greater risk with a score of 8.2. Being under 20, 60 or older, and having no previous ESRD therapy are each of moderate importance. Neither sex nor race appear to have much impact independently on probability of dying while on CAPD. Since these risk scores are determined without accounting for other characteristics, they are liable to vary when considered in the multivariate setting, in the presence of one another.

In order to identify possible interactions to be included in the Cox model, Table 2 presents an examination of the impact of each factor, within patient subgroups, on time to death while on CAPD. Note that even though the risk scores for sex and race were low, the possible variation among subgroups is examined to determine whether these characteristics may be influencing the risk of dying while on CAPD in

TABLE 1. Risk Scores of Subgroup A / Subgroup B for Each of Six Factors that May be Related to Death While on CAPD

FACTOR RELATIVE RISK		RISK SCORE	TOTAL NUMBER OF PATIENTS*
Previous ESRD Therapy			3747
No Previous ESRD Therapy		-4.1	2237
Race:	Black		996
	White	1.5	4610
Sex:	Female		2655
	Male	0.9	3329
Living Arrangement:	Without Family		1050
	With Family	8.2	4934
Renal Disease:	Diabetic**		1345
	Non-Diabetic	9.7	4639
Age:	Under 20		321
	20-59	3.3	3673
Age:	60 & over		1949
	20-59	4.4	3673

*Number of patients in Subgroup A
Number of patients in Subgroup B

**Primary renal disease is Diabetic Glomerulosclerosis

selected subgroups. Because of the limited number of young patients, the variation in risk among subgroups of patients under age 20 was not analyzed.

Examination of Table 2 discloses the presence of 10 potential interactions, two of which are large in magnitude. Patients with prior therapy who are diabetic are at an increased risk of death while on CAPD as compared to patients with no prior therapy (risk score of 6.2 in column 2), whereas patients with prior therapy who are non-diabetic are at a decreased risk (risk score of -6.3 in column 2). Diabetic patients living with family are at an increased risk compared to non-diabetic patients (risk score of 12.1 in column 4), whereas diabetic patients living apart from family are at a somewhat lower risk (risk score of − 1.7 in column 4). The other possible interactions apparent from Table 2 are: race and sex, race and diabetic status, race and sex, race and living arrangement, prior therapy and living arrangement, diabetic status and sex, and living arrangement and sex.

(b) Stage Two Analyses

Terms for seven individual variables (diabetic status, age < 20, age ≥ 60, prior ESRD therapy, race, sex, and living arrangement) and the

TABLE 2.   Risk Scores for Various Characteristics When Examined within Individual Subgroups

SUBGROUP	BLACK WHITE (1)	PRIOR THERAPY NO PRIOR THERAPY (2)	60 AND OLDER 20-59 (3)	DIABETIC* NON-DIABETIC (4)	FEMALE MALE (5)	NO FAMILY FAMILY (6)
White		-4.1**	4.4	10.5	1.6	8.4
Black		-3.8**	3.6	4.5 b	-2.3**c	4.5 d
No Previous ESRD Tx	1.7		6.5 e	2.1	0.2	11.4
Previous ESRD Tx	1.9		2.8	15.0 f	1.4	6.3 g
Under 20 Years of Age	-4.2**	0.6		***	-5.0**	***
20-59 Years	2.6 a	-3.0** e		10.4	0.7	8.6
60 Years and Older	1.7	-6.6**		11.8	2.7	7.0
Non-Diabetic	3.1	-6.3**	5.3		-0.1**	11.1
Diabetic	-3.5** b	6.2 f	7.0		4.0 h	-2.3** i
Male	3.3	-4.6**	3.6	7.9		10.0
Female	-0.7** c	-3.5**	5.8	11.9 h		6.1 j
Lives With Family	1.7	-3.4**	4.6	12.1	1.3	
Lives Without Family	-1.7** d	-7.1** g	3.5	-1.7**i	-2.3**j	

*Renal Disease is diabetic glomerulosclerosis.

**The group in the numerator is at lower risk than the group in the denominator.

***Insufficient patients for calculation to be reliable.

ten interactions noted above were included in a Cox model. The resulting fit of the first model (primarily intended to identify interactions to be eliminated) indicated that only four interactions (prior therapy × age < 20, prior therapy × age ≥ 60, prior therapy × diabetic status, and living arrangement × diabetic status) were statistically significant and therefore were worth considering in further models. A second model constructed with these four interactions, as well as the seven individual factors, led to elimination of several terms because of lack of statistical importance in the presence of all other terms.

The terms to be included in the final model were race, age < 20, age ≥ 60, diabetic status, prior therapy, and interactions of age < 20 and age ≥ 60 with prior therapy. The values of the parameters so obtained, as well as the standard errors and p-values for a test that each parameter value is different from zero appear in Table 3. All parameters were found to be statistically significant; being over 60 years of age and having diabetes are the most important factors when all factors are considered jointly.

In Table 4, the effects are assessed in terms of the percent of additional risk compared to a baseline patient. The baseline patient is white, 20–59 years of age, non-diabetic, and without prior therapy for ESRD. Each variation from one of these factors adds some additional

TABLE 3.   Parameter Estimates and Standard Errors of Jointly
Considered Prognostic Variables Obtained Through
the Use of Final Cox Proportional Hazards Model

VARIABLE	PARAMETER ESTIMATE	STANDARD ERROR	P-VALUE*
Age < 20	.821	.236	.0005
Age ≥ 60	1.202	.123	<.0001
Race (Effect of black race)	.225	.102	.027
Diabetic**	.816	.077	<.0001
Prior ESRD Therapy	.398	.115	.0005
Under 20 Years Old and Prior Therapy (Interaction)	-.917	.368	.013
Over 60 Years Old and Prior Therapy (Interaction)	-.485	.150	.001

*If the p-value is < .05, the parameter estimate is unlikely to
differ from zero because of chance

**Primary renal disease is diabetic glomerulosclerosis

TABLE 4.   Additional Risks (%) of Deaths While on CAPD, for Patients with Various Characteristics as Compared with a "Baseline Patient"

		TRAIT			% ADDITIONAL RISK
	DIABETIC STATUS	AGE	RACE	Prior ESRD Therapy	
"Baseline Patient"	Non-Diabetic	20-59	White	No	0.0*
Patients differing from "baseline patient" with respect to traits listed on each line. (1)	Diabetic				126.1
(2)		<20			127.3
(3)		≥60			232.6
(4)			Black		25.2
(5)				Yes	48.9
(6)	Diabetic	<20			414.0
(7)	Diabetic	≥60			652.3
(8)	Diabetic		Black		183.2
(9)	Diabetic			Yes	236.7
(10)		<20	Black		184.6
(11)		<20		Yes	35.3
(12)		≥60	Black		316.6
(13)		≥60		Yes	205.0
(14)			Black	Yes	86.5
(15)	Diabetic	<20	Black		543.7
(16)	Diabetic	<20		Yes	205.9
(17)	Diabetic	≥60	Black		842.2
(18)	Diabetic	≥60		Yes	589.6
(19)		<20	Black	Yes	69.4
(20)		≥60	Black	Yes	281.9
(21)	Diabetic		Black	Yes	321.6
(22)	Diabetic	<20	Black	Yes	283.1
(23)	Diabetic	≥60	Black	Yes	763.7

*By definition of a "baseline patient"

risk to the baseline patient's chance of dying while on CAPD. Being over 60 adds 233% additional risk all by itself, whereas being under 20 adds 127% additional risk. Compared with the 'baseline patient,' other additional risks shown in the table range from 25.2% for blacks without other differing traits to 842.2% for black diabetics who are over 60. As indicated in Table 3, the interaction terms each have a negative value, which somewhat offsets the effect of having both of the risk factors they pertain to. For example, a black patient who is over 60 with diabetes is at a higher risk than the same person who has also had prior therapy. This is the result of the mathematical effect of the separate factors balancing against the interactions, which probably reflects clinical criteria used in selecting patients for CAPD therapy. It may also reflect considerations involved in transferring patients off CAPD following early complications. An illustration of this effect, and the method for computing the percent of additional risk is found in a previous report [1].

Discussion

It is not surprising to note that being over 60 is more closely associated with the risk of death than is any other variable. This age effect was included not to assess age impact but rather to see how greatly the other factors are associated with the outcome when the age of the person is taken into account. To have excluded age from the model might not have correctly gauged the importance of other factors such as race, diabetes, or prior therapy.

In addition to the noted importance of age, the effect of diabetes is also profound. If over the age of 60, a diabetic maintained by CAPD has more than 6 times the additional chance of dying as compared with a person who is between 20 and 59 years old and non-diabetic. A non-diabetic person over 60 on CAPD has a risk of dying which is 45% that of a diabetic over 60. Age and diabetes together are a much greater risk than age by itself. The effects of race and prior therapy are of less consequence and only moderately increase the risk associated with age and diabetes.

It is interesting to compare the CAPD population with the general population. Among the patients in this study, the average age of those 20–59 years was 43 years. The average age of patients 60 years of age and older was 68 years. In the general population of white persons, the one year probability of dying for persons 68 years of age is almost 10 times as large as for persons 43 years of (2.56% vs 0.27%) [4]. This age differential in mortality risk in the general population is larger than the age differential observed among CAPD patients (the risk among white patients 60 years of age and older was 3.3 times the risk in patients 20–59 years of age).

It is not surprising that diabetes with its many systemic complications is associated with an increased risk of death. Mechanisms whereby race contributes to death are not clear. Patients who come to CAPD from a prior therapy may be, at least in part, patients with many medical problems and a poor prognosis on any form of therapy to see if they will do better.

In considering the findings of this analysis the limitations of the available data must be borne in mind. Since the Registry is limited to patients placed on CAPD, information is not available on the characteristics and death rates of patients with ESRD maintained by means of other modalities. Numerous recent reports in the literature attempt to compare patient survival on different modalities [4–12]. Recognizing the effects of age and diabetes on survival, these reports have focused primarily on results in nondiabetic patients between the ages of 20 and

60. Even in the face of such analyses of restricted 'low risk' populations, the experiences are widely scattered and there is no consistent superiority of patient survival on CAPD or center hemodialysis over the other. Patient survivals on home hemodialysis, however, tend to be consistently in the very high range of the scatter. Home hemodialysis populations are usually very compliant patients with a trainable partner and an acceptable home situation. These analyses are all uncontrolled; there are no randomized prospective comparisons of patient survivals with different dialysis therapies and anecdotal experiences vary greatly even in restricted populations.

The information provided in this report should not be used to decide whether to place high risk patients on CAPD. First, as mentioned above, the same risk factors may be just as significant with other forms of therapy. Secondly, Registry information is limited to those deaths which occur during CAPD therapy or within 2 weeks of transfer. Thirdly, information is not available on the criteria used in selecting patients for CAPD and the variation in criteria among treatment centers. Our study only presents findings from one modality and the alternative treatments need to be analyzed in a similar manner before the important decisions regarding patient placement on a particular modality can be made. More appropriately, identification of patient characteristics associated with a high mortality risk while on CAPD may be useful in formulating more effective patient follow-up policies and in interpreting patient survival data.

References

1. Report of the National CAPD Registry of the National Institutes of Health: Characteristics of participants and selected outcome measures for the period January 1, 1981 through August 31, 1984. NIADDK, 1985.
2. Mantel N. Evaluation of survival data and two new rank order statistics arising in its consideration. Cancer Chemother Rep 1966; 50:163–170.
3. Cox DR. Regression models and life tables (with discussion). J Royal Stat Soc (B) 1972; 34:187–220.
4. National Center for Health Statistics. Vital statistics of the United States, 1980, Vol. II, Sec. 6, Life Tables. DHHS Pub. No. (PHS) 84–1104. Public Health Service, Washington. U.S. Government Printing Office, 1984.
5. Capelli JP, Camiscioli TC, Vallorani RD. Comparative analysis of survival on home hemodialysis, in-center hemodialysis and chronic peritoneal dialysis (CAPD-IPD) therapies. Dial & Transplant 1985; 14:38–52.
6. Blagg CR, Wahl PW, Lamers JY. Treatment of chronic renal failure at the Northwest Kidney Center, Seattle, from 1960–1982. ASAIO 1983 Oct-Dec; 6(4):170–175.
7. Shapiro FL, Umen A. Risk factors in hemodialysis patient survival. ASAIO 1983 Oct-Dec; 6(4):176–184.

208

8. Khanna R, Wu G, Vas S, Oreopoulos DG. Mortality and morbidity on continuous ambulatory peritoneal dialysis. ASAIO 1983 Oct-Dec; 6(4):197–204.

9. Mion CM, Mourad G, Canaud B, et al. Maintenance dialysis: A survey of 17 years' experience in Langueddoc-Roussillon with a comparison of methods in a 'standard population'. ASAIO 1983 Oct-Dec; 6(4):205–213.

10. Wing AJ, Broyer M, Brunner FP, et al. The contribution of continuous ambulatory peritoneal dialysis in Europe. ASAIO 1983 Oct-Dec; 6(4): 214–219.

11. Nolph KD, Pyle WK, Hiatt M. Mortality and morbidity in continuous ambulatory peritoneal dialysis: Full and selected Registry populations. ASAIO 1983 Oct-Dec; 6(4):220–226.

12. Kramer P, Broyer M, Brunner FP, Brynger H, Oules R, Rizzoni G, Selwood NH, Wing AJ, Balas EA. Combined report of regular dialysis and transplantation in Europe, XIV, 1983. Proc of EDTA 1984; 21:2–68.

D. Trends in the Occurrence of Complications and of Treatment Outcomes*

Introduction

The basic report contains data on the probability over time of the first occurrence of peritonitis, exit site/tunnel infection, catheter replacement, and of hospitalization for CAPD-related complications (see Figures 3 and 4, Tables 14 and 15, 1986 Registry Report). The probability of dying while on CAPD is presented in Figure 2 and Table 8 (see 1986 Registry Report). This analysis examines the changes that have occurred among patients who started on CAPD in successive years, 1981 through 1985.

Methods and Results

The data for this special report are based on all 7,377 Class 1 patients in the Registry who started on CAPD between 1981 and 1985. Forty Class 1 patients who began therapy late in 1980 are excluded. All Class 2 patients are also excluded, because of the lack of complete information on events occurring prior to their first follow-up. Some of the Class 1 patients were reported by centers that have only recently joined the Registry, and others are from centers that have ceased participation before 1985. A comparison was conducted in order to determine whether changes in outcome observed in cohorts of patients beginning CAPD in different years are indicative of actual trends, independent of whether the patients were from centers with lengthy or short participation periods. Twelve month probabilities of peritonitis, catheter replace-

* The material contained in this report has been published as follows:
  Nolph KD, Cutler SJ, Steinberg SM, Novak JW. Special studies from the NIH Registry.
  Peritoneal Dial Bull 6:28–35, 1986.

TABLE 1.   Probability (%) of First Event Occurring within 12 Months
of Starting CAPD, by Year Started CAPD

Type of Event	1981	1982	1983	1984
A. All Class 1 Patients				
Peritonitis	67.7	63.9	57.8	59.8
Exit Site/Tunnel Infection	37.5	39.1	36.9	29.5
Catheter Replacement	20.6	19.2	19.8	19.9
CAPD-Related Hospitalization	57.5	54.5	49.9	40.9
Dying while on CAPD	12.1	12.8	12.5	14.5
Number of Patients Started CAPD	896	2,115	1,823	1,936
B. Class 1 Patients at Veteran Centers *				
Peritonitis	66.8	63.3	57.7	59.1
Exit Site/Tunnel Infection	38.0	39.0	36.6	30.0
Catheter Replacement	20.7	19.7	19.6	20.6
CAPD-Related Hospitalization	57.0	54.4	50.0	41.2
Dying while on CAPD	14.7	14.7	15.1	19.0
Number of Patients started CAPD	782	1,848	1,629	1,659

* Currently active centers that entered the registry program in 1981 or 1982.

ment, exit site/tunnel infection, hospitalization, and death were computed by year began CAPD, for all Class 1 patients, and for Class 1 patients at Veteran Centers (currently active centers that entered the Registry program in 1981 or 1982).

Examination of the data in Table 1, indicates that the trends are the same regardless of which set of data is used. A similar comparison of 18–month probabilities confirmed this finding. Curves are presented based on all Class 1 patients, and trends for each of the years may be discussed without concern regarding possible biases due to variation in the length of time clinics have participated in the Registry program.

Two figures are presented indicating probabilities of events occurring over time as a function of the year patients began CAPD. Figure 1 presents the probabilities for peritonitis and exit site/tunnel infection as a function of the year patients began CAPD, while Figure 2 presents similar probabilities for first CAPD-related hospitalization and for death while on CAPD. Supporting data for these figures are presented in Tables 2, 3, 5 and 6.

The upper set of curves in Figure 1 portray the trend in the probability of the first episode of peritonitis. There was a downward trend from 1981 through 1983, but the curve for 1984 was somewhat higher than for 1983. Preliminary data for 1985 suggest that the trend may be stabilizing at about the 1984 level (see Table 2). It is noteworthy that the curves for the four cohorts converge as length of follow-up

FIGURE 1.   Probability of First Peritonitis and of First Exit Site/Tunnel Infection
By Year Started CAPD

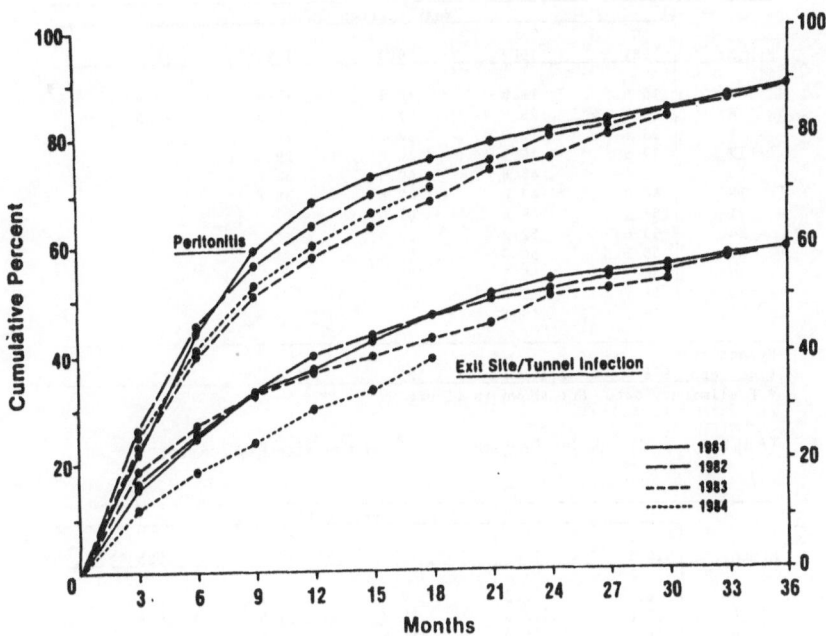

Note: Probability of first catheter replacement not shown because of
minimal variation among the four calendar cohorts.

TABLE 2.   Data for Figure 1: Cumulative Probability of First
Episode of Peritonitis

| | Year Started CAPD | | | | |
Months	1981	1982	1983	1984	1985 *
3	22.0	26.3	23.1	25.3	23.6
6	44.3	45.5	39.5	40.8	40.6
9	58.7	56.5	50.8	52.5	
12	67.7	63.9	57.8	59.8	
15	72.9	70.2	63.5	66.1	
18	76.4	72.8	68.0	71.3	
21	78.9	76.4	74.1		
24	81.3	79.6	76.4		
27	83.2	82.0	79.9		
30	84.9	84.8	83.5		
33	87.3	86.7			
36	88.6	88.8			
Number at time zero	896	2,115	1,823	1,936	607

* Preliminary data. Not shown in figure.

increases. By the 30th month after starting on CAPD, the cumulative
probabilities for 1981, 1982, and 1983 are all close to 85 percent.

The lower set of curves in Figure 1 pertain to the probability of the
first exit site/tunnel infection. The curves for 1983 and 1984 suggest a

TABLE 3.   Data for Figure 1: Cumulative Probability of First
            Episode of Exit Site/Tunnel Infection

Months	Year Started CAPD				
	1981	1982	1983	1984	1985 *
3	15.6	16.8	18.9	11.5	9.4
6	25.1	25.7	27.3	18.5	21.5
9	33.1	32.9	32.7	24.0	
12	37.5	39.1	36.9	29.5	
15	42 6	43.6	40.3	33.6	
18	46.9	47.0	42.8	38.8	
21	51.1	49.6	45.6		
24	53.6	52.2	50.5		
27	55.1	54.0	52.4		
30	56.2	55.3	53.3		
33	58.1	57.7			
36	59.1	59.1			
Number at time zero	896	2.115	1.823	1.936	607

* Preliminary data. Not shown in figure.

TABLE 4.   Cumulative Probability of First Catheter Replacement

Months	Year Started CAPD				
	1981	1982	1983	1984	1985 **
3	6.6	8.3	7.7	6.1	5.3
6	12.0	12.0	11.3	11.5	9.8
9	16.9	15.2	15.5	15.5	
12	20.6	19.2	19.8	19.9	
15	24.2	22.5	23.4	23.4	
18	27.8	26.3	26.2	25.0	
21	31.8	29.9	30.5		
24	33.6	32.9	33.4		
27	37.3	35.5	36.3		
30	38.8	38.0	38.4		
33	40.4	41.2			
36	42.3	43.7			
Number at time zero	896	2.115	1.823	1.936	607

 * Data not shown graphically because of minimal variation over time.
** Preliminary data.

TABLE 5.   Data for Figure 2: Cumulative Probability of First
            Hospitalization for CAPD-Related Complications

Months	Year Started CAPD				
	1981	1982	1983	1984	1985 *
3	20.6	23.6	23.1	15.2	13.7
6	35.4	38.5	35.6	24.9	21.6
9	48.7	47.7	43.0	32.7	
12	57.5	54.5	49.9	40.9	
15	63.9	60.3	54.0	47.2	
18	69.4	64.9	57.2	49.5	
21	73.4	68.8	60.9		
24	76.2	70.8	63.8		
27	78.1	73.0	67.5		
30	79.1	74.9	71.6		
33	81.1	77.9			
36	82.1	79.1			
Number at time zero	896	2.115	1.823	1.936	607

* Preliminary data. Not shown in figure.

TABLE 6.   Data for Figure 2: Cumulative Probability of Dying
            While on CAPD

Months	Year Started CAPD				
	1981	1982	1983	1984	1985 *
3	0.9	1.2	2.0	1.3	0.5
6	4.6	5.3	5.3	5.3	1.5
9	8.0	9.3	9.1	9.5	
12	12.1	12.8	12.5	14.5	
15	15.4	16.4	16.9	19.0	
18	17.5	18.5	20.4	22.9	
21	19.7	21.0	23.7		
24	23.6	23.3	27.6		
27	26.5	25.8	31.7		
30	29.3	28.1	37.1		
33	34.3	31.6			
36	36.9	33.6			
Number at time zero	896	2,115	1,823	1,936	607

* Preliminary data. Not shown in figure.

FIGURE 2.   Probability of First Hospitalization for CAPD-Related Complications
             and of Dying While on CAPD by Year Started CAPD

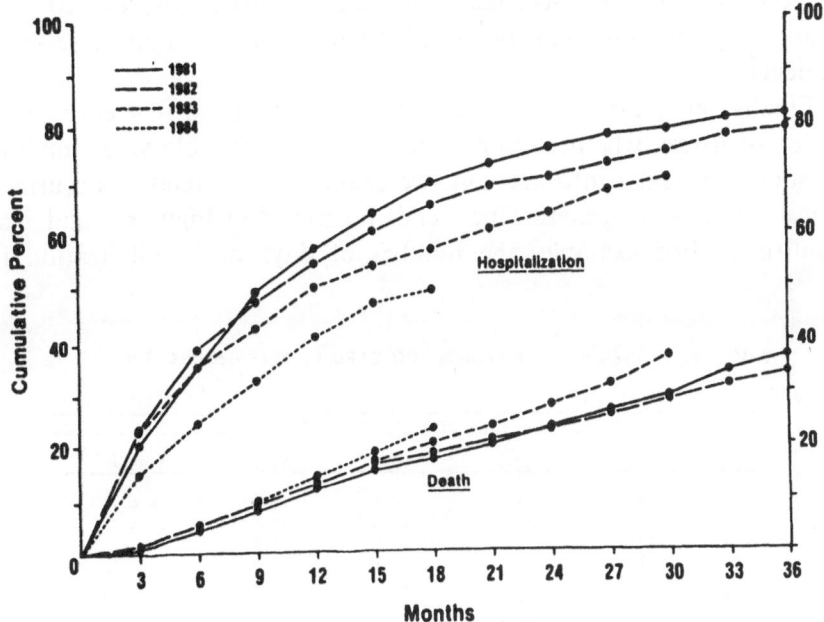

definite downward trend, with 1984 indicating a more substantial improvement.

It is also of interest to examine the probability of first catheter replacement. These data were not plotted, however, because of the minimal changes observed. For example, as shown in Table 4, very little, if any trend is evident, and no graphical representation is required.

The trend in the probability of first hospitalization for CAPD-related complications, as shown in the upper part of Figure 2, indicates improvement, and may have been influenced by a variety of factors. The probability of hospitalization within 18 months of starting CAPD decreased from 69 percent in 1981 to 50 percent in 1984, for example. This marked change appears concurrently with an increase in the probability of dying while on CAPD (lower set of curves). The 18–month probability of dying increased from 18 percent in 1981 to 23 percent in 1984.

Table 7 contains data for the probability of transfer by year began CAPD. The data indicate a downward trend, which is consistent with the downward trends in the probabilities for peritonitis and exit site/tunnel infection (Figure 1). The observed increase in the probability of dying while on CAPD could be associated with the decrease in the probability of transfer. With declining complication rates, it appears that patients are being continued on CAPD for longer periods; thus, there is an increased potential for death while on CAPD. It is of interest to note that life tables calculated for those patients who are 20 to 59 years of age and non-diabetic exhibit similar patterns as do those for all patients.

Finally, since the data in Figure 1 and 2 pertain to first episodes, in order to assess whether similar trends are discernable when multiple episodes are taken into account, we examined the trend in occurrence rates (Table 8). In general, the trends portrayed in Figures 1 and 2 are confirmed. For example, the number of days of hospitalization for

TABLE 7.   Probability of Transfer Off CAPD by Year Began CAPD

	Year Started CAPD				
Months	1981	1982	1983	1984	1985 *
3	5.2	6.4	6.1	5.9	6.4
6	11.0	10.7	10.5	10.4	13.8
9	17.2	15.9	14.5	15.6	
12	21.9	21.3	19.2	18.9	
15	26.8	25.3	22.7	22.9	
18	29.5	28.8	25.2	32.2#	
21	33.2	31.9	27.8		
24	37.0	34.4	31.6		
27	40.7	36.6	33.8		
30	42.1	39.8	36.7		
33	44.4	42.5			
36	45.3	44.0			
Number at time zero	896	2.115	1.823	1.936	607

* Preliminary data.

The 95% confidence interval for this probability is 19–49%. Thus, the apparent sharp increase from 22.9% at 15 months to 32.2% at 18 months may be due to chance variation.

TABLE 8.   Rates of Occurrence per Patient Year of Observation, for Class 1 CAPD
Patients, by Year Began Therapy

	YEAR BEGAN CAPD					
Rate Under Consideration	1981	1982	1983	1984	1985	All Patients
Peritonitis	1.44	1.37	1.33	1.34	1.25	1.36
Exit Site/Tunnel Infection	0.60	0.60	0.62	0.52	0.53	0.59
Catheter Replacement	0.25	0.26	0.27	0.27	0.23	0.26
CAPD-Related Hospitalization (days per patient-year)	9.2	8.3	7.6	6.9	5.4	8.0
All Hospitalization (days per patient-year)	20.8	20.5	20.3	19.8	17.6	20.4
Number of Patients	896	2,115	1,823	1,936	607 *	7,417 **
Patient-Year of Observation	1,535.2	3,121.3	2,186.6	1,392.6	146.8	8,451.5

* Reflects a lag in reporting

** Exceeds sum of patients in years 1981-1985 since 40 patients who began
CAPD very late in 1980 are included.

CAPD-related complications decrease from 9.2 per patient-year in 1981
to 6.9 in 1984. Preliminary data for 1985 suggest continuation of this
trend. A similar, though more gradual trend occurred with respect to
hospital days for all causes.

In summary, there are trends showing improvement over time in
patients' experience with peritonitis, exit site/tunnel infection, and
CAPD-related hospitalization. There are also small increases in the
probability of dying while on CAPD, which may be associated with the
decreasing probability of transfer off CAPD.

E. Variation in Treatment Outcome According to Center Size*

Introduction

It is of interest to explore whether a relationship exists between the amount of experience a treatment center has had with CAPD and the resulting treatment outcome. This can be addressed by examining the experience of the 204 centers that entered the Registry program in 1981 or 1982 and currently are active participants. For this analysis the centers were grouped into eight size categories. The term 'size' refers to the number of CAPD patients each center has registered and followed since 1981.

Methods and Results

Among the 333 centers that have ever participated in the Registry, 204 began following patients in 1981 or 1982, and are still actively providing patient data in 1985. These centers have provided 6,431 of the 7,417 (87%) Class 1 CAPD patients followed by the Registry. Analyses in this report will be restricted to these 6,431 Class 1 patients in order to eliminate biases that may result from the inclusion of centers that have participated in the Registry program over differing periods of time.

   The eight size categories were constructed so as to put approximately equal numbers of centers in each, utilizing size boundaries divisible by five. Charts labeled Figure 1, 2, and 3, respectively present the minimum, maximum, median, and the 25 and 75 percentile points of the rates for peritonitis, exit site/tunnel infection, and CAPD-related hospi-

* The material contained in this report has been published as follows:
   Nolph KD, Cutler SJ, Steinberg SM, Novak JW. Special studies from the NIH Registry. *Peritoneal Dial Bull* 6:28–35, 1986.

FIGURE 1. Peritonitis Rate Per Patient-Year According to Center Size;
Active Veteran Centers; Class 1 Patients

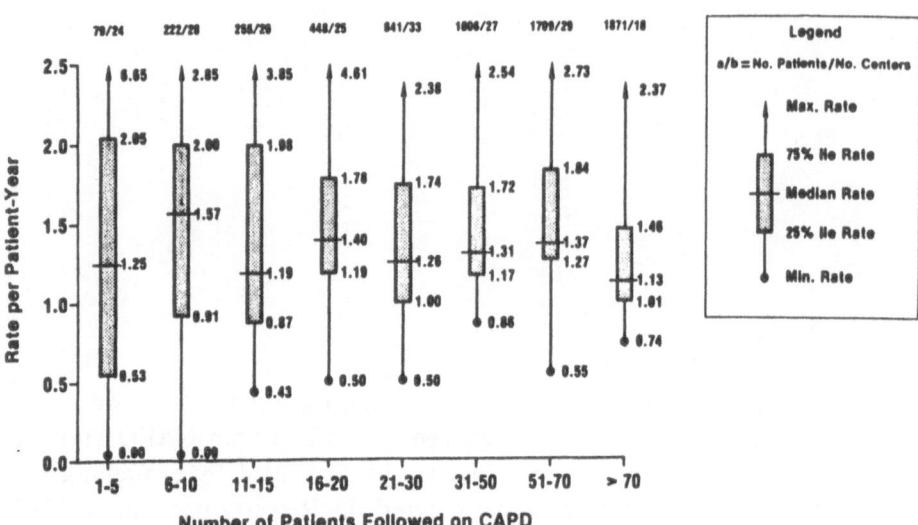

FIGURE 2. Exit Site/Tunnel Infection Rate Per Patient Year According to Center Size;
Active Veteran Centers; Class 1 Patients

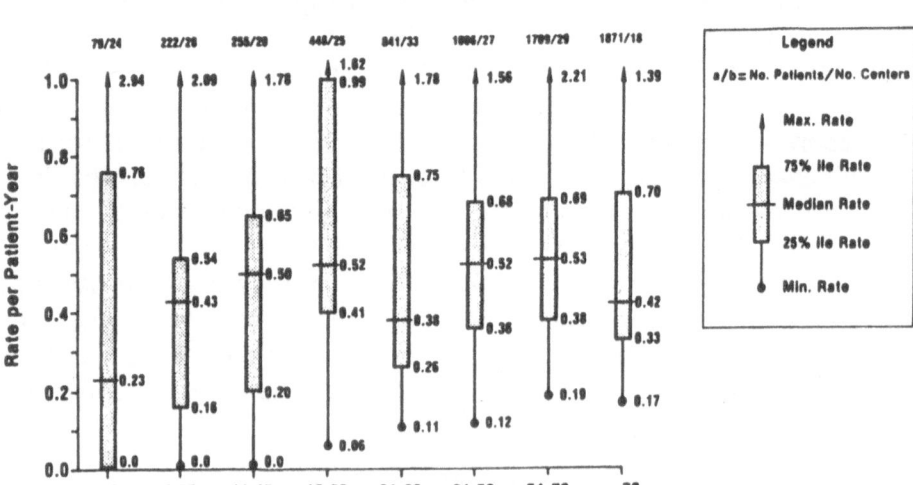

FIGURE 3. Days Hospitalized Per Patient Year for CAPD-Related Complications According to Center Size; Active Veteran Centers; Class 1 Patients

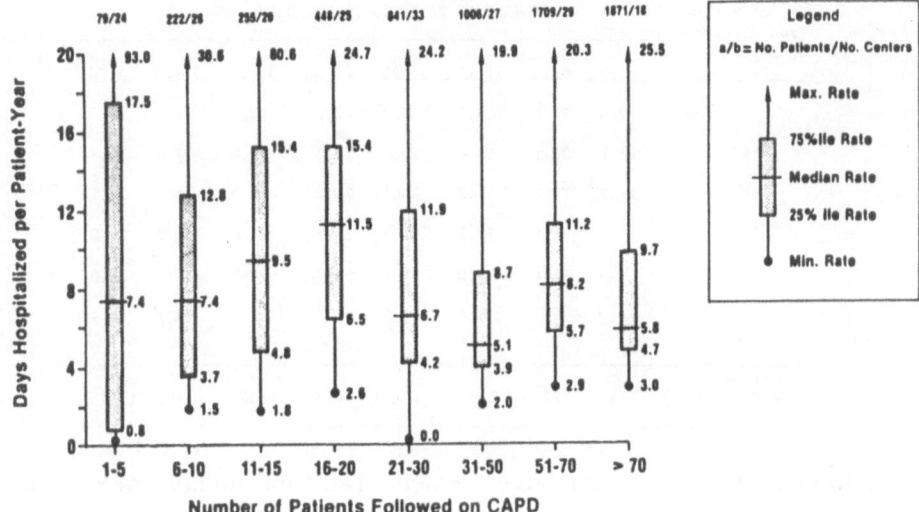

TABLE 1. Probability of Transfer According to Center Size; Active Veteran Centers; Class 1 Patients

No. of Months From Placement On CAPD	NUMBER OF PATIENTS FOLLOWED ON CAPD							
	1-5	6-10	11-15	16-20	21-30	31-50	51-70	> 70
6	14.9	10.2	12.5	12.1	9.7	10.4	12.4	9.1
12	29.5	22.1	24.6	22.4	18.8	19.3	22.1	18.8
18	36.5	29.3	33.4	30.9	24.6	26.6	29.2	25.3
24	--	37.4	39.5	36.4	31.0	31.9	37.2	30.9
30	--	42.1	44.1	41.7	40.0	37.4	42.2	35.7
36	--	--	--	--	47.5	41.7	45.7	40.2
Number at Time Zero	79	223	255	448	841	1,005	1,709	1,873

talization within each size category. The thin rectangular regions in each Class represent the middle 50% of the rates for each category. The rates for the smaller centers are subject to considerable chance variation because of limited numbers of patients per center. The large 'interquantile' ranges depicted by the rectangles for centers with under 5 patients illustrate this. Rates for the smaller centers should be interpreted more

220

TABLE 2. Probability of Dying While on CAPD According to Center Size;
Active Veteran Centers; Class 1 Patients

No. of Months From Placement On CAPD	NUMBER OF PATIENTS FOLLOWED ON CAPD							
	1-5	6-10	11-15	16-20	21-30	31-50	51-70	> 70
6	6.4	10.0	8.7	8.2	7.2	7.6	9.1	8.7
12	13.8	22.1	16.0	15.4	14.3	15.4	17.4	16.3
18	16.5	27.0	21.2	24.3	21.2	21.0	24.3	22.5
24	--	31.8	25.2	31.2	27.5	24.0	30.3	29.0
30	--	35.4	29.0	39.9	31.7	29.1	36.2	34.0
36	--	--	37.9	46.1	35.6	33.9	43.7	39.9
Number at Time Zero	79	223	255	448	841	1,005	1,709	1,873

cautiously than those for larger centers. The total number of patients used to develop the rate for a size category is presented in the numerator of each fraction at the top of each chart, while the denominator indicates the number of centers in each category.

It is also of interest to examine the probability of transferring off CAPD or of dying while on CAPD as a function of center size. These probabilities are presented in Tables 1 and 2.

As can be seen in Figure 1, the median peritonitis rate is lowest for the largest size category: 1.13 for the 18 centers that registered and followed more than 70 CAPD patients each. However, there is no discernable trend among the other seven size categories. The occurrence rates for exit site/tunnel infection shown in Figure 2 do not exhibit any systematic trend. Finally, the number of days hospitalized for CAPD-related complications depicted in Figure 3, shows that the rate for the largest size category (5.8) is at the low end of the range of medians, but it is not the lowest. The lowest rate was 5.1 for centers in the 31–50 patient category. The rate for the category between these two size groups (51–70 patients) was 8.2. Thus, no clear relationship between center size and hospitalization is discernible.

The probability of transfer to hemodialysis or IPD, presented in Table 1, is relatively low for the largest size category, e.g., 30.9 percent by 24 months, 35.7% by 30 months, and 40.2% by 36 months. However, there is no definite relationship between center size and the probability of transfer off CAPD. In examining Table 2, we find that no size category is 'unique' with respect to the probability of patients dying while on CAPD.

In summary, the data in this analysis indicate that the amount of experience a center has had with CAPD, as measured by total Class 1 patients treated in 4 to 5 years, has little relationship to rates of complication or hospitalization, or to probabilities of dying while on CAPD or transferring off CAPD.

F. Variation in Treatment Outcome According to Treatment and Patient Characteristics*

Introduction

While a variety of patient and treatment characteristics have been reported since the Registry began in 1981, other characteristics have only been obtained on patients who entered the program during 1984 or 1985. It is of interest to examine these additional characteristics and their effects on treatment outcomes. Specifically, treatment characteristics, such as number of exchanges per day, hypertonic exchanges per day, volume per exchange, type of equipment and use of insulin, and patient characteristics, such as use of a partner, performance status, visual status, and prior kidney transplant or home dialysis experiences will be related to peritonitis, exit site/tunnel infection, catheter replacements, and days hospitalized.

Methods and Results

Revised registration and status (follow-up) forms introduced to the Registry program in 1984 were designed to collect information on a wide variety of patient and treatment characteristics that had not been previously addressed. Information from these forms has been accumulating for over 18 months, and is now sufficiently mature for analysis and presentation. The analyses provided will be restricted to Class 1 patients who were registered via the revised registration form and followed exclusively on the revised status form. Thus, the analyses will only include patients whose entire experience on CAPD is described on

* The material contained in this report has been published as follows:
  Nolph KD, Cutler SJ, Steinberg SM, Novak JW. Special studies from the NIH Registry. *Peritoneal Dial Bull* 6:28–35, 1986.

the revised forms. A total of 2,336 Class 1 patients fitting this description are available for analysis.

Various outcomes measured for these patients are presented in Table 1, for differing characteristics of treatment, and in Table 2 for differing characteristics of the patients themselves. Results pertaining to treatment characteristics presented in Table 1 are as follows:

Exchanges per Day

Nearly 80 percent of patients performed 4 CAPD exchanges per day. These patients experienced higher complication rates than did those who performed 3 exchanges or those who performed 5 or more exchanges per day. The 4-exchange group was also hospitalized for a larger average number of days for CAPDrelated complications. Patients who varied the number of exchanges per day since starting on CAPD had a much higher occurrence rate for exit site/tunnel infections. Further experience

TABLE 1. Rates of Occurrence Per Patient-Year for Class 1 CAPD Patients by Characteristic of Therapy

Characteristic	Peritonitis	Exit Site/Tunnel Infection	Catheter Replacement	Days Hospitalized CAPD Related	Days Hospitalized All Reasons	Number of Patients	Patient-Years of Observation
Exchanges Per Day:							
3	1.08	0.40	0.11	5.3	22.8	166	85.1
4	1.34	0.55	0.26	6.7	18.3	1,570	990.8
5-9	1.15	0.18	0.23	2.8	16.2	41	21.8
Varied	1.30	1.46	0.23	5.7	15.0	238	198.9
Hypertonic (4.25% dextrose) Exchanges Per Day:							
0	1.18	0.52	0.24	5.4	16.9	811	485.2
1	1.35	0.44	0.22	6.9	19.5	479	260.7
2	1.68	0.67	0.45	15.0	28.0	136	64.3
≥3	3.21	1.05	0.56	19.0	30.1	39	14.3
Varied	1.32	0.53	0.24	5.5	17.2	553	472.5
Average Volume Per Exchange (liters):							
<1.0	1.66	0.79	1.05	13.1	41.7	20	11.4
1.0	1.52	0.32	0.19	4.2	10.6	68	37.1
1.5	1.08	0.33	0.17	4.4	14.6	252	143.8
2.0	1.35	0.54	0.24	6.6	17.7	1,507	961.3
2.5/3.0	1.60	1.09	0.80	9.3	15.2	11	3.7
Varied	1.22	0.59	0.29	6.5	25.8	162	140.5
Type of Equipment:							
Manual	1.23	0.57	0.24	5.9	17.7	1,405	887.8
U.V.	1.26	0.43	0.25	8.2	17.7	329	171.4
All Other (incl. S.C.D., filter, varied)	1.65	0.40	0.28	7.0	20.1	280	236.3
Non-diabetic	1.29	0.52	0.25	6.0	14.7	1,346	842.1
Diabetic:	1.34	0.52	0.24	7.0	24.8	671	454.7
No Insulin	1.69	0.44	0.15	3.3	15.3	66	33.7
Insulin SubQ	1.53	0.42	0.24	7.6	23.3	133	86.7
Insulin IP	1.23	0.68	0.33	7.5	28.0	292	187.7
IP & SubQ	1.09	0.66	0.22	5.7	28.9	21	9.2
Changed	1.31	0.37	0.13	7.0	23.5	159	137.4

is required to assess whether this observation may have been due to chance variation, since this is a relatively small group (238 patients).

Hypertonic (4.25 percent dextrose) Exchanges per Day

There is a definite direct relationship between complication rates, CAPD-related hospitalization, and the number of hypertonic exchanges per day. For example, the number of days hospitalized for CAPD-related complications increased from 16.9 for the group without daily hypertonic exchanges to 30.1 for patients with 3 or more such exchanges per day. Clinical information indicates that 4.25% dextrose dialyzing fluid is often used by patients with a higher infection risk, and this higher infection risk may increase the duration of hospitalization.

Average Volume per Exchange

The complication rates and hospitalization rates for patients receiving less than one liter of fluid per exchange were higher than for any other group. This observation reflects the high rates among children. Of the patients receiving less than one liter exchanges, 40 percent were under 5 years of age, 34 percent were 5–9 years of age, and 14 percent were 10–14 years of age. The complication and hospitalization rates for the other exchange volume groups did not vary significantly.

Type of Equipment

The available data do not indicate any advantage in the use of any nonstandard equipment with regard to the rate of occurrence of complications.

Use of Insulin

Diabetic patients were hospitalized for a greater average number of days than were non-diabetics, particularly when all reasons for hospitalization are combined. However, the occurrence rates for CAPD-related complications were about the same in the two groups. When the diabetic patients are characterized with respect to the use of insulin and the route of insulin administration, some variation in occurrence rates is discernible. Patients who use intraperitoneal infusion of insulin had a lower peritonitis rate. However, the same patients had higher rates for exit site/tunnel infection and catheter replacement.

Specific results pertaining to patient characteristics are presented in Table 2 for Class 1 patients, and are as follows:

Age and Use of Partner

The patient population was divided into three age groups for this analysis: under 15 years, 15–59 years, and 60 years and older. These three age groups differ markedly with respect to the proportion of patients utilizing a partner in performing CAPD exchanges—under 15: 78 percent; 15–59: 11 percent; and 60 and older: 21 percent. The influence of a partner on the occurrence of complications and hospitalization among patients under 15 years of age is difficult to assess from the data at hand, since there were only 16 patients in this age group who

TABLE 2. Rates of Occurrence Per Patient-Year for Class 1 Patients by Selected Patient Characteristics

				RATE UNDER CONSIDERATION			
Characteristic	Peritonitis	Exit Site/ Tunnel Infection	Catheter Replacement	Days Hospitalized CAPD - Related	Days Hospitalized All Reasons	Number of Patients	Patient - Years of Observation
Age and Use of Partner:							
Under 15 years	1.64	0.65	0.47	7.8	25.0	74	40.2
Partner	1.54	0.78	0.56	7.4	26.7	58	28.5
No Partner *	1.89	0.35	0.26	8.9	21.1	16	11.7
15-59 years	1.34	0.55	0.25	6.4	17.7	1,445	875.1
Partner	1.35	0.37	0.28	11.9	35.6	166	89.0
No Partner	1.34	0.57	0.25	5.8	15.7	1,279	786.1
60 years and older	1.26	0.43	0.25	8.0	23.1	792	428.3
Partner	1.12	0.34	0.24	7.7	26.8	264	126.6
No Partner	1.32	0.47	0.25	8.0	21.6	528	301.7
Performance Status							
Fully Active	1.22	0.58	0.23	4.7	10.2	675	399.3
Ambulatory <50% bedridden,	1.46	0.55	0.27	6.7	16.4	458	264.9
unable to work	1.39	0.47	0.28	9.7	30.4	213	111.9
>50% bedridden, limited self-care	1.59	0.59	0.19	11.4	39.3	75	30.8
Completely bedridden	2.16	0.14	0.0	17.3	86.7	24	7.0
Worsened during follow-up	1.28	0.49	0.23	7.6	26.3	328	292.9
Improved during follow-up	1.25	0.45	0.24	4.2	12.4	245	190.4
Vision							
Blind	1.44	0.36	0.31	7.6	24.5	155	83.5
Not Blind	1.34	0.53	0.26	6.9	19.6	2,179	1,262.1
Prior Kid. Transplant							
yes	1.47	0.67	0.30	8.2	20.5	173	118.3
no	1.33	0.51	0.26	6.8	19.8	2,146	1,231.7
Prior Home Dialysis							
yes	1.08	0.59	0.28	6.1	18.6	181	112.6
no	1.37	0.51	0.26	7.0	20.0	2,155	1,238.3

* Rates subject to considerable chance variation due to small number of patients (16) in this group.

did not use a partner. Consequently, the observed rates were subject to substantial chance variation.

Among patients 15–59 years of age there was no difference in the rate of occurrence of peritonitis and catheter replacement between the 'partner' and 'no partner' groups, whereas exit site/tunnel infections occurred more frequently in the 'no partner' group. A marked difference was observed with respect to hospitalization. Patients using partners for exchanges had a higher average number of days of hospitalization for CAPD-related complications than did patients not using partners (11.9 vs 5.8 days). A similar difference was observed between these two groups with respect to hospitalization for all reasons (35.6 vs 15.7 days). This observation suggests that in this age group, patients using partners are probably in poorer health than those not using partners. This is also reflected by differences in performance status, as 86 percent of patients 15–59 not requiring a partner are fully active or ambulatory as compared with 39 percent of patients 15–59 who use a partner in performing exchanges.

Among patients 60 years of age and older, those utilizing a partner had somewhat lower infection rates, but had higher hospitalization rates for nonCAPD-related reasons.

Performance Status

Performance status was obtained throughout follow-up and may remain constant, or may worsen or improve through time. Although there is no relationship between performance status at initiation of CAPD and complication rates, there is a definite relationship between performance status and hospitalization. Days hospitalized per patient-year for CAPD-related complications increased steadily from 4.7 among 'fully active' patients to 17.3 among 'completely bedridden' patients. Hospitalization for all reasons showed a similar trend; from 10.2 to 86.7 days. Patients who exhibited an improvement in performance status while on CAPD (any improvement from first follow-up to most recent follow-up) had lower hospitalization rates than did patients whose performance status had worsened.

Other Patient Characteristics

The complication and hospitalization rates were generally somewhat higher among blind patients as compared with patients without impaired vision, which may be related to the fact that over 80 % of blind patients are diabetic. The rates are also higher among patients with a kidney transplant prior to starting CAPD as compared to patients with no prior transplant. There was little difference between patients with and those without experience with some form of home dialysis prior to starting CAPD.

G. Some Additional Factors Associated with Transfer off CAPD*

Introduction

Patients registered in 1984 and 1985 had information supplied to the Registry regarding their use of a partner in performing exchanges, their use of prior home dialysis or receipt of a prior kidney transplant, their performance status, and travel time to their CAPD treatment center. This analysis presents the relationship between these newly available patient characteristics, and time to transfer off CAPD onto hemodialysis or IPD.

Methods and Results

As discussed in Special Report F, revised registration and status forms introduced in 1984 permitted collection of additional information on patient and treatment characteristics. The same 2,336 Class 1 patients first monitored by the new forms, and discussed in the previous special report, are included in this analysis of transfer probabilities. The first analysis relates the use of a partner (and patient current age) to probability of transfer, the second describes transfer experience of patients who have received a prior transplant or previous home dialysis (particularly, home hemodialysis), the third relates patient performance status (categorized as either worsened, improved, or stable over time within one of five descriptive categories) to the probability of transfer, and the final analysis relates travel time to the CAPD treatment center to probability of transfer. The specific findings for each of these four characteristics are as follows:

* The material contained in this report has been published as follows:
  Nolph KD, Cutler SJ, Steinberg SM, Novak JW. Special studies from the NIH Registry. *Peritoneal Dial Bull* 6:28–35, 1986.

230

TABLE 1.   Probability (%) of Transfers Off CAPD by Age Group and Use of Partner in Performing Exchange

Months	With Partner			Without Partner		
	0-14	15-59	60+	0-14	15-59	60+
3	4.7	8.1	7.2	6.7	4.4	7.8
6	8.5	13.0	10.4	6.7	9.8	12.1
9	18.4	15.8	16.5	6.7	14.9	16.7
12	18.4	19.6	20.3	6.7	19.9	18.3
15	18.4	33.4	20.3	6.7	24.6	24.2
Number at time zero	58	166	264	16	1,279	528

Age and Use of Partner

Among patients under 15 years of age, those who use a partner to perform CAPD exchanges appear to be more likely to be transferred off CAPD than those who do not use a partner (Table 1). However, the data for the latter group are based on only 16 patients and are statistically not reliable. Among patients 15–59 years of age, those using partners were more likely to be transferred than patients who do not use partners (33 vs 25 percent within 18 months). This observation is consistent with the finding in the preceding section, which indicated that, in this age group, patients with partners had a higher hospitalization rate for CAPD-related complications. Among patients 60 years of age or older, there was little difference in the probability of transfer between patients with and without partners. This finding is also consistent with the findings in the previous section with regard to hospitalization.

Prior ESRD Therapy

Of the 2,336 patients who started CAPD and were registered in 1984 and early 1985, 971 had had no prior ESRD Therapy while 1,365 did have a prior therapy. The ones with prior therapy were more likely to transfer within 18 months of initiating CAPD—38 percent of patients with prior therapy compared to 26 percent of patients with no prior therapy. When the group with prior therapy is sub-divided into two categories (only prior in-center hemodialysis or IPD, 1,077 patients; and transplant or home dialysis, 288 patients) a marked difference in transfer probability becomes evident. At 18 months, the transfer probability for the hemodialysis or IPD sub-group is 41%, whereas for the transplant or home dialysis group the same probability is only 20 percent (Table 2).

TABLE 2. Probability of Tranfer According to Type of Prior
ESRD Therapy

Months	None	Prior Therapy		
		Any	In center IPD or Hemodialysis	Transplant or Home Dialysis
3	5.2	6.3	6.1	6.7
6	8.8	11.9	12.1	11.5
9	13.6	17.2	18.0	15.0
12	17.3	21.2	22.4	17.4
15	21.8	26.6	28.6	20.4
18	25.6	38.3	41.2	20.4
Number at time zero	971	1,365	1,077	288

There is no difference in transfer probabilities for patients with prior transplants compared to those who have exposure to a prior home dialysis technique.

Performance Status

Patients whose performance status worsened while on CAPD were more likely to transfer than patients whose performance status improved (18 percent transferring vs 10 percent at 18 months, Table 3). Among patients with an unchanged performance status while on CAPD, the data suggest that patients in poorer condition may be likely to transfer somewhat sooner, but the relationship is not clear.

TABLE 3. Probability of Transfer Off CAPD by Performance Status
at Last Report

Months	Worsened	Performance Status Codes *					Improved
		Unchanged					
		1	2	3	4	5	
3	0.0	1.4	3.4	5.0	5.9	0.0	1.3
6	2.0	4.4	10.3	9.0	18.2	10.0	2.2
9	6.0	9.4	19.8	15.7	31.1	32.5	3.4
12	14.5	12.9	22.4	15.7	31.1	-	5.6
15	18.2	17.7	30.1	15.7	31.1	-	9.7
Number at time zero	328	675	458	213	75	24	245

* 1 = Fully Active
  2 = Ambulatory, capable of light work
  3 = In bed less than 50% of time, capable of self-care but not work activities
  4 = In bed over 50% of time, capable of only limited self-care
  5 = Completely bedridden

TABLE 4. Probability of Transfer Off CAPD by Travel Time to CAPD Center

	Travel Time (hours)			
Months	<1 hr.	1-2 hrs.	2-3 hrs.	>3 hrs.
3	6.4	4.4	5.0	6.1
6	12.3	6.8	9.2	7.4
9	17.6	11.4	17.0	9.2
12	21.8	14.4	21.1	13.0
15	28.1	19.3	21.1	13.0
Number at time zero	1.525	532	160	112

Travel Time to CAPD Center

Patients who have to travel more than three hours to a treatment center are less likely to transfer off CAPD (Table 4). Long travel time may be associated with lower transfer due to a reluctance to place patients onto center hemodialysis who live great distances away. This is also consistent with the finding that compared with those living closer, a slightly higher proportion of patients living more than two hours from their treatment center have had prior experience with another form of home dialysis.

H. Characteristics of Patients Who Received a Kidney Transplant, Whose Kidney Funciton Returned, or Who Discontinued CAPD without Return of Kidney Function*

Introduction

While a great deal of attention has been focused on characteristics of patients that transfer to other maintenance dialysis therapies, the Registry had not focused on patients who received kidney transplants, who left dialysis without return of kidney function, or whose kidney function returned. This report presents a brief description of demographic and primary renal disease characteristics of those patients.

Methods and Results

Among 11,865 CAPD patients followed by the Registry, 956 left CAPD upon receipt of a functioning kidney, 111 had return of kidney function, and 61 left all forms of dialysis without return of kidney function. When considered together, these patients represent approximately 10% of the entire Registry, but the smallest of these groups represent only 0.6% of all patients. The age distribution of each of these patient groups, according to sex, is presented in Table 1, and the primary renal disease is presented in 2. Findings relating to each last reported status are as follows:

Received Kidney Transplant

The sex distribution of patients who discontinued CAPD because they received a kidney transplant was similar to that for the total CAPD

---

* The material contained in this report has been published as follows:
  Nolph KD, Cutler SJ, Steinberg SM, Novak JW. Special studies from the NIH Registry. *Peritoneal Dial Bull* 6:28–35, 1986.

234

TABLE 1. Current Age, and Sex of CAPD Patients, by Whether Left Dialysis without Return of Kidney Function, Kidney Function Returned, or Received Kidney Transplant

Age Group In Years	Received Transplant						Kidney Function Returned						Left Dialysis Without Return Of Kidney Function						All CAPD	
	Male		Female		Total		Male		Female		Total		Male		Female		Total			
	No.	%	No.	%	No.	%	No.	%	No.	%	No.	%	No.	%	No.	%	No.	%	No.	%
≤ 10	31	5.7	24	5.8	55	5.8	4	6.2	1	2.1	5	4.5	2	8.7	0	0.0	2	3.4	198	1.7
11-20	55	10.2	34	8.2	89	9.3	1	1.6	2	4.3	3	2.7	1	4.4	0	0.0	1	1.7	369	3.2
21-30	105	19.4	99	23.9	204	21.4	2	3.1	6	12.8	8	7.2	1	4.4	2	5.6	3	5.1	919	7.9
31-40	150	27.8	146	35.2	296	31.0	4	6.3	7	14.9	11	9.9	2	8.7	2	5.6	4	6.8	1,770	15.1
41-50	118	21.9	61	14.7	179	18.7	6	9.4	5	10.6	11	9.9	0	0.0	3	8.3	3	5.1	1,842	15.8
51-60	68	12.6	43	10.4	111	11.6	9	14.1	9	19.1	18	16.2	4	17.4	9	25.0	13	22.0	2,540	21.7
61-70	13	2.4	8	1.9	21	2.2	27	42.2	10	21.3	37	33.3	4	17.4	8	22.2	12	20.3	2,674	22.9
71-80	0	0.0	0	0.0	0	0.0	11	17.2	7	14.9	18	16.2	6	26.1	10	27.8	16	27.1	1,227	10.5
81-90	0	0.0	0	0.0	0	0.0	0	0.0	0	0.0	0	0.0	3	13.0	2	5.6	5	8.5	150	1.3
Total	540		415		955		64		47		111		23		36		59		11,689	100.0
Percent By Sex		56.5		43.5		100.0		57.7		42.3		100.0		39.0		61.0		100.0		
Percent By Race																				
White					81.1						79.3						79.7			76.2
Black					11.6						16.2						16.9			17.2
Other					7.3						4.5						3.4			6.7

TABLE 2. Primary Renal Disease of CAPD Patients, by Whether Left Dialysis without Return of Kidney Function, Kidney Function Returned, or Received Kidney Transplant

RENAL DISEASE	Received Transplant		Kidney Function Returned		Left Without Return Of Kidney Function		All Patients	
	No.	Percent	No.	Percent	No.	Percent	No.	Percent
Chronic Glomerulonephritis	210	23.5	14	12.7	6	10.9	2,201	19.6
Diabetic Glomerulosclerosis	213	23.8	7	6.4	14	25.5	2,593	23.1
Hypertensive Renal Disease	69	7.7	19	17.3	10	18.2	1,724	15.3
Polycystic Kidney(s)	57	6.4	1	0.9	4	7.3	774	6.9
Chronic Pyelonephritis	27	3.0	2	1.8	4	7.3	537	4.8
Systemic Immunological Disease with Renal Involvement	34	3.8	7	6.4	2	3.6	340	3.0
Interstitial Nephritis	23	2.6	3	2.7	1	1.8	302	2.7
Obstructive Uropathy	28	3.1	4	3.6	1	1.8	243	2.2
Rapidly Progressing Glomerulonephritis	30	3.4	7	6.4	0	0.0	250	2.2
Familial Nephritis	19	2.1	0	0.0	0	0.0	123	1.1
Aplastic/Hypoplastic Kidney(s)	13	1.5	0	0.0	1	1.8	68	0.6
Stone-Forming Renal Disease	3	0.3	1	0.9	0	0.0	59	0.5
Amyloidosis with Renal Involvement	2	0.2	0	0.0	1	1.8	61	0.5
Renal Infarct, Secondary to Vascular Occlusion	1	0.1	6	5.5	0	0.0	55	0.5
Nephrectomy, Secondary to Cancer	2	0.2	0	0.0	1	1.8	43	0.4
Gouty Nephropathy	3	0.3	0	0.0	0	0.0	25	0.2
Bilateral Cortical Necrosis	0	0.0	2	1.8	0	0.0	11	0.1
Other	125	14.0	32	29.1	6	10.9	1,143	10.2
Unknown	35	3.9	5	4.6	4	7.3	691	6.1
TOTAL	894	100.0	110	100.0	55	100.0	11,244	100.0

population in the Registry: 56.5% male, 43.5% female. The race distribution was also similar: 81% of the transplant group was white compared to 76% of the total population. However, the age distribution was clearly different. Sixty-eight percent of the transplant group was 40 years of age or younger compared to 30% of all CAPD patients in the registry.

The distribution with respect to primary renal disease was essentially similar except for a deficiency of patients with hypertensive renal disease in the transplant group: 7.7% compared to 15.3% in the total CAPD Registry. This may be due to the smaller percentage of young patients with hypertensive renal disease: 16% 40 years of age or younger compared to 30% in the total CAPD population.

Kidney Function Returned

The sex and race distributions of patients whose kidney function returned while on CAPD were similar to the distributions for the total CAPD population. There were more elderly people among those whose kidney function returned: 52% over the age of 60 compared to 35% in the total CAPD registry.

Among patients whose kidney function returned there were proportionately fewer patients with chronic glomerulonephritis, diabetic glomerulosclerosis, and polycystic kidneys compared to the total CAPD population. There were relatively more patients whose primary renal disease was reported as 'Other' than the 16 specific types listed in Table 2: 29% compared to 10% in the total registry.

Left Dialysis without Return of Kidney Function

This is a small group: 59 patients out of 11,865 in the CAPD Registry, so the observed percentages are subject to considerable chance variation. Nevertheless, the available information is informative. The proportion of male patients in this group was 39% compared to 56% in the total CAPD population. The percentage of black patients was similar to that in the total registry. There were more patients over 70 years of age: 36% compared to 12% in the total CAPD population. There were fewer patients with chronic glomerulosclerosis: 11% compared to 20% in the total CAPD population.

I. Comparison of outcomes for patients with and without prior ESRD therapy*

Introduction

Of the patients who began CAPD therapy at time of entry to the Registry program, 2,850 had received no prior ESRD therapy (Class 1A) and 4,567 had some form of prior ESRD therapy (Class 1B). This analysis explores whether these two groups differ with respect to the probability of developing major treatment outcomes.

Results

Data on the probability of first peritonitis, presented in Table 1, indicates that patients with prior ESRD therapy are likely to develop the first episode of peritonitis a little sooner. For example, at 12 months the probability is 55.5% for Class 1B patients compared to 52.0% for Class 1A. At 24 months, the respective figures are 80.3% and 75.5%. Table 13A in the basic report indicates that the relationship is similar when repeat episodes are taken into account. The peritonitis occurrence rates were 1.4 episodes per patient year for Class 1B and 1.3 for Class 1A patients.

Patients with prior ESRD therapy are likely to be hospitalized for CAPD-related complications somewhat sooner than patients with no prior therapy (Table 2). For example, at 12 months the probability of first hospitalization was 51.4% for Class 1B and 46.8% for Class 1A. The relationship is similar to the one for peritonitis. However, when repeat hospitalization is taken into account (Table 13A of the 1986

* The material contained in this report has been published as follows:
Nolph KD, Cutler SJ, Steinberg SM, Novak JW. Special studies from the NIH Registry. *Peritoneal Dial Bull* 6:28–35, 1986.

238

TABLE 1. Probability of First Episode of Peritonitis by Class of Case*

	Case	
Months	1A	1B
6	41.2	42.5
12	59.8	63.0
18	68.5	73.0
24	75.5	80.3
30	81.1	85.4
36	85.2	89.3
42	87.0	92.5
Number at time zero	2,850	4,567

*1A – No prior ESRD Therapy; new to CAPD at first follow-up.
1B – Some prior ESRD Therapy; new to CAPD at first follow-up.

TABLE 2. Probability of First CAPD-Related Hospitalization by Class of Case*

	Case	
Months	1A	1B
6	30.9	33.7
12	46.8	51.4
18	57.4	61.5
24	64.6	68.2
30	69.8	73.0
36	74.7	77.4
42	79.8	80.1
Number at time zero	2,850	4,567

*1A – No prior ESRD Therapy; new to CAPD at first follow-up.
1B – Some prior ESRD Therapy; new to CAPD at first follow-up.

Registry Report) no difference between these two groups of patients is evident.

The probability of transfer from CAPD to hemodialysis or IPD is somewhat higher for patients with prior therapy. For example, 36.3% of patients with prior ESRD therapy transferred within 24 months of staring CAPD compared to 29.5% of patients with no prior therapy.

TABLE 3.   Transfer Probability by Class of Case*

Months	Case	
	1A	1B
6	8.5	12.0
12	16.5	22.7
18	22.6	30.2
24	29.5	36.3
30	34.4	41.9
36	39.0	45.8
42	45.6	49.7
Number at time zero	2,850	4,567

*1A - No prior ESRD Therapy; new to CAPD at first follow-up.
 1B - Some prior ESRD Therapy; new to CAPD at first follow-up.

TABLE 4.   Probability of Dying While on CAPD by Class of Case*

Months	Case	
	1A	1B
6	8.6	8.7
12	16.4	16.1
18	22.4	22.9
24	28.4	28.3
30	33.9	33.5
36	40.1	39.6
42	46.3	45.5
Number at time zero	2,850	4,567

*1A - No prior ESRD Therapy; new to CAPD at first follow-up.
 1B - Some prior ESRD Therapy; new to CAPD at first follow-up.

Patients with prior experience with another form of therapy may be less inclined to continue accepting the logistics and complications involved in CAPD therapy (Table 3).

As shown in Table 4, the probability of dying while on CAPD is similar for Class 1A and Class 1B patients.

SECTION NINE

Special Report—1985

A. Prognostic Factors Associated with the First Episode of Peritonitis*

Introduction

Peritonitis is the most common and perhaps the most bothersome complication associated with Continuous Ambulatory Peritoneal Dialysis (CAPD). The National CAPD Registry[1] reports that 43% of patients receiving CAPD for End- Stage Renal Disease (ESRD) experience their first episode of peritonitis within six months of beginning treatment, and that 63% of patients experienced an episode within 12 months. The purpose of this study is to examine the relationship between the time to the first episode of peritonitis and a number of patient characteristics for which information is available in the Registry. Specifically, the role of patients' age, sex, race, living arrangement (with or without family), history of diabetes, and prior therapy for ESRD are examined to determine whether they are associated with the development of peritonitis. The relationship between those variables and repeated episodes of peritonitis are beyond the scope of this analysis.

Subjects and Methods

Fifty-nine hundred, eighty-four (5,984) of the 8,829 CAPD patients with follow-up information in the National CAPD Registry comprise the study group. All study patients were followed by the Registry from the time they began CAPD—either as first ESRD therapy, or after transfer

* The material contained in this report has been published as follows:
  Steinberg SM, Cutler SJ, Novak JW, Nolph KD. Prognostic factors associated with the first episode of peritonitis in patients with continuous ambulatory peritoneal dialysis (CAPD). *ASAIO J* 8:238–243, 1985.
  Steinberg SM, Cutler SJ, Novak JW, Nolph KD. Prognostic factors associated with peritonitis among patients on continuous ambulatory peritoneal dialysis (CAPD). *Trans Am Soc Artif Int Organs* 31:565–567, 1985

off another treatment modality, or after failure of transplant graft. The 2,845 Registry patients not included in this study started CAPD therapy prior to registration; the lack of information regarding these patients' early experience on CAPD required their exclusion from the present study. Demographic information (age, race, living arrangement, sex), the nature of the patients' primary renal disease, and whether there was prior ESRD therapy were available for all patients included in the study.

In order to determine the relationship between time to first peritonitis and the other variables studied, a two-stage analysis was employed. In the first stage, the Mantel-Haenszel[2] procedure was used to determine the presence of association between each variable and time to first peritonitis. For each of the six variables, the patients were classified into two subgroups and the Mantel-Haenszel technique was used to estimate the relative risk of the first peritonitis episode in each subgroup relative to the other. This method was first applied to the total study population to find the overall risk associated with each factor. The same method was then applied within each subgroup, in order to identify possible interactions between the variables being studied.

This approach may best be explained through an example. The relative risk of peritonitis was first assessed for each variable, (e.g., diabetics vs non-diabetics) and then separately with various subgroups (e.g., with respect to age). If results obtained varied considerably for the subgroups, an interaction between the variable divided into subgroups and the one under study was suggested.

Estimates of the relative risks were next converted into risk scores by multiplying the common logarithms of the relative risks by 100. The resulting risk scores are such that if two subgroups (e.g. male and female) had identical risks of developing first peritonitis by a certain time, the risk score will be zero (0). In such a case, we might reasonably conclude that sex had no impact on outcome. A risk score of 8 to 12 corresponds to an excess risk of first peritonitis (for example, for blacks as compared to whites) of 20 to 30 percent more first episodes of peritonitis during a defined follow-up period. Variables characterized by risk scores larger than 12 are likely to be noticed in a moderate size nephrology practice and, therefore, considered of importance. Scores of 8 to 12, implying a 20 to 30 percent excess risk may be clinically meaningful, but may be unrecognized in an individual clinic. Risk scores as small as 4 or 5 may indicate a 'statistically' significant difference in a large patient population; however, since these scores are indicative of excess risks of only 10 to 12 percent, they need to be interpreted more conservatively.

In the second stage of the analysis, the individual factors and the potentially important interactions are evaluated simultaneously - through the use of a multivariate mathematical model. Specifically, the Proportional Hazards Method of Cox[3] was used to evaluate the impact of each selected factor on time to first peritonitis, while adjusting for the influence of the other variables included in the model. With this technique, changes in risk attributable to each factor are calculated while taking account of other pertinent characteristics. The resulting parameter estimate for each factor represents its individual prognostic importance. For example, the risk associated with living with family vs living without family on development of first peritonitis may be examined by mathematically holding effects of sex, age, race, disease, and treatment history fixed at some level. The results of such an analysis should provide a clearer picture of the influence of each of the variables studied on development of first peritonitis.

In summary, the results of applying the Cox model makes possible a description of the risk of developing peritonitis for patients with a variety of characteristics as compared to a 'baseline' patient group. To implement the model, it is customary to select as a baseline, a set of characteristics associated with a presumed low risk patient. In this analysis, the baseline group was defined to possess the following traits: white, 20–59 years of age, non-diabetic, no prior ESRD therapy, and living apart from family. The risk for all other patient groups is expressed as 'percent additional risk' relative to the baseline group.

Results

(a) Stage One Analyses

Table 1 provides summary information on the risk scores associated with each of the factors studied. Patients' race, which had a risk score of 12.0, appears to be more closely linked to time to first peritonitis than the other factors studied; and the presence of diabetic glomeruloslerosis, with a risk score of 4.9, was found to rank second in importance. Age under 20 (vs 20–59 years of age) and living arrangement ranked third and fourth. In this analysis, previous ESRD therapy, sex, and age 60 and over (vs 20–59 years of age) did not appear to influence the risk of developing peritonitis.

The impact of each factor on time to first peritonitis within the various patient subgroups is provided in Table 2, in order to identify possible interaction terms to be included in the Cox model. Note that,

TABLE 1.   Risk Scores for Each of Six Factors in Development
            of First Peritonitis of <u>Subgroup A</u>
                                     <u>Subgroup B</u>

FACTOR RELATIVE RISK		RISK SCORE	TOTAL NUMBER OF PATIENTS*
<u>Previous ESRD Therapy</u>			<u>3747</u>
No Previous ESRD Therapy		1.1	2237
Race:	<u>Black</u>		<u>996</u>
	White	12.0	4610
Sex:	<u>Female</u>		<u>2665</u>
	Male	0.3	3329
Living Arrangement:	<u>Without Family</u>		<u>1050</u>
	With Family	3.7	4934
Renal Disease:	<u>Diabetic**</u>		<u>1345</u>
	Non-Diabetic	4.9	4639
Age:	<u>Under 20</u>		<u>321</u>
	20-59	4.1	3673
Age:	<u>60 & over</u>		<u>1949</u>
	20-59	1.3	3673

*<u>Number of patients in Subgroup A</u>
 Number of patients in Subgroup B

**Primary renal disease is Diabetic Glomerulosclerosis

even though the risk score for ages 60 and over (vs ages 20–59) was low, the possible variation of risk among subgroups is examined to determine whether it may be clinically operative in selected subgroups. The variation in risk among subgroups of patients under age 20 was not analyzed, because of the limited number of young patients.

The effect of race (black vs white) within individual subgroups is presented in Column 1 of Table 2. The risk scores are generally 10 or higher, indicating that race is a noteworthy prognostic factor, with respect to time to first peritonitis; among patients living with family, blacks are at substantially higher risk than whites (risk score of 13.7). In contrast, among patients living apart from family, the risk score for blacks is only 4.7.

The effect of ages 60 and over (vs ages 20–59) is noticeable within two subgroups: patients with diabetic glomerulosclerosis (score of 7.2) and among black patients (score of 4.6); see Column 2, Table 2. The effect of diabetic glomerulosclerosis is pronounced among patients 60 years of age and older, and is noteworthy among black patients, patients with a history of ESRD therapy prior to initiation of CAPD, and among patients living with family; see Column 3, Table 2. The risk scores for

TABLE 2.   Risk Scores for Various Characteristics When Examined within Individual Subgroups

SUBGROUP	BLACK WHITE (1)	OVER 60 20-60 (2)	DIABETIC # NON-DIABETIC (3)	NO FAMILY FAMILY (4)
Race:				
White		1.7	4.7	4.8
Black		4.6	7.2	-4.8*
Age:				
Under 20	9.5		**	**
20-60	11.6		4.0	3.9
60+	14.8		10.3	4.3
Primary Renal Disease:				
Non-Diabetic	11.5	0.9		4.8
Diabetic #	14.6	7.2		-0.3*
Living Arrangement:				
With Family	13.7	1.4	5.8	
W/o Family	4.7	1.7	0.6	
Treatment History:				
No Previous ESRD Tx	10.2	3.2	3.5	4.6
Previous ESRD Tx	12.9	0.3	6.4	3.2

*The group in the numerator is at lower risk than the group in the denominator.

**Insufficient patients for calculation to be reliable.

#Diabetic Glomerulosclerosis

living arrangement (Column 4) are all less than 5, suggesting that living with or apart from family has relatively little influence on the risk of developing peritonitis. There is, however, a marked difference in the risk scores for white and black patients: +4.8 among whites compared to −4.8 among blacks. Such scores suggest that among white patients, living apart from family is associated with an increased risk, while among black patients, the opposite is true.

In summary, the results of the first stage analysis, provided in Tables 1 and 2 suggest that, except for sex, the factors considered in this analysis should be included in the Cox model. Further, the interaction between race and living arrangement appears to be potentially important and, likewise, should be included in the analysis model to be developed.

(b) Stage Two Analyses

Terms for six individual variables (diabetic status, age < 20, age ≥ 60, prior ESRD therapy, race, and family present) and one interaction (race × family) were included in the proportional hazards model. The parameter values obtained for each are presented in Table 3. Each of the variables was evaluated for its effect on the risk of developing peritonitis, while accounting for the influence of the other characteristics.

All terms included in the model are statistically significant in the presence of one another, with the exception of race. The diminished statistical significance of race in the multivariate analysis (Cox model) compared to the univariate analysis (Mantel-Haenszel method) is accounted for by the interaction between race and living arrangement. Each of the variables listed in Table 3 increases the risk of peritonitis, while the interaction term (white patients living with family) decreases the risk (parameter $= -.323$). The parameter values in Table 3 are used to estimate the additional risk of developing peritonitis for patients with various combinations of characteristics. Additional risk is calculated as a percentage compared to the risk for a 'baseline patient', and the arithmetic procedure for using the parameters in Table 3 to produce the risk estimates in Table 4 is described in the Technical Note.

There is one type of patient with a risk lower than that for the 'baseline patient': a white patient, 20–59 years of age, non-diabetic,

TABLE 3. Parameter Estimates of Jointly Considered Prognostic Variables, Obtained Through Use of Cox Proportional Hazards Model

VARIABLE	PARAMETER ESTIMATE	P-VALUE*
Diabetic**	.128	.004
Age, < 20	.178	.024
Age, ≥ 60	.115	.003
Prior ESRD Therapy	.088	.020
Race (Effect of Black Race)	.135	.194
Family Present	.270	.007
Race x Family Interaction (whites living with family)	-.323	.005

*If the p-value is <.05, the parameter estimate is unlikely to differ from zero because of chance.

**Primary renal disease is diabetic glomerulosclerosis.

TABLE 4.   Examples of Additional Risks (%) of Developing First Peritonitis, for Patients with Various Characteristics as Compared with a "Baseline Patient"

			TRAIT			% ADDITIONAL RISK
	DIABETIC STATUS	AGE	RACE	LIVING ARRANGEMENT	PRIOR ESRD THERAPY	
"BASELINE PATIENT"	Non-Diabetic	20-59	White	Without Family	No Prior Therapy	0.0*
(1)				With Family		-5.2
(2)			Black			14.5
(3)		<20				19.5
(4)		≥60				12.2
Patients Differ- (5)					Prior Therapy	9.2
ing from (6)			Black	With Family		49.9
Characteristics (7)		≥60	Black			28.4
of "Baseline (8)		≥60		With Family		6.4
Patient" with (9)		≥60	Black	With Family		68.2
respect to (10)		≥60	Black	With Family	Prior Therapy	83.7
traits listed (11)	Diabetic					13.6
on each line (12)	Diabetic	≥60				27.5
(13)	Diabetic	≥60	Black			45.9
(14)	Diabetic		Black	With Family		70.4
(15)	Diabetic	≥60	Black	With Family		91.2
(16)	Diabetic	≥60	Black	With Family	Prior Therapy	108.8

*By definition of a "baseline patient"

with no prior ESRD therapy, and *living with family* (see line 1, Table 4). This is a result of the interaction between race and living arrangement. In all other cases, traits that differ from those of the 'baseline patient' result in an increased risk of peritonitis. In general, the more traits that differ, the greater the increase in risk. This is well illustrated in the additional risks for patients described on lines 11 through 16, for whom the additional risks range from 13.6 percent to 108.8 percent.

Discussion

Information available in the National CAPD Registry was examined to identify and assess the relative importance of patient characteristics on the risk of developing peritonitis. In this analysis, attention was limited to the time from initiation of CAPD to the first episode of peritonitis. The factors considered were sex, race, age, ESRD therapy prior to initiation of CAPD, living arrangement, and primary renal disease (i.e., diabetic glomerulosclerosis vs all others.)

An exploratory, univariate analysis (Mantel-Haenszel method) revealed that of the six factors under study, only sex appeared to have no influence on the risk of peritonitis. This analysis also indicated that there was a potentially meaningful interaction between race and living arrangement. Whereas living with family appeared to decrease the risk of peritonitis for white patients, it appeared to increase the risk for black

250

patients. The latter finding was unexpected and may reflect criteria used in selecting black patients for CAPD, e.g., stricter criteria might be used in selecting black patients living apart from family. However, the possible negative influence on patient well-being of the home environment in black families cannot be ruled out. Information is not available on specific living arrangements, such as number and ages of household members.

A multivariate analysis (Cox model) was used to assess the relative importance of the five factors identified as having an effect on the risk of peritonitis, plus the interaction between race and living arrangement. The analysis identified one group with a risk that was a little lower than the baseline; namely, white patients with all the characteristics of the baseline group, except that they lived with family. Patients less than 20 years of age and patients 60 years of age and older were at a higher risk than patients in the baseline age range—20–59 years. As shown in Table 4, the analysis identified seven groups with additional risks ranging between 45.9 and 108.8 percent, whereas the other sets of traits produced additional risks below 30%. The strong race and living arrangement interaction is also clearly identifiable in this analysis.

In considering the findings of this analysis, the limitations of the available data must be borne in mind. The Registry is limited to patients placed on CAPD and, therefore, information is not available on the characteristics and experience of patients with ESRD maintained by means of other modalities. Similarly, information is not available on the criteria used in selecting patients for CAPD and the variation in criteria among treatment centers. The importance of these two conditions cannot be overemphasized. As a result, the data that have been analyzed reflect the identifiable factors that are related to the observed experiences. Even with this limitation, these findings should be useful in selecting patients for CAPD, developing training programs for different groups of patients, and for developing monitoring programs for them. In addition, these findings may be useful in identifying questions for further study.

References

1. Report of the National CAPD Registry of the National Institutes of Health: Characteristics of Participants and Selected Outcome Measures for the Period January 1, 1981, through August 31, 1984. NIADDK, 1985.
2. Mantel, N. Evaluation of survival data and two new rank order statistics arising in its consideration. Cancer Chemother Rep 1966; 50:163–170.
3. Cox, D.R. Regression models and life tables (with discussion). J Royal Stat Soc (B) 1972; 34:187–220.

Technical note on calculation of additional risks presented in Table 4

Table 4 contains additional risk percentages for various sets of characteristics compared with characteristics for a "baseline patient." The parameter estimates presented in Table 3 are used to compute effects of characteristics that differ from those of a baseline patient.

Steps involved in such computations are as follows:

(1) Determine the patients' characteristics in terms of the five variables examined.

(2) Identify the traits which differ from those of the baseline patient.

(3) Using Table 3, write down the parameter estimate for each trait(s) which differ(s) from that of the baseline patient. Be sure to include the parameter estimate for the interaction (-.323) if the patient is white *and* living with family.

(4) Sum the values from the previous step.

(5) Compute:

Z = 2.71828 (sum of parameter estimates)

where 2.71828 = e, the base of the natural logarithm

(6) Calculate:

(Z - 1) 100%, which is the percentage of additional risk as compared to that of a "baseline patient."

Two examples will illustrate the technique:

Example 1: Baseline patient, except living *with* family.

Steps	Baseline Patient	Example 1 Patient	Parameter Estimate
(1), (2), (3)	Non-Diabetic	(same)	0
	20-60	(same)	0
	White	(same)	0
	Without Family	With Family	.270-.323
			(interaction since *white*)
	No Prior Therapy	(same)	0
(4)			-0.053
(5)	2.71828-0.053 = .948		
(6)	(.948 - 1) × 100% = -5.2% (lower risk than baseline)		

Example 2: Baseline patient, except *black* and *living with family*

Steps	Baseline Patient	Example 2 Patient	Parameter Estimate
(1), (2), (3)	Non-Diabetic	(same)	0
	20-60	(same)	0
	White	(Black)	.135
	Without Family	With Family	.270
			(interaction since *black*)
	No Prior Therapy	(same)	0
(4)			-0.053
(5)	$2.71828.405 = 1.499$		
(6)	$(1.499 - 1) \times 100\% = 49.9\%$ (additional risk compared with baseline)		

Special Report—1984

A. Considerations in Analysis of Complications

This is a special report on the normally recognized complications of CAPD. Its purpose is to describe the patterns of complications which individuals and groups of patients experience while on CAPD. All sections of the report emphasize peritonitis because this is the major complication reported and merits special attention.

A. Variation in Patient Experience: Case Studies

The complication rates presented in the Chapter IV of the 1984 report are useful summary indices. However, since they are averages, they do not provide insight into the variation in experience among patients; some remain on CAPD for an extended period of time, whereas others are transferred to hemodialysis or die within a few weeks or months after initiation of CAPD. Some patients experience many complications, while others do not.

In order to provide some insight into the variation in experience among patients, a sample of 50 patients was chosen via a random procedure and their experience is portrayed in Figure 1. The sample was selected in the following manner:

1. All patients who were first followed by the registry within a few weeks of starting CAPD (Class 1A and 1B) were identified, and those with an initial status report pertaining to the fourth calendar quarter of 1981 were initially selected. This quarter was selected because it was the quarter during which the Registry program went into full operation.
2. Patients from 'pilot centers' were excluded because their experience might be unrepresentative. The 15 pilot centers began reporting at the beginning of 1981. Also excluded were patients from 'inactive centers', i.e., centers that submitted no patient status reports pertaining to the third and/or fourth calendar quarters of 1983.

256

3. A total of 501 patients were retained and their records were ordered according to social security number. Beginning with a random number (in this case 7), the seventh record and every tenth record thereafter was selected, for a total of 50.

All patients in this sample had the potential of being followed through the end of 1983 (1983Q4). The initial status report for all 50 patients pertained to the fourth quarter of 1981 (1981Q4), but about half of them had started on CAPD in the preceding quarter (1981Q3).

Since the Patient Status Reports, on which Figure 1 is based, provide information by calendar quarter, exact dates are not reported. The legend to the figure indicates the symbols used for each type of

FIGURE 1.   Variation of Patient Experience: Sample of 50 Patients

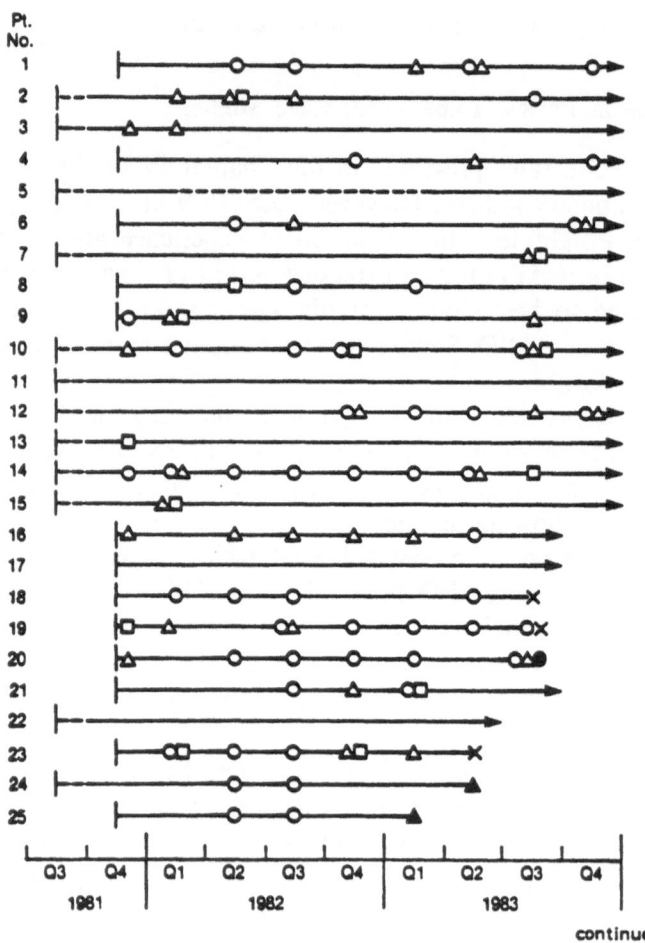

continued

FIGURE 1 - continued

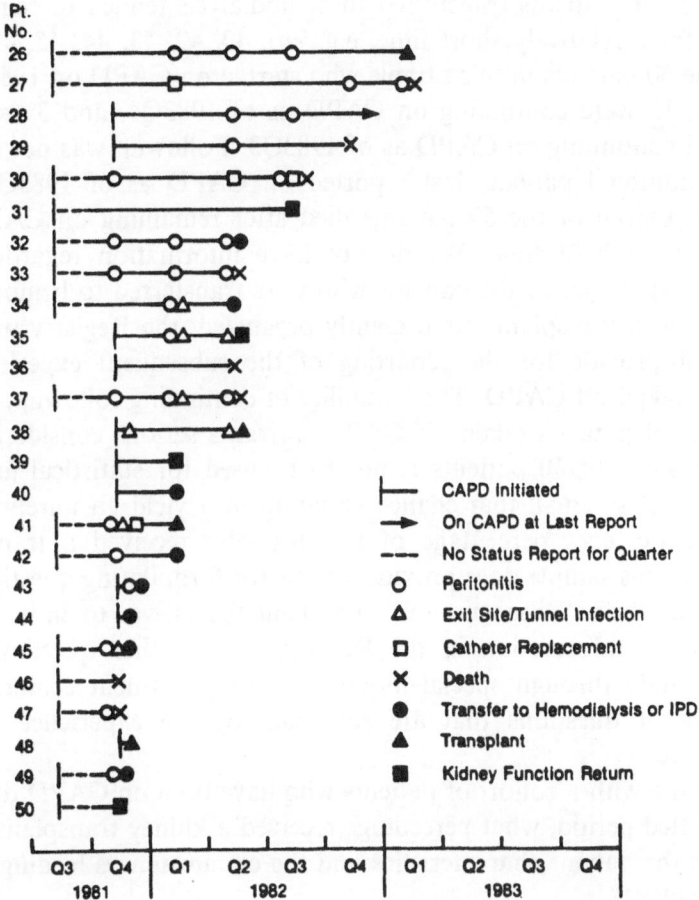

complication and for each type of outcome. If more than one type of complication was reported for a calendar quarter, all are shown. However, multiple reports of the same type of complication within a calendar quarter are represented by the same symbol as single reports. Thus, the chart portrays, for each patient, the quarter in which no complications were reported and the quarters in which one, two, or three types of complications occurred.

The patients are ordered in the chart by length of followup, beginning with those followed the longest. Within each length of followup group, the patients are shown in the random order in which they were selected.

Examination of Figure 1 indicates that complications are common, although a few patients had none or very few, e.g., patients no. 3, 11, 13,

15. The chart reveals that several patients who had a series of complications remained on CAPD for more than two years, e.g., patients no. 1, 2, 10, 12, 14. Patients transferred to hemodialysis tended to remain on CAPD for a relatively short time, e.g., no. 40, 42, 43, 44, 45, 49.

Of the 50 patients in this sample who started on CAPD on 1981Q3 or 1981Q4, 15 were continuing on CAPD as of 1983Q4, and 3 were last reported continuing on CAPD as of 1983Q3. Followup was not current for 2 additional patients last reported on CAPD as of 1983Q2, and 1982Q4. Eleven of the 50 patients died after remaining on CAPD for varying lengths of time. We do not have information regarding the survival experience of the patients who were transferred to hemodialysis or received a transplant. As presently organized, the Registry program does not provide for the reporting of the subsequent experience of patients taken off CAPD. The feasibility of continuing followup, via the Registry, of patients taken off CAPD warrants serious consideration.

The sample of 50 patients is not to be used for statistical analysis, because it is so small that chance variation may yield an unrepresentative statistic, e.g., percentage of patients who received a transplant. However, this sample does provide a basis for formulating questions for further analyses. Some questions may lend themselves to investigation through the information in the Registry, while other questions may require study through special inquiries to the treatment centers. Two examples of questions that are suggested by the experience of this sample are:

1. Starting with a cohort of patients who have been on CAPD during a specified period, what percentage received a kidney transplant; what were the patient characteristics and the circumstances leading to the transplant?

2. What were the characteristics and what was the experience of patients who remained on CAPD for two years or longer compared to patients who were transferred to hemodialysis or IPD within six months of starting CAPD? (Note: In the sample of 50 patients, those who remained on CAPD for extended periods generally did experience repeated complications.)

B. Life Table Analysis of Successive Complications

In this section, consideration is given to the probabilities of successive complications, i.e., from the first to the second, from the second to the third, and from the third to the fourth. Times between complications are estimated because of two characteristics of the reporting system in use through the end of 1983. (1) exact dates of occurrence were not reported; only whether one or more events occurred during a calendar quarter; and (2) no specific definition was available for the clearing up of one complication, such as peritonitis, and the occurrence of a second episode. In the calculation of occurrence rates, presented in Section IVE (see page 32, 1984 Report), all episodes of each type of complication were counted as reported. On the basis of the data in Table 12 (see page 33, 1984 Report), it was suggested that the degree of possible overstatement was not great.

FIGURE 2.   Probability of Successive Complications: Either Peritonitis, or Exit Site/Tunnel Infections, or Catheter Replacement as a Function of the Complications Previously Experienced

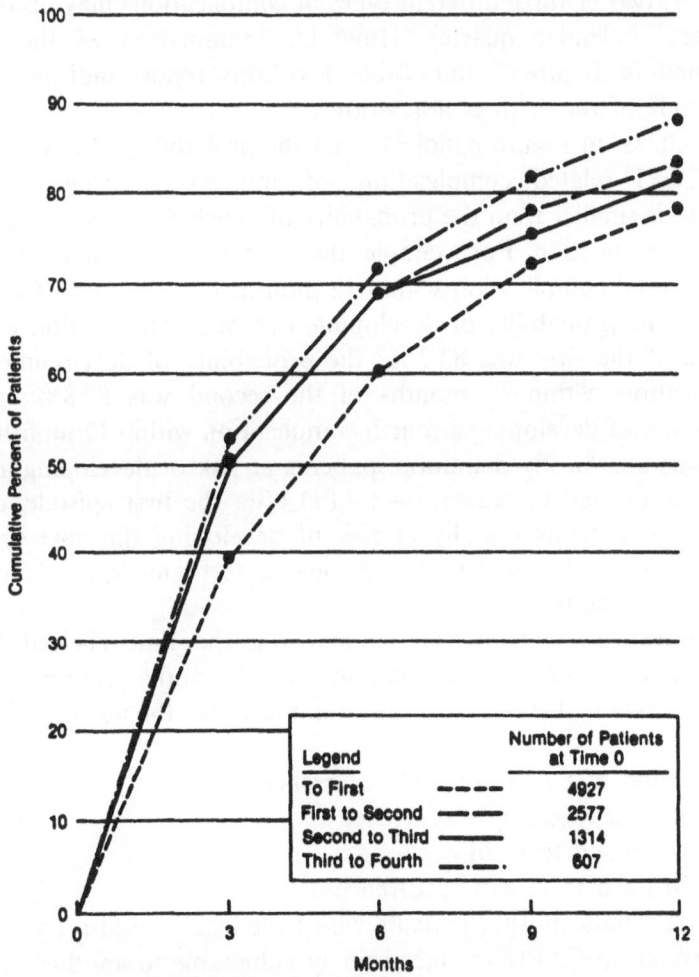

Note: Two or more complications reported for the same calendar quarter were treated as one complication.

In this life table analysis of the probability of successive episodes of complications, two or more complications reported for one calendar quarter were counted only once. On the basis of the data in Table 12, it is suggested that in considering individual types of complications the time from one episode to the next may be overstated, but that the degree of overstatement is small. For example, peritonitis is the complication that occurs most frequently, but two or more episodes of peritonitis were reported in only 5.7% of the patient-calendar quarters of observation. On the other hand, in considering successive episodes of any CAPD-related complication, whatever the type, the degree of overstatement of the time between successive episodes may be more than trivial. This is because two or more complications of some type were reported in 11.9% of the patient calendar quarters of observation. As shown in Figure 1, two or three different types of complications may occur within the same calendar quarter. However, examination of the findings presented in Figure 2 and Table 1 of this report indicate that the magnitude of the error is not serious.

The curves in Figure 2 indicate that the probability of developing the first CAPD-related complication, of any type, during a specified interval, is smaller than the probability of developing a second, third or fourth complication. For example, the probability of a patient developing an initial complication within 12 months of starting on CAPD was 78.8%. The probability of developing a second complication within 12 months of the first was 83.7%; the probability of developing a third complication within 12 months of the second was 82.8%; and the probability of developing a fourth complication within 12 months of the third was 88.3%. By definition, patients at risk of developing a second complication had to remain on CAPD after the first episode, etc. The number of patients initially at risk of developing the next successive complication is shown as part of the legend to Figure 2, i.e., 'number of patients at time 0.'

A convenient statistic for summarizing the time elapsed between successive episodes is the 'median number of months between episodes.' This is shown in Table 1. For 'any complication' the median times were as follows:

— Initiation of CAPD to first occurrence   4.5 months
— From first to second occurrence   3.0 months
— From second to third occurrence   3.0 months
— From third to fourth occurrence   2.7 months

These data indicate that patients who have experienced a complication and remain on CAPD are increasingly vulnerable to another complication. In view of the magnitude of the median values, the situation appears to be clinically serious in spite of the possible understatement of

TABLE 1. Median Number of Months Between Successive Episodes of CAPC
Related Complications, by Type of Complications

TYPE OF COMPLICATIONS	NO. MONTHS	NO. PATIENTS AT TIME ZERO
ANY COMPLICATION		
Time to first occurrence	4.5	4,927
Time from first to second occurrence	3.0	2,577
Time from second to third occurrence	3.0	1,314
Time to fourth occurrence	2.7	607
CATHETER REPLACEMENT		
Time to first catheter change	>24	4,920
Time from first to second change	>24	613
Time from second to third change	>24	86
EXIT SITE/TUNNEL INFECTION ("infection")		
Time to first infection	17.7	4,939
Time from first to second infection	7.0	1,250
Time from second to third infection	5.4	435
Time from third to fourth infection	4.8	153
PERITONITIS		
Time to first peritonitis	7.3	4,966
Time from first to second peritonitis	4.6	2,042
Time from second to third peritonitis	4.2	864
Time from third to fourth peritonitis	3.7	326

these medians resulting from the method used in handling the available data.

Figure 3 summarizes the experience of Registry patients regarding successive catheter replacements. The probability of a patient requiring a catheter replacement within 12 months of initiation of therapy is relatively low − 20.2%. Consequently, relatively few patients were available for analysis regarding successive episodes. Nevertheless, the data do indicate an upward shift. The probability of a patient requiring a second replacement within 12 months of the first or of requiring a third replacement within 12 months of the second was between 30 and 40 percent.

Figure 4 summarizes patient experience with respect to successive episodes of exit site/tunnel infection. A very definite trend is evident. As shown in Table 16, the successive median number of months between successive episodes were:
— To first infection   17.7 months
— First to second infection   7.0 months
— Second to third infection   5.4 months
— Third to fourth infection   4.8 months
Figure 5 pertains to successive episodes of peritonitis. The trend is not as dramatic as for exit site/tunnel infections, but it is present. The successive median values were:
— To first peritonitis   7.3 months

FIGURE 3. Probability of Successive Catheter Replacements as a Function of the Number Previously Replaced

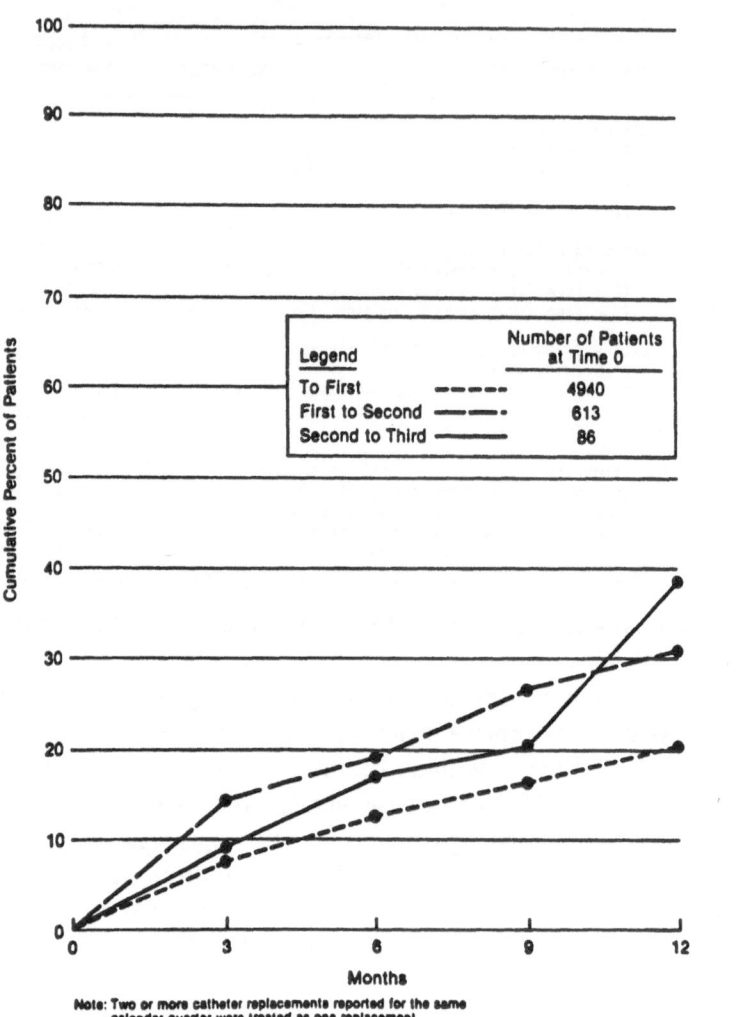

Note: Two or more catheter replacements reported for the same calendar quarter were treated as one replacement.

— First to second peritonitis	4.6 months
— Second to third peritonitis	4.2 months
— Third to fourth peritonitis	3.7 months

Thus, the median time from the third to the fourth episode is approximately half that to the first episode. As many patients experienced multiple episodes of peritonitis, these values are quite reliable.

In view of the importance of peritonitis as a complication of CAPD and the frequency with which successive episodes occur, an analysis of the risk of peritonitis in various patient groups is discussed in the next section.

FIGURE 4.   Probability of Successive Exit/Tunnel Infections as a Function of the Number Previously Experienced

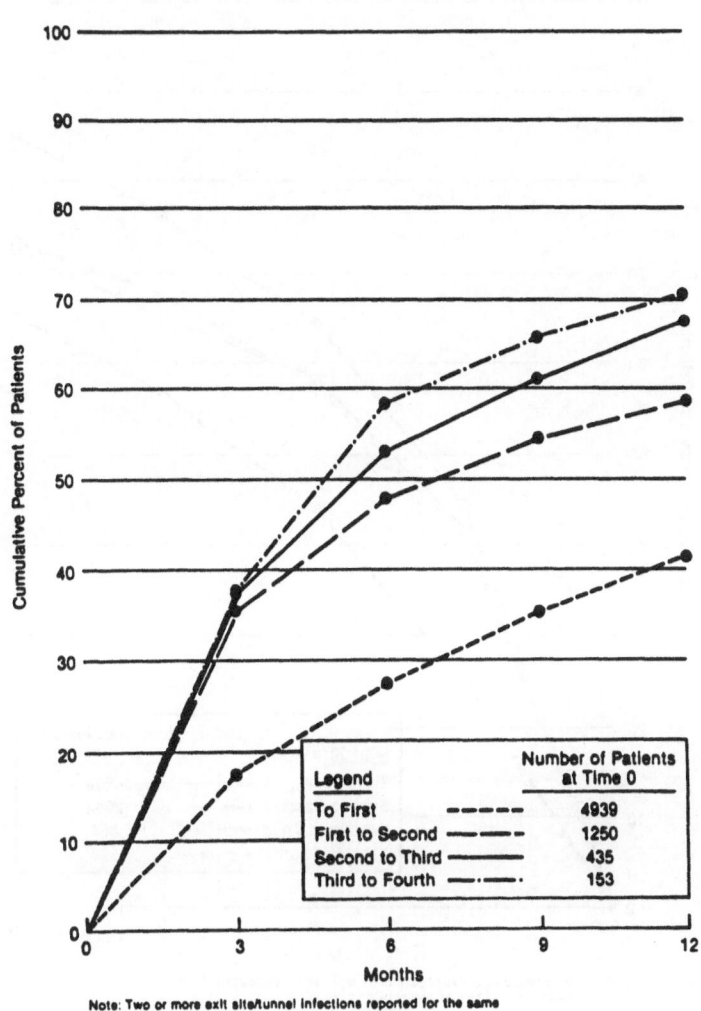

Note: Two or more exit site/tunnel infections reported for the same calendar quarter were treated as one infection.

C. Probability of First Episode of Peritonitis for Selected Patient Groups

Since peritonitis is the most common and perhaps the most bothersome complication of CAPD, lifetable analyses of time to event were undertaken for a number of subgroups to determine if any had prognostic value. These analyses considered different renal disease, age, sex, and

FIGURE 5. Probability of Successive Episodes of Peritonitis as a Function of the Number Previously Experienced

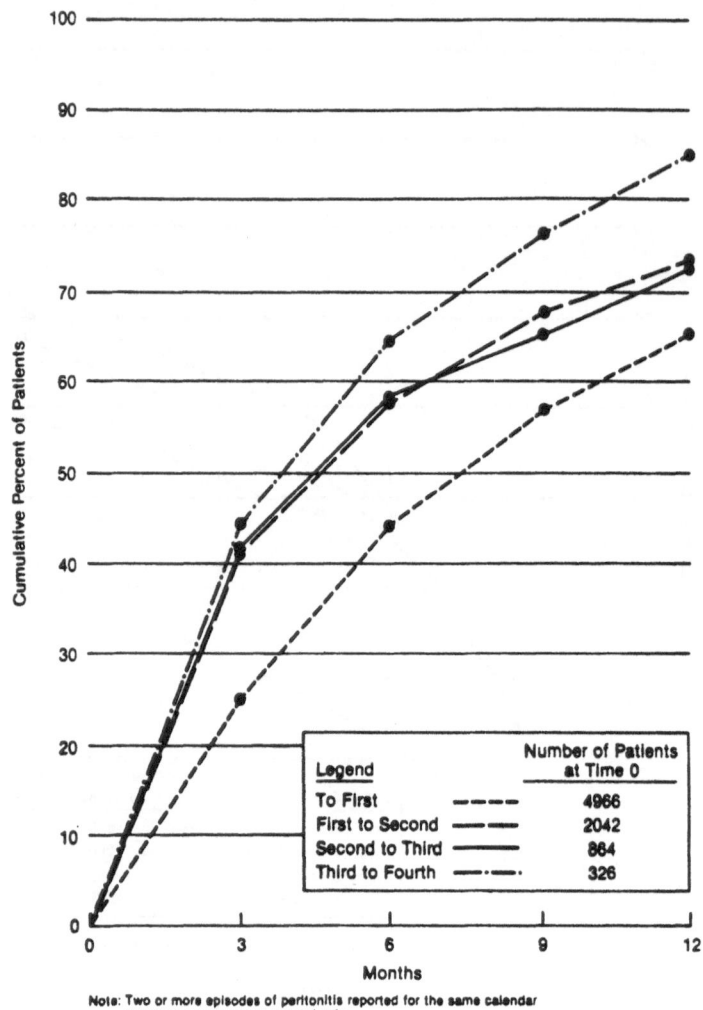

Note: Two or more episodes of peritonitis reported for the same calendar quarter were treated as one episode.

race categories, as well as last reported status and the year CAPD was started. No attempt was made to examine interactions between these variables (except for age and race). As well, no formal analysis was performed to determine whether apparent differences in lifetable probabilities are statistically significant. Thus, the findings contained in this report are meant to be descriptive and not conclusive. In a future report, analyses will be undertaken to examine the prognostic significance of the factors mentioned and whether the factors interact in special ways to influence outcomes.

The lifetable analyses conducted are as follows:

FIGURE 6.   Probability of First Episode of Peritonitis as a Function of Primary Renal Disease

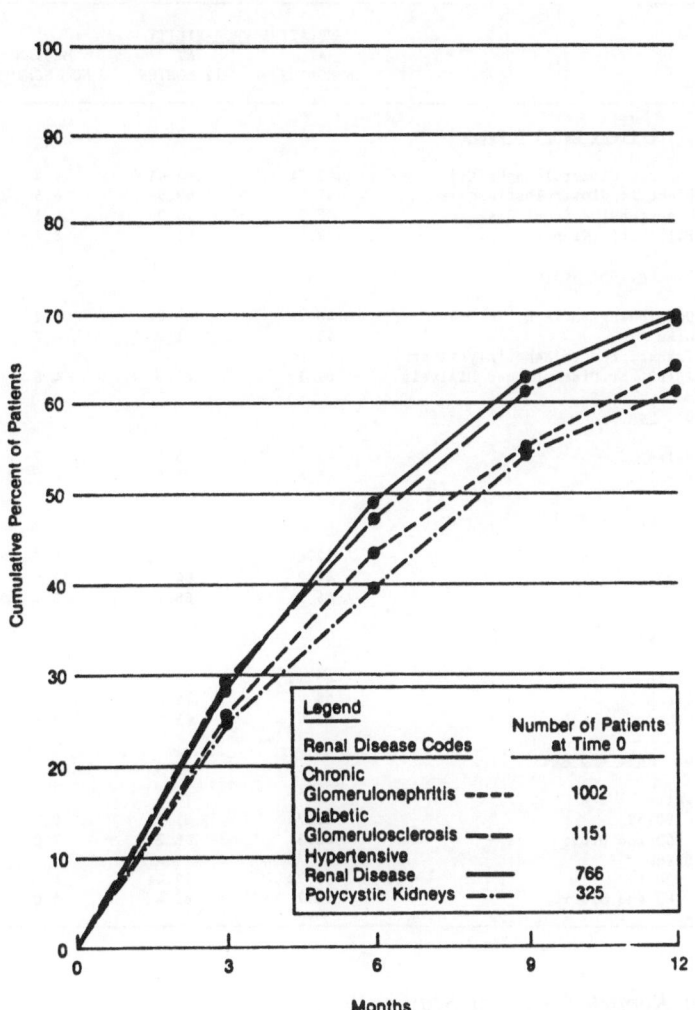

1. Primary Renal Disease

Variation in the probability of developing peritonitis according to the patient's primary renal disease is portrayed in Figure 6. Supporting data are contained in Table 2. There is a clear difference in the median time to the first episode of peritonitis for patients with diabetic glomerulosclerosis (6.5 months), hypertensive renal disease (6.3 months), chronic glomerulonephritis (7.4 months), or polycystic kidneys (8.2 months).

TABLE 2.   Probability of First Episode of Peritonitis for Selected
             Patient Groups

	CUMULATIVE PROBABILITY		
	AT 6 MONTHS	AT 12 MONTHS	MEDIAN NO. MONTHS
1. Primary Renal Disease			
Chronic Glomerulonephritis	43.7%	64.4%	7.4
Diabetic Glomerulosclerosis	47.8	69.9	6.5
Hypertensive Renal Disease	49.3	70.0	6.3
Polycystic Kidney(s)	39.9	61.5	8.2
2. Patient Status			
Continuing on CAPD	40.7%	61.0%	8.2
Died	49.2	71.9	6.2
Transferred to Hemodialysis or IPD, or Discontinued Dialysis	61.1	84.0	4.6
3. Sex			
Males	45.2%	65.6%	7.2
Females	45.6	66.8	6.7
4. Age (years)			
< 20	52.6%	70.6%	5.7
20-59	44.2	64.8	7.4
60+	46.3	68.1	6.7
5. Race			
White	46.7%	63.5%	7.0
Black	58.9	78.6	4.8
Other	41.9	65.2	7.9
6. Race and Age			
White			
20-59	40.7%	61.5%	8.3
60 and older	45.3	66.2	7.0
Black			
20-59	59.7%	77.4%	4.7
60 and older	55.7	83.4	5.0

2. Last Reported Patient Status

The separation among the curves portraying time to the first episode of
peritonitis according to patients' last reported status is very marked.
Patients who were transferred to hemodialysis or IPD or discontinued
CAPD without return of kidney function developed peritonitis relatively
soon after initiation of the therapy — 61.1% within 6 months, 84.0%
within 12 months. In contrast, the comparable figures for patients last
reported to be continuing on CAPD were 40.7% at 6 months and
61.0% at 12 months. The curve for patients who died on CAPD is
approximately midway between the other two (see Figure 7 and Table
2).

FIGURE 7.   Probability of First Episode of Peritonitis as a Function of Last Reported Status

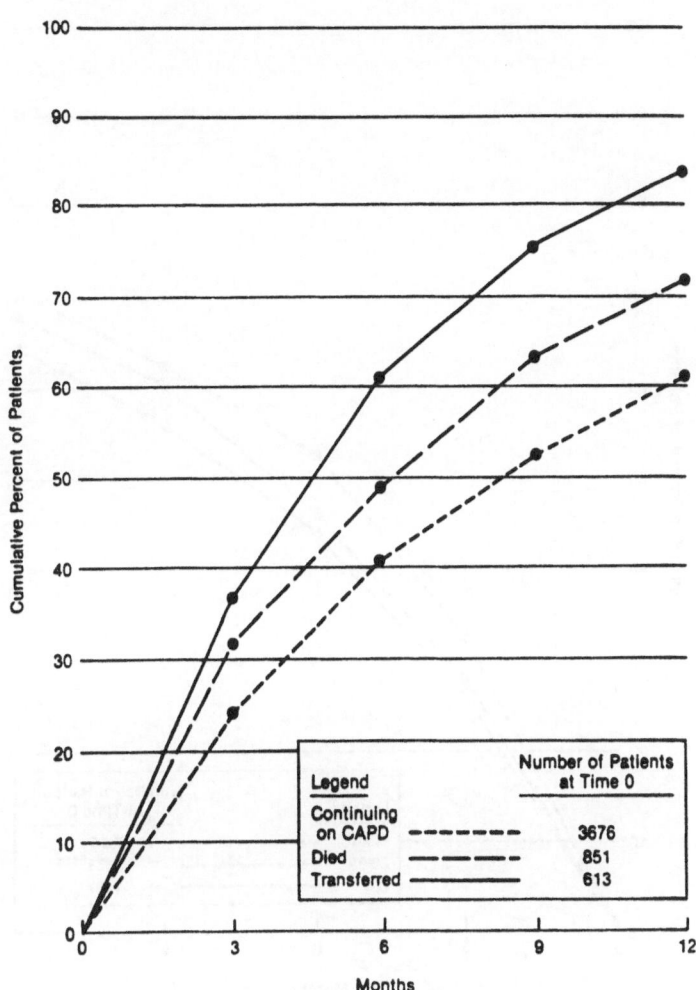

3. Sex

There is virtually no difference in the experience of male and female patients with respect to time to the first episode of peritonitis (see Table 2).

4. Age

The principal difference by age with respect to time to first peritonitis is between patients 20 years of age or younger and adult patients. The

FIGURE 8.   Probability of First Episode of Peritonitis as a Function of Age

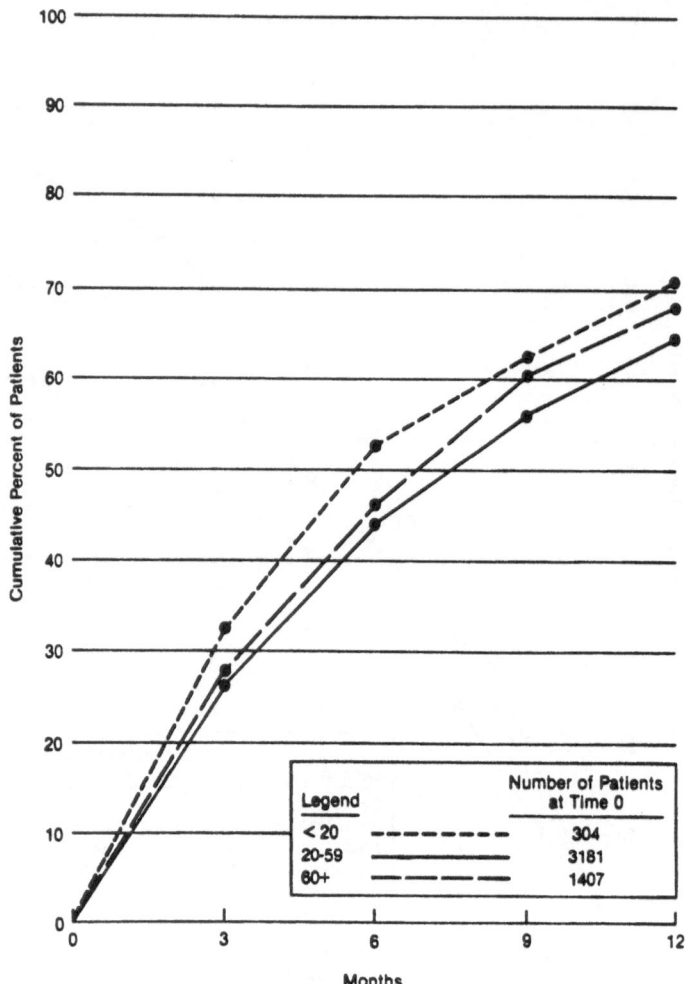

Legend	Number of Patients at Time 0
< 20	304
20-59	3181
60+	1407

median times were 5.7 months for the youngest of the three age groups and 7.4 and 6.7 months for the two older groups (see Figure 8 and Table 2).

5. Race

There is a marked difference between the curves in Figure 13 for white and black patients which portray time to first peritonitis. The median times were 7.0 and 4.8 months respectively (see Figure 8 and Table 2).

The number of other nonwhite patients is small, but the available data indicate that their experience was similar to that of the white patients.

6. Race and Age

When the patients are subdivided with respect to race and age, the effect of age on time to first peritonitis among white adults shows up more clearly than it did in Figure 7, which dealt with age for all races combined. A clear difference is evident between the curves for patients 20-59 years of age and for patients 60 years of age and older (see Figure 9 and Table 2).

FIGURE 9.　Probability of First Episode of Peritonitis as a Function of Race

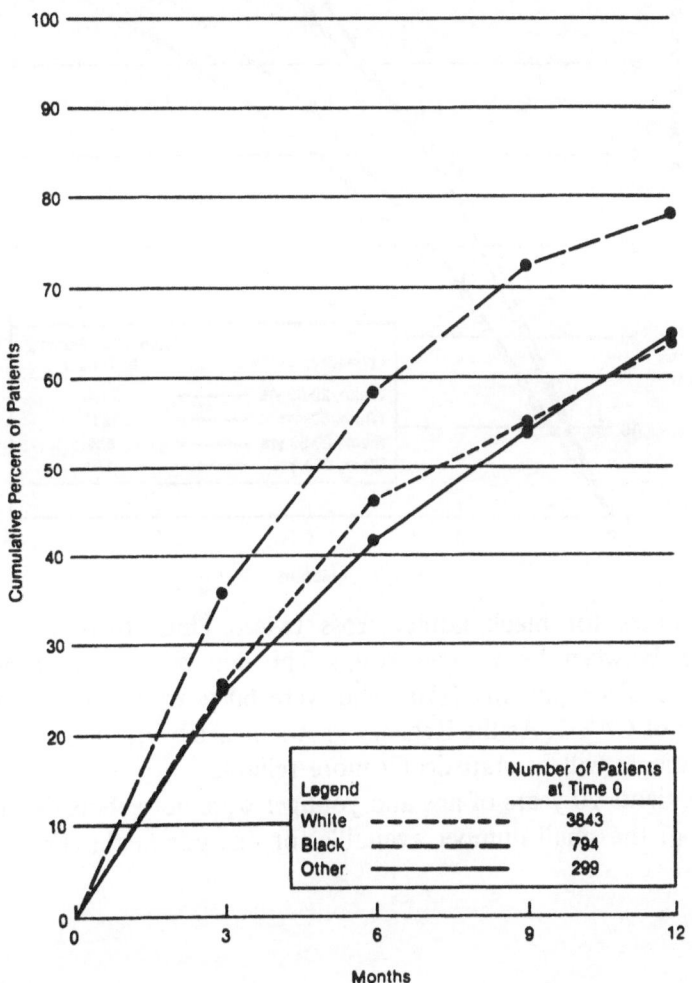

Months

FIGURE 10.   Probability of First Episode of Peritonitis as a Function of
Age and Race

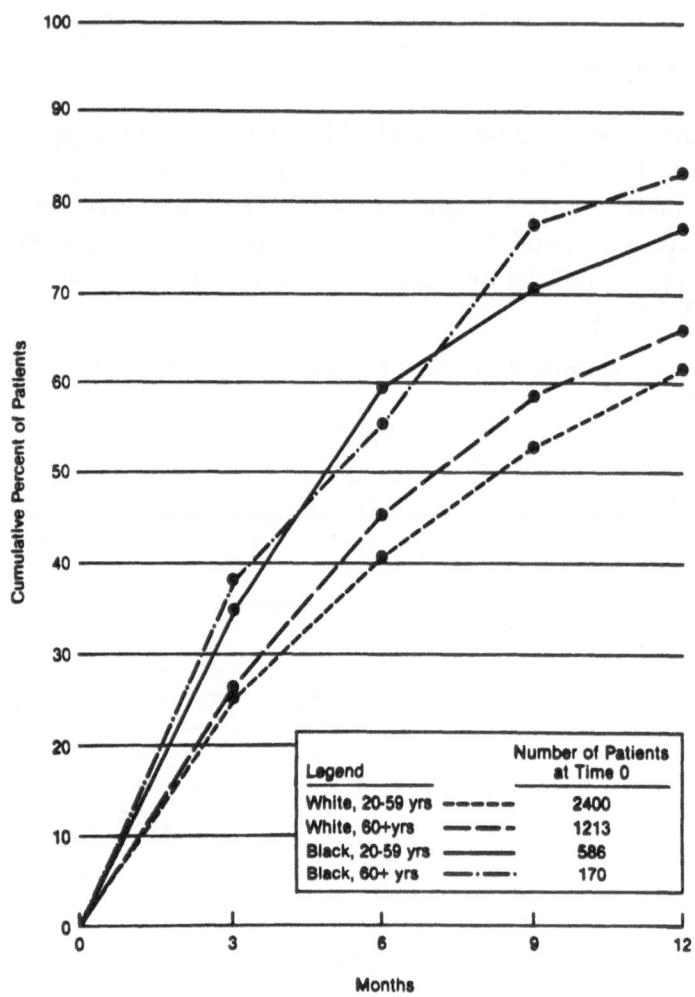

The curves for black adults cross twice. Thus, there is no clear difference between the two age groups. This may be because of the small number of black patients (170) who were 60 years of age or older at initiation of CAPD. As the Registry grows in size over time, the data for black patients will be statistically more reliable.

The patients 20 years of age and younger were not subdivided by race because of the small number available for analysis at this time.

7. Year CAPD Initiated

Time to first peritonitis was examined for patients who started on CAPD in 1981, 1982, and 1983. The curves for the three calendar cohorts were virtually superimposed one upon another (not shown).

D. Successive Episodes of Peritonitis in Various Patient Groups

As previously indicated, peritonitis is the most frequently occurring complication associated with CAPD. It is of interest to assess the pattern of successive episodes of peritonitis in various subgroups; is there a common general pattern. Characterization of patients with respect to various parameters indicates that the time between the first and second episodes of peritonitis is shorter than the time from initiation of CAPD to the first episode. Also, the time from the second to the third episode is shorter than between the first and second episodes. The specific patterns for specific subgroups of patients are discussed below.

In Table 3, comparison is made with respect to the last reported status for each patient. Within each status category, the median number of

TABLE 3.   Time to Successive Episodes of Peritonitis by Last Report Status

LAST REPORTED STATUS	MEDIAN NO. MONTHS	NO. PATIENTS AT TIME ZERO
Continuing on CAPD		
Time to: First Episode	8.2	3,076
First to Second	5.7	1,228
Second to Third	5.5	525
Third to Fourth	4.8	199
Transferred*		
Time to: First Episode	4.6	851
First to Second	2.9	399
Second to Third**	2.7	174
Died		
Time to: First Episode	6.2	613
First to Second	3.2	254
Second to Third**	2.6	95

*Transferred to hemodialysis or IPD, or left dialysis without return of kidney function.

**Insufficient number of patients remained on CAPD for calculation of time from the third to the fourth episode.

months between events decreases as the sequence number of the event increases. For example, among patients last reported to be continuing on CAPD, the time to the first episode of peritonitis was 8.2 months; from first to second, 5.7 months; from second to third, 5.5 months; and from third to fourth, 4.8 months.

The time between episodes was consistently longer among patients remaining on CAPD than for the two other groups. The time to the first episode was shorter for patients transferred off CAPD than for patients who died while on CAPD. However, after the first episode there was little difference between these two groups.

Patients with different primary renal diseases are compared in Table 4. For each disease group, the time to the first episode was longer than the time between subsequent episodes. However, the pattern of intervals between the first and second, and the second and third episodes was not consistent among the four disease groups.

Variation with respect to age and race is described in Table 5. Comparison of patients 20-59 years of age and patients 60 and older indicates consistency in two respects: (1) In each age group the interval between events decreases as the sequence number of the event increases; and (2) the time between any two events is shorter among patients 60 years and older than among patients between 20 and 59 years of age.

TABLE 4.   Time to Successive Episodes of Peritonitis by Primary Renal Disease

PRIMARY RENAL DISEASE	MEDIAN NO. MONTHS	NO. PATIENTS AT TIME ZERO
Chronic Glomerulonephritis		
Time to: First Episode	7.4	1,002
First to Second	5.8	427
Second to Third	4.3	169
Diabetic Glomerulosclerosis		
Time to: First Episode	6.5	1,151
First to Second	4.3	463
Second to Third	4.4	197
Hypertensive Renal Disease		
Time to: First Episode	6.3	766
First to Second	4.1	346
Second to Third	4.3	148
Polycystic Kidney(s)		
Time to: First Episode	8.2	325
First to Second	4.5	144
Second to Third	3.0	67

TABLE 5.   Time to Successive Episodes of Peritonitis by Age and
           Race

AGE AND RACE	MEDIAN NO. MONTHS	NO. PATIENTS AT TIME ZERO
Ages 20-59 Years		
Time to: First Episode	7.4	3,181
First to Second	5.0	1,307
Second to Third	4.7	555
Ages 60 and Over		
Time to: First Episode	6.7	1,407
First to Second	4.5	585
Second to Third	3.8	243
White Patients		
Time to: First Episode	7.0	3,843
First to Second	4.8	1,514
Second to Third	4.8	627
Black Patients		
Time to: First Episode	4.8	794
First to Second*	3.7	391

*Insufficient number of black patients remained on CAPD for
calculation of time from the second to the third episode.

A similar consistency of pattern is evident in comparing white and black patients, with longer intervals among the whites. The available data were also examined with respect to the time between the first and second episodes, and between the second and third episodes, according to the time from initiation of CAPD to the first episode of peritonitis. A moderate trend was discerned. Among patients who developed peritonitis within 3 months of starting on CAPD, or between 3 and 6 months, the time between subsequent intervals was approximately 4.5 months. Among patients who developed peritonitis for the first time 6 to 9 months after starting on CAPD, the time between subsequent intervals was approximately 5 months.

Appendices

Appendix I

Executive Advisory Committee of the National CAPD Registry of the National Institutes of Health

Steven R. Alexander, M.D.
University of Texas Health Center at Dallas
Dallas, TX

Christopher R. Blagg, M.D.
Northwest Kidney Center
Seattle, W.A.

John A. Goffinet, M.D.
VA Hospital
West Haven, CT

Richard J. Hamburger, M.D.
Indiana University Medical Center
Indianapolis, IN

Robert W. Hamilton, M.D.
Bowman Gray School of Medicine
Winston-Salem, NC

Joanne J. Hoover, M.D., MPH
University of Washington
Seattle, WA

John F. Maher, M.D.
Uniformed Services University of Health Sciences
Bethesda, MD

George W. Williams, Ph.D.
Cleveland Clinic Foundation
Cleveland, OH

NIH Project Officer

Gladys Hirschman, M.D.
Chronic Renal Disease Program
Kidney-Urology Branch (DKUHD)
NIDDK
Bethesda, Maryland

Appendix II

Participating Centers of the National CAPD Registry of the National Institutes of Health

AFFILIATED HOSPITALS DIAL. CTR
CREVE COEUR   MO   63141

ALBANY MED. CTR--PEDIATRIC UNIT
ALBANY   NY   12208

ALBANY MEDICAL CENTER HOSPITAL
ALBANY   NY   12208

ALBERT EINSTEIN MEDICAL CENTER
PHILADELPHIA   PA   19141

ALL CHILDRENS HOSPITAL
ST. PETERSBURG   FL   33701

ALLEGHANY DIALYSIS FACILITY
COVINGTON   VA   24426

ALLEGHENY GENERAL HOSPITAL
PITTSBURGH   PA   15212

AMERICAN DIALYSIS CENTER, INC
MIAMI   FL   33175

ANTELOPE VALLEY DIAL. FACILITY
LANCASTER   CA   93534

ARKANSAS CHILDRENS HOSPITAL
LITTLE ROCK,   AR   72202-3591

ARTIFICIAL KID. FOUND. OF CA.
ANAHEIM   CA   92803

ARTIFICIAL KIDNEY MED. CLINIC
STOCKTON,   CA   95204

ASHEVILLE KIDNEY CENTER
ASHVILLE,   NC   28801

ATHENS DIALYSIS FACILITY, INC.
ATHENS   GA   30610

AUGUSTA COUNTY DIAL. FACILITY
STAUNTON   VA   24401

AUGUSTA DIALYSIS CENTER
AUGUSTA   GA   30909

AULTMAN HOSPITAL
CANTON,   OH   44710

AUSTIN DIAGNOSTIC CLINIC
AUSTIN   TX   78705

BALL MEMORIAL HOSPITAL
MUNCIE   IN   47303

BAPTIST MEDICAL CENTER
OKLAHOMA CITY   OK   73112

BAPTIST MEMORIAL HOSPITAL
MEMPHIS   TN   38104

BAUMRITTER KIDNEY CENTER
BRONX   NY   10461

BAYSIDE DIALYSIS, INC
BERKELEY   CA   94704

BEAUMONT RENAL CENTER
ROYAL OAK   MI   48072

BERKLEY DIALYSIS INC.
BERKELEY   CA   94705

BERKSHIREM MEDICAL CENTER
PITTSFIELD,   MA   01201

BIOMEDICAL ARTIFICIAL KID. CTR
SAN DIEGO   CA   92111

BIOMEDICAL COMMUNITY DIAL. UNIT
NATIONAL CITY   CA   92050

BIRMINGHAM VA MEDICAL CTR
BIRMINGHAM   AL   35233

BISHOP CLARKSON MEMORIAL HOSP
OMAHA   NE   68105

BMA DIALYSIS OF OAKLAND
OAKLAND   CA   94623

BMA EUREKA
EUREKA   CA   95501

BMA GREENSBORO
GREENSBORO   NC   27401

BMA LOUISVILLE
LOUISVILLE   KY   40202

BMA OF DETROIT
DETROIT   MI   48201

BMA OF WESTERN PENNSYLVANIA
PITTSBURGH   PA   15224

BMA-BAKERSFIELD
BAKERSFIELD   CA   93301

BMA-DECATUR VALLEY DIALYSIS
DECATUR   AL   35601

BMA-DEKALB-GWINNETT
DECATUR   GA   30030

BOCA RATON ARTIFICIAL KID CTR
BOCA RATON   FL   33432

BOOTH MEMORIAL SATELLITE DIAL.
FLUSHING   NY   11355

BORGESS HOSPITAL
KALAMAZOO   MI   49001

BRADENTON ARTIFICIAL KIDNEY CTR
BRADENTON   FL   33529

BRAZOS KIDNEY DISEASE CENTER
WACO   TX   76708

BROCKTON DIALYSIS CENTER
BROCKTON,   MA   02401

BRONSON METHODIST HOSPITAL
KALAMAZOO,   MI   49007

BRONX-LEBANON HOSPITAL CENTER
BRONX,   NY   10456

BROOKE ARMY MEDICAL CENTER
FORT SAM HOUSTON TX   78234

BROOKHAVEN MEMORIAL HOSPITAL
E. PATCHOQUE,   NY   11772

BRYN MAWR HOSPITAL
BRYN MAWR   PA   19010

CAPD UNIT WACC 515B
BOSTON   MA   02114

CENTRAL FLORIDA KIDNEY CENTER
ORLANDO   FL   32806-2980

CENTRAL GEORGIA DIALYSIS CENTER
MACON   GA   31201

CENTRAL MARYLAND DIALYSIS
LUTHERVILLE   MD   21093

CENTRE COMMUNITY HOSPITAL
STATE COLLEGE   PA   16803

CHALMETTE DIALYSIS CTR.
CHALMETTE   LA   70043

CHARLOTTE HUNGERFORD HOSPITAL
TORRINGTON   CT   06790

CHILDRENS HOSP OF WI DIAL PRO
MILWAUKEE,   WI   53201

CHILDRENS HOSP. OF LOS ANGELES
LOS ANGELES   CA   90027

CHILDRENS HOSPITAL MEDICAL CTR.
CINCINNATI,   OH   45229

CHILDRENS HOSPITAL OF BUFFALO
BUFFALO,   NY   14222

CHILDRENS HOSPITAL OF MICHIGAN
DETROIT   MI   48201

CHILDRENS MEDICAL CENTER
DALLAS   TX   75235

CHILDRENS MEDICAL HOSPITAL
CHICAGO   IL   60614

CHROMALLOY AMERICAN KIDNEY CTR
ST. LOUIS   MO   63110

CLEVELAND CLINIC
CLEVELAND   OH   44106

CLEVELAND DIAL. FACILITY, INC.
CLEVELAND   TN   37311

CLINESHARE DIALYSIS NETWORK
VAN NUYS   CA   91405

CLINISHARE DIALYSIS NETWORK
LONG BEACH   CA   90806

COASTAL BEND RENAL DIALYSIS CTR
CORPUS CHRISTI   TX   78404

COBB DIALYSIS, INC
MARIETTA   GA   30090

COMM. DIAL. SERV. OF NORTHLAND
N. KANSAS CITY,   MO   64116

COMM. DIAL. SERVICES OF INGELWOOD
INGLEWOOD,   CA   90307

COMMUNITY DIAL. SERV. OF DOTHAN
DOTHAN   AL   36301

COMMUNITY DIAL. SERV. OF TAMPA
TAMPA   FL   33612

COMMUNITY DIAL. SERV., VALLEJO
VALLEJO,   CA   94590

COMMUNITY DIALYSIS SERVICE
MEDFORD   OR   97501

COMMUNITY DIALYSIS SERVICES
PACOIMA   CA   91331

COMMUNITY DIALYSIS SERVICES
BRUNSWICK   GA   31520

CONEJO VALLEY RENAL CENTER
THOUSAND OAKS   CA   91360

COSTAL DIALYSIS & MED. CLINIC
SAVANNAH,   GA   31404

COVENANT MED. CTR.-ST. FRANCIS
WATERLOO,   IA   50702

CUMBERLAND VALLEY DIALYSIS
CHAMBERSBURG   PA 17201

CUYAHOGA COUNTY HOSPITAL
CLEVELAND   OH 44109

DAKOTA HOSPITAL
FARGO,   ND 58103

DALY CITY DIALYSIS
DALY CITY   CA 94015

DANBURY HOSPITAL
DANBURY   CT 06810

DANVILLE UROLOGIC CLINIC
DANVILLE,   VA 24543

DEACONESS HOSPITAL
ST. LOUIS   MO 63139

DEERS HEAD CENTER
SALISBURY   MD 21801

DESERT DIALYSIS
TUCSON   AZ 85719

DIAGNOSTIC CLINIC OF HOUSTON
HOUSTON   TX 77030

DIAL. FOUNDATION OF SO. ARIZONA
TUCSON   AZ 85712

DIAL. NETWORK INTER., PASADENA
PASADENA   CA 91103

DIAL. NETWORK INTER., VAN NUYS
VAN NUYS   CA 91405

DIALYSIS CENTER OF UPLAND
UPLAND   CA 91786

DIALYSIS CLIN. INC. KANSAS CITY
KANSAS CITY,   MO 64114

DIALYSIS CLINIC INC.
COLUMBIA   MO 65202

DIALYSIS CLINIC INC. S. (DCI S.)
LEXINGTON,   KY 40503

DIALYSIS CLINIC INC.-PIEDMONT
ATLANTA,   GA 30303

DIALYSIS CLINIC OF LEXINGTON
LEXINGTON   KY 40508

DIALYSIS CLINIC, INC
CHATTANOOGA   TN 37404

DIALYSIS CLINIC, INC
KNOXVILLE   TN 37920

DIALYSIS CLINICS, INC.
CINCINNATI   OH 45206

DIALYSIS CLINICS,INC
ALBUQUERQUE   NM 87106

DIALYSIS CORP. OF HARRISBURG
LEMOYNE   PA 17043

DIALYSIS CTRS. OF VENTURA COUNTY
OXNARD   CA 93030

DIALYSIS HOME TEACHING
PHOENIX   AZ 85006

DIALYSIS INSTITUTE OF INDIANA
INDIANAPOLIS   IN 46202

DIALYSIS SERV. OF NEW HAMPSHIRE
CONCORD   NH 03301

DIVINE PROVIDENCE HOSPITAL
WILLIAMSPORT   PA 17701

DOBSON MEMORIAL DIAL. FACILITY
MESA   AZ 85202

DR. PAUL LATOUR
NASHVILLE   TN 37211

DUKE UNIVERSITY MEDICAL CENTER
DURHAM   NC 27710

DUPONT CIRCLE DIALYSIS CENTER
WASHINGTON,   DC 20036

DWIGHT D. EISENHOWER MED. CTR.
AUGUSTA   GA 30905

EAST BAY DIALYSIS
HAYWARD   CA 94541

EAST LOS ANGELES KIDNEY CENTER
LOS ANGELES   CA 90022

EAST VALLEY DIALYSIS
MESA   AZ 85206

EASTERN CASCADE DIALYSIS CENTER
BEND   OR 97701

EASTERN MAINE MED. CTR.
BANGOR,   ME 04401

EL CAMINO DIALYSIS SERVICE
MOUNTAIN VIEW   CA 94040

EL PASO DIALYSIS CENTER
EL PASO   TX 79936

ERIE COUNTY MEDICAL CENTER
BUFFALO   NY 14215

F.B. SMITH DIALYSIS CENTER
SYRACUSE,   NY 13203

FITZSIMONS ARMY MEDICAL CENTER
AURORA   CO 80045

FLORIDA KIDNEY CENTER
FT. LAUDERDALE   FL 33313

FORT SANDERS KIDNEY CENTER
KNOXVILLE   TN 37916

FOUR CORNERS DIALYSIS
BRONX   NY 10457

FOUR CORNERS DIALYSIS UNIT
FARMINGTON   NM 87401

FOUR STATE REGIONAL DIAL. CTR
JOPLIN   MO 64804

FOX VALLEY REGIONAL DIAL. CTR
NEENAH   WI 54956

FRANCIS SCOTT KEY MEDICAL CTR
BALTIMORE   MD 21224

FRANKLIN DIALYSIS CENTER
PHILADELPHIA   PA 19106

FRESNO COMMUNITY HOSP. DIALYSIS
FRESNO   CA 93715

FROEDTERT MEM. LUTHERAN HOSP.
MILWAUKEE   WI 53226

GARFIELD HEMODIALYSIS CENTER
MONTEREY PARK   CA 91754

GEISINGER MEDICAL CENTER
DANVILLE   PA 17822

GEORGETOWN UNIVERSITY HOSPITAL
WASHINGTON   DC 20007

GLENDALE HEMODIALYSIS FACILITY
GLENDALE   CA 91206

GLENDALE PERITONEAL DIALYSIS
GLENDALE,   AZ 85301

GLENDORA ARTIFICIAL KIDNEY CTR
GLENDORA   CA 91740

GLENS FALLS RENAL CENTER
GLENS FALLS   NY 12801

GOOD SAMARITAN HOSPITAL
PORTLAND   OR 97210

GOOD SAMARITAN HOSPITAL
CINCINNATI   OH 45220

GOOD SAMARITAN HOSPITAL
VINCENNES,   IN 47591

GRAD HOSP MED ASSOC DIAL CTR
PHILADELPHIA,   PA 19146

GRADY MEMORIAL HOSPITAL
ATLANTA   GA 30303

GRATIOT COMMUNITY HOSPITAL
ALMA   MI 48801

GREENFIELD HEALTH SYSTEM
DETROIT   MI 48202

GREENFIELD HEALTH SYSTEMS CORP.
TOLEDO   OH 43614

GREENVILLE DIALYSIS CENTER
GREENVILLE   NC 27834

GROSSMONT/EAST COUNTY DIALYSIS
LA MESA   CA 92041

HACKENSACK MEDICAL CENTER
HACKENSACK,   NJ 07601

HARRISONBURG HEMO UNIT
HARRISONBURG   VA 22801

HARTFORD DIALYSIS
HARTFORD   CT 06115

HATTIESBURG CLINIC, PROF ASSN
HATTIESBURG   MS 39401

HAVERFORD DIALYSIS UNIT
PHILADELPHIA,   PA 19151

HEALTH SYSTEMS INTERNATIONAL
BRYAN   TX 77802

HEARTLAND HOSPITAL WEST DIALYSIS
ST. JOSEPH   MO 64051

HIGHLAND PARK HOSP. RENAL UNIT
HIGHLAND,   IL 60035

HILLCREST MEDICAL CENTER
TULSA   OK 74104

HOLY NAME HOSPITAL/CAPD UNIT
TEANECK   NJ 07621

HOUSTON NORTHWEST MED CTR.
HOUSTON,   TX 77090

HOWARD COUNTY DIALYSIS FACILITY
COLUMBIA   MD 21044

HUNTINGTON ARTIFICIAL KID. CTR
HUNTINGTON STAT NY 11746

HURLEY MEDICAL CENTER
FLINT   MI 48502

INDIANA KIDNEY CENTER
INDIANAPOLIS,   IN 46219

INDIANA UNIVERSITY MEDICAL CTR
INDIANAPOLIS   IN 46202

JERSEY SHORE MEDICAL CENTER
NEPTUNE,   NJ 07753

JOHNS HOPKINS PEDIATRIC PD CTR
BALTIMORE,   MD 21205

JOHNSON COUNTY DIALYSIS, INC.
LENEXA,   KA 66214

KAISER FOUNDATION HOSPITAL
LOS ANGELES   CA 90027

KANSAS CITY DIALYSIS UNIT
KANSAS CITY   MO 64110

KANSAS UNIVERSITY MEDICAL CTR
KANSAS CITY   KS 66103

KID. DIAL. FAC. TIFTON GEN HOSP
TIFTON,   GA 31794

KIDNEY CARE, INC
JACKSON   MS 39216

KIDNEY CTR. DELAWARE CTY, LTD
CHESTER,   PA 19013

KOLFF DIALYSIS CENTER
SALT LAKE CITY   UT   84112

KUAKINI
HONOLULU   HI   96817

LAC/USC MEDICAL CENTER
LOS ANGELES   CA   90033

LACROSSE LUTHERAN HOSPITAL
LACROSSE   WI   54601

LAKEVIEW MED. CENTER
DANVILLE,   IL   61832

LANCASTER GENERAL HOSPITAL
LANCASTER   PA   17603

LANKENAU HOSPITAL
PHILADELPHIA   PA   19151

LENOX HILL HOSPITAL
NEW YORK   NY   10021

LESTER E. COX MEDICAL CENTER
SPRINGFIELD   MO   65802

LETTERMAN ARMY MEDICAL CENTER
SAN FRANCISCO   CA   94129-6700

LIMA MEMORIAL CAPD UNIT
LIMA   OH   45804

LINCOLIN PARK DIALYSIS
CHICAGO   IL   60614

LINCOLN DIALYSIS CENTER
PHOENIX   AZ   85020

LOMA LINDA DIALYSIS SERVICES
LOMA LINDA   CA   92350

LONG ISLAND COLLEGE HOSPITAL
BROOKLYN   NY   11201

LONG ISLAND JEWISH HOSPITAL
NEW HYDE PARK   NY   11042

LOS ALAMITOS HEMODIALYSIS CTR
LOS ALAMITOS   CA   90720

LOVELACE MEDICAL CENTER
ALBUQUERQUE,   NM   87108

LOW COUNTRY DIALYSIS FACILITY
BEAUFORT   SC   29902

LUTHER HOSPITAL
EAU CLAIRE   WI   54701

LUTHERAN HOSPITAL
FORT WAYNE   IN   46807

LUTHERAN MEDICAL CENTER
BROOKLYN   NY   11220

MAC NEAL RENAL LIFELINE SERVICE
BERWYN,   IL   60402

MACON DIALYSIS FACILITY, INC
MACON   GA   31211

MADISON COUNTY MEDICAL CENTER
MADISONVILLE   TX   77864

MANSFIELD KIDNEY CENTER
MANSFIELD   OH   44905

MARIAN HEALTH CENTER DIALYSIS
SIOUX CITY   IA   51101

MARICOPA COUNTY GENERAL HOSP.
PHOENIX   AZ   85008

MARQUETTE GENERAL HOSPITAL
MARQUETTE   MI   49855

MARY GREELEY MEMORIAL HOSPITAL
AMES   IA   50010

MARY IMOGENE BASSETT HOSPITAL
COOPERSTOWN   NY   13326

MAYO FOUNDATION CLINIC
ROCHESTER   MN   55905

MCGUIRE V. A. MED. CTR (111D)
RICHMOND   VA   23249

MED ARTS CLINIC ASSOC DIAL CTR
CORSICANA,   TX   75110

MED. CTR. CLINIC DIALYSIS CTR.
PENSACOLA,   FL   32514

MEDICAL CENTER HOSP. OF VERMONT
BURLINGTON   VT   05401

MEDICAL CENTER OF GARDEN GROVE
GARDEN GROVE   CA   92643

MEDICAL COLLEGE OF VIRGINIA
RICHMOND   VA   23298

MEDICAL PARK PROFESSIONAL BLDG.
WHEELING   WV   26003

MEDICAL PLAZA DIALYSIS/CAPD UNIT
OKLAHOMA CITY   OK   73112

MELBOURNE KIDNEY CENTER
MELBOURNE   FL   32901

MEMORIAL MEDICAL CENTER
SPRINGFIELD   IL   62781

MERCY HOSPITAL
MUSKEGON,   MI   49443

METABOLISM ASSOCIATES
NEW HAVEN   CT   06511

METHODIST HOSPITAL
MINNEAPOLIS   MN   55440

METROLINA KIDNEY CENTER
CHARLOTTE,   NC   28204

MIAMI VALLEY HOSPITAL
DAYTON   OH   45409

MIDDLESEX MEMORIAL HOSPITAL
MIDDLETOWN   CT   06457

MIDSHORE DIALYSIS CENTER
EASTON   MD 21601

MILLS MEM HOSP RENAL DIAL CTR
SAN MATEO,   CA 94401

MINNEAPOLIS V. A. MEDICAL CTR
MINNEAPOLIS   MN 55417

MONMOUTH MEDICAL CENTER
LONG BRANCH   NJ 07740

MONT. NEPHROLOGY REFERRAL CTR
MONTGOMERY   AL 36104-4477

MOSES TAYLOR HOSPITAL
SCRANTON,   PA 18510

MOUNT AIRY KIDNEY CENTER
PHILADELPHIA   PA 19119

MOUNT CARMEL MEDICAL CENTER
COLUMBUS,   OH 43222

MOUNT DIABLO HOSP. MED. CTR
CONCORD   CA 94520

MOUNT SINAI MEDICAL CENTER
MILWAUKEE   WI 53201

MT ZION HOSPITAL MED CTR
SAN FRANCISCO   CA 94120

MT. CARMEL HOSP. KIDNEY CTR.
DETROIT   MI 48235

MT. SINAI HOSPITAL
HARTFORD   CT 06112

MT. VERNON KIDNEY CENTER
MT. VERNON,   IL 62864

N.W. FLORIDA A.K.C.
PENSACOLA   FL 32501

NAPA VALLEY COMMUNITY DIAL. CTR
NAPA   CA 94558

NEOMEPICA DIALYSIS CTR. INC.
CHICAGO,   IL 60611

NEOPHRON
BREA   CA 92621

NEW BRITAIN GENERAL HOSPITAL
NEW BRITAIN   CT 06050

NEW ENGLAND DEACONESS HOSPITAL
BOSTON   MA 02215

NEW HAVEN CAPD UNIT
NEW HAVEN,   CT 06510

NEW WEST DIALYSIS
CHICO   CA 95926

NEW WEST DIALYSIS - YUBA
YUBA CITY   CA 95991

NEW WEST DIALYSIS-CARMICHAEL
CARMICHAEL   CA 95608

NEW WEST DIALYSIS-REDDING
REDDING   CA 96001

NEW WEST DIALYSIS-SACRAMENTO
SACRAMENTO   CA 95823

NEW YORK V.A. MEDICAL CENTER
NEW YORK   NY 10010

NEWARK BETH ISRAEL MEDICAL CTR
NEWARK   NJ 07112

NORTH ALABAMA NEPHROLOGY CENTER
HUNTSVILLE   AL 35801

NORTH CAROLINA MEMORIAL HOSP.
 CARRBORO   NC 27510

NORTH CENTRAL DIAL. CTR. LTD.
CHICAGO,   IL 60602

NORTH COUNTY DIALYSIS CENTER
ESCONDIDO   CA 92025

NORTH SHORE UNIVERSITY HOSP.
MANHASSET,   NY 11030

NORTHERN COLORADO KIDNEY CENTER
FORT COLLINS   CO 80524

NORTHERN LOUISIANA DIALYSIS CTR
MONROE   LA 71201

NORTHERN MICHIGAN HOSPITALS
PETOSKEY   MI 49770

NORTHERN ROCKIES KIDNEY CENTER
BILLINGS   MT 59103

NORTHSIDE DIALYSIS CENTER
ATLANTA   GA 30342

NORTHWEST KIDNEY CENTER
SEATTLE   WA 98122

NORTHWESTERN DIALYSIS FACILITY
LENOIR   NC 28645

NORTHWESTERN MEMORIAL HOSPITAL
CHICAGO   IL 60611

NORWALK HOSPITAL
NORWALK   CT 06856

NORWOOD CLIN. DIAL. FACILITY
BIRMINGHAM,   AL 35283

OCHSNER CLINIC DIALYSIS CENTER
NEW ORLEANS   LA 70121

OGDEN LIMITED CARE DIALYSIS
OGDEN   UT 84403

OHIO STATE UNIV. HOSP. CLINIC
COLUMBUS   OH 43210

OKLAHOMA CHILDRENS MEM. HOSP.
OKLAHOMA CITY   OK 73190

OKLAHOMA MEMORIAL HOSPITAL
OKLAHOMA CITY   OK 73126

OKLAHOMA OSTEOPATHIC HOSPITAL
TULSA   OK 74127

OLYMPIC PENINSULA KIDNEY CTR.
BREMERTON   WA 98310

ORANGE COUNTY DIALYSIS
ANAHEIM   CA 92801

OREGON HEALTH SCIENCES
PORTLAND   OR 97201

OREGON KIDNEY CENTER
PORTLAND   OR 97213

ORLANDO ARTIFICIAL KIDNEY CTR
ORLANDO   FL 32804

OWENSBORO DAVIESS CO. HOSPITAL
OWENSBORO   KT 42301

PANAMA CITY ARTIFICIAL KID. CTR
PANAMA CITY   FL 32402

PENN DIALYSIS CLINIC OF READING
WYOMISSING   PA 19610

PHOENIX ARTIFICIAL KIDNEY CTR
PHOENIX,   AZ 85345

PHYSIOLOGICAL SYSTEMS
LAS VEGAS   NV 89102

PIEDMONT DIALYSIS CENTER
WINSTON-SALEM   NC 27103

PIEDMONT HOSPITAL DIALYSIS UNIT
ATLANTA   GA 30309

PIKES PEAK DIALYSIS CENTER
COLORADO SPRNGS CO 80909

POLYCLINIC MEDICAL CENTER
HARRISBURG   PA 17105

PORTLAND V. A. MEDICAL CENTER
PORTLAND   OR 97201

PRESBYTERIAN DENVER HOSPITAL
DENVER   CO 80218

PROVIDENCE MEDICAL CENTER
PORTLAND   OR 97213

PROVIDENCE VA MEDICAL CENTER
PROVIDENCE   RI 02908

REGIONAL KIDNEY DISEASE PROGRAM
MINNEAPOLIS   MN 55415

RENAL CARE CENTERS
WILMINGTON   DE 19806

RENAL CARE OF ERIE, INC
ERIE   PA 16514

RENAL CARE OF ILLINOIS
BELLEVILLE   IL 62223

RENAL CENTERS OF JOHNSON CITY
JOHNSON CITY   TN 37604

RENAL DIALYSIS CTR OF LAS VEGAS
LAS VEGAS   NV 89109

RHODE ISLAND RENAL INST. WESTERLY
WESTERLY   RI 02891

RHODE ISLAND RENAL INSTITUTE
WARWICK   RI 02886

RICHARDSON MEMORIAL DIALYSIS CTR.
EMPORIA   VA 23847

RICHMOND KIDNEY CENTER
STATEN ISLAND,   NY 10301

RILEY HOSPITAL FOR CHILDREN
INDIANAPOLIS,   IN 46223

RIVERSIDE GENERAL HOSPITAL
RIVERSIDE   CA 92501

RIVERSIDE HOSPITAL
NEWPORT NEWS   VA 23601

RIVERSIDE HOSPITAL CAPD CENTER
JACKSONVILLE   FL 32204

RIVERSIDE METHODIST HOSPITAL
COLUMBUS   OH 43214

RIVERSIDE/SAN BERNARDINO HEMO.
RIVERSIDE   CA 92501

RMCH DIALYSIS - CAPD
GALLUP   NM 87301

ROBERT PACKER HOSPITAL
SAYRE   PA 18840

ROBERT WOOD JOHNSON UNIV. HOSP.
NEW BRUNSWICK,   NJ 08901

ROCHESTER GENERAL HOSPITAL
ROCHESTER   NY 14621

ROCKFORD MEMORIAL HOSPITAL
ROCKFORD   IL 61101

ROCKVILLE GENERAL HOSPITAL
ROCKVILLE   CT 06066

ROCKWOOD DIALYSIS CLINIC
RICHMOND   VA 23235

ROCKY MOUNTAIN KIDNEY CENTER
DENVER,   CO 80220

ROSEVILLE DIALYSIS CENTER
ROSEVILLE,   CA 95678

RUSH-PRES. ST. LUKES MED. CTR
CHICAGO   IL 60612

S. BROOKLYN NEPHROLOGY CTR.
BROOKLYN,   NY 11234

S. BROWARD ARTIFICIAL KID. CTR
HOLLYWOOD   FL 33021

SACRED HEART GENERAL HOSPITAL
EUGENE   OR 97401

SAINT FRANCIS HOSP.& MED. CTR
HARTFORD   CT 06105

SALINAS VALLEY DIAL. SERVICES
SALINAS   CA 93901

SAMARITAN RENAL CENTER
DETROIT   MI 48214

SAN ANTONIO KIDNEY DISEASE CTR.
SAN ANTONIO   TX 78212

SAN BERNARDINO VALLEY DIAL. CTR
SAN BERNARDINO   CA 92404

SAN FERNANDO-WEST KIDNEY CENTER
CANOGA PARK   CA 91307

SAN FRANCISCO PERITONEAL DIAL.
SAN FRANCISCO   CA 94115

SAN LUIS OBISPO GENERAL HOSP.
SAN LUIS OBISPO   CA 93406

SAT. DIAL. CENT. INC.-WATSONVILLE
WATSONVILLE,   CA 95076

SATELLITE DIALYSIS CENTER
MENLO PARK   CA 94025

SATELLITE DIALYSIS CENTER
SAN JOSE   CA 95123

SATELLITE DIALYSIS, INC
MODESTO   CA 95355

SCOTT & WHITE MEMORIAL HOSPITAL
TEMPLE   TX 76508

SCOTTSDALE DIALYSIS
SCOTTSDALE   AZ 85251

SHANDS HOSPITAL
GAINESVILLE   FL 32610

SHANDS TEACHING HOSP & CLIN INC
GAINESVILLE   FL 32610

SIOUX VALLEY HOSP. DIAL. UNIT
SIOUX FALLS   SD 57105

SOUTH FL ARTIFICIAL KIDNEY CTR.
MIAMI,   FL 33176

SOUTH PALM BEACH DIALYSIS CTR.
LANTANA,   FL 33462

SOUTH PHOENIX DIALYSIS
PHOENIX   AZ 85003

SOUTH PLAINS DIALYSIS CENTER
LUDBOCK,   TX 79410

SOUTH PLAINS KIDNEY DISEASE CTR
LUBBOCK   TX 79416

SOUTH SUBURBAN KIDNEY UNIT
OLYMPIC FIELD   IL 60461

SOUTHEASTERN DIALYSIS CENTER
WILMINGTON,   NC 28401

SOUTHERN CT OUT-OF-HOSP DIAL.
BRIDGEPORT   CT 06606

SOUTHERN HILLS DIALYSIS CLINIC, INC
NASHVILLE   TN 37211

SOUTHWEST HOUSTON DIALYSIS CENTER
HOUSTON   TX 77071

SOUTHWESTERN DIALYSIS CENTER
DALLAS   TX 75235

SPOHN HOSPITAL
CORPUS CHRISTI   TX 78404

ST ALEXIUS MEDICAL CENTER
BISMARCK,   ND 58502

ST ALPHONSUS REGIONAL MED. CTR
BOISE   ID 83706

ST BARNABAS HOSPITAL
LIVINGSTON   NJ 07039

ST BERNARDS REGIONAL MED. CTR.
JONESBORO,   AK 72401

ST CHRIS. HOSP. FOR CHILDREN
PHILADELPHIA   PA 19133

ST CLAIR RENAL CENTER
DETROIT   MI 48236

ST CLAIR RENAL CTR. SATELITE
PORT HURON,   MI 48060

ST ELIZABETH HOSPITAL
LAFAYETTE   IN 47904

ST ELIZABETH HOSPITAL
YAKIMA   WA 98902

ST FRANCIS HOSPITAL
MIAMI BEACH   FL 33141

ST FRANCIS HOSPITAL
PEORIA   IL 61637

ST FRANCIS HOSPITAL
TULSA   OK 74136

ST FRANCIS HOSPITAL & MED. CTR
TOPEKA   KS 66606

ST FRANCIS MEDICAL CENTER
HONOLULU,   HI 96817

ST JOHNS HOSPITAL
SAN ANGELO   TX 76902-5741

ST JOSEPH HOSP HEALTH CARE CTR
TACOMA,   WA 98401

ST JOSEPH HOSPITAL
MARSHFIELD   WI 54449

ST JOSEPH HOSPITAL
ORANGE   CA   92668

ST JOSEPH HOSPITAL
OMAHA   NE   68131

ST JOSEPH HOSPITAL
LOWELL   MA   01854

ST JOSEPH MEDICAL CENTER
SOUTH BEND   IN   46634

ST JOSEPHS HOSPITAL
PARKERSBURG   WV   26101

ST JOSEPHS MED. CENTER
YONKERS,   NY   10701

ST LOUIS CHILDRENS HOSPITAL
ST LOUIS   MO   63178

ST LUKES HOSPITAL
KANSAS CITY   MO   64111

ST LUKES HOSPITAL
BETHLEHEM   PA   18015

ST LUKES HOSPITAL
DAVENPORT   IA   52803

ST MARGARET HOSPITAL
HAMMOND,   TN   46320

ST MARY CORWIN HOSPITAL
PUEBLO   CO   81004

ST MARY HOSPITAL
LIVONIA   MI   48154

ST MARYS HOSPITAL
GRAND RAPIDS   MI   49503

ST MARYS HOSPITAL
MILWAUKEE   WI   53211

ST MARYS MEDICAL CENTER
LONG BEACH   CA   90801

ST MICHAELS HOSPITAL
STEVENS POINT   WI   54481

ST PATRICK HOSPITAL
MISSOULA   MT   59802

ST PAUL RAMSEY MED. CENTER
ST. PAUL,   MN   55101

ST PETERS COMMUNITY HOSPITAL
HELENA   MT   59601

ST VINCENT HOSPITAL
GREEN BAY   WI   54301

ST VINCENT MEDICAL CENTER
TOLEDO   OH   43608

ST VINCENTS DIALYSIS CENTER
LOS ANGELES   CA   90057

ST VINCENTS HOSPITAL
INDIANAPOLIS   IN   46260

ST. JOHN HOSPITAL
CLEVELAND,   OH   44102

ST. JOSEPH HOSP. AND HEALTH CARE
KOKOMO   IN   46902

ST. MARY'S HOSPITAL DIALYSIS UNIT
LANGHORNE   PA   19047

ST. MICHAEL HOSPITAL
MILWAUKEE,   WI   53209

ST. PATRICK REGIONAL DIALYSIS
LAKE CHARLES   LA   70601

STANFORD UNIVERSITY DIAL. CTR
STANFORD   CA   94035

SUTTER GENERAL HOSPITAL
SACRAMENTO   CA   95816

TARRANT COUNTY NEPHROLOGY CTR
FT. WORTH   TX   76104

TEMPLE UNIV. HEALTH SCIEN. CTR
PHILADELPHIA   PA   19140

THE ALLENTOWN HOSPITAL
ALLENTOWN   PA   18102

THE ALTOONA HOSPITAL
ALTOONA   PA   16603

THE CHILDRENS HOSPITAL
BIRMINGHAM   AL   35233

THE CHRIST HOSPITAL
CINCINNATI   OH   45219

THE GOOD SAMARITAN HOSPITAL
BALTIMORE   MD   21239

THE GREATER MILWAUKEE DIAL. CTR.
MILWAUKEE,   WI   53233

THE KIDNEY CENTER
BOSTON,   MA   02215

THE MEDICAL CENTER HOSPITAL
COLUMBUS   GA   31994

THE MEMORIAL HOSPITAL
CUMBERLAND,   MD   21502

THE METHODIST HOSPITAL
HOUSTON   TX   77030

THE UNIVERSITY HOSPITAL
ST. LOUIS,   MO   63104

THE WESTERN PENNSYLVANIA HOSP
PITTSBURGH   PA   15224

THOMAS JEFFERSON UNIV. HOSPITAL
PHILADELPHIA,   PA   19107

TOURO INFIRMARY
NEW ORLEANS   LA   70115

TRI-STATE DIALYSIS
DUBUQUE,   IA   52001

TRISTATE RENAL DISEASE CENTER
EVANSVILLE   IN   47750

TUFTS NEW ENGLAND MEDICAL CTR
BOSTON   MA   02111

U. OF IOWA HOSPITALS & CLINICS
IOWA CITY,   IA   52242

U.S. NAVAL REGIONAL MED. CTR
PORTSMOUTH   VA   23708

UCLA CENTER FOR HEALTH SCIENCES
LOS ANGELES   CA   90024

UCLA CTR FOR HEALTH SCIENCES
LOS ANGELES   CA   90024

UNION HOSPITAL
TERRE HAUTE   IN   47804

UNIV OF MISSOURI/ PEDIATRICS
COLUMBIA,   MO   65212

UNIV. OF PENNSYLVANIA HOSPITAL
PHILADELPHIA   PA   19104

UNIV. OF VIRGINIA HOSPITALS
CHARLOTTESVILLE VA 22908

UNIV. OF WISC. HOSP. & CLINICS
MADISON   WI   57792

UNIVERSITY HOSPITAL
ANN ARBOR   MI   48109

UNIVERSITY HOSPITAL
SAN DIEGO   CA   92103

UNIVERSITY HOSPITAL
JACKSONVILLE,   FL   32209

UNIVERSITY HOSPITAL OF ARKANSAS
LITTLE ROCK   AR   72205

UNIVERSITY HOSPITAL-BOSTON
BOSTON,   MA   02118

UNIVERSITY OF ALABAMA HOSPITAL
BIRMINGHAM   AL   35233

UNIVERSITY OF CALIF. RENAL CTR
SAN FRANCISCO   CA   94110

UNIVERSITY OF CALIFORNIA-IRVINE
ORANGE   CA   92668

UNIVERSITY OF CHICAGO HOSPITAL
CHICAGO,   IL   60615

UNIVERSITY OF COLORADO
DENVER   CO   80262

UNIVERSITY OF ILLINOIS HOSP
CHICAGO   IL   60612

UNIVERSITY OF LOUISVILLE
LOUISVILLE   KY   40292

UNIVERSITY OF MARYLAND HOSPITAL
BALTIMORE   MD   21201

UNIVERSITY OF PITTSBURGH
PITTSBURGH   PA   15261

UNIVERSITY PHYSICIANS FOUND.
MEMPHIS   TN   38105

UPSTATE MEDICAL CENTER
SYRACUSE,   NY   13210

USHAWL, INC
LOS ANGELES   CA   90011

USHAWL, INC
LOS ANGELES   CA   90048

UTAH DIALYSIS LAB
SALT LAKE CITY,   UT   84102

UTAH DIALYSIS LAB/LDS HOSPITAL
SALT LAKE CITY,   UT   84102

V. A. MED. CTR./ANN ARBOR, MI
ANN ARBOR   MI   48105

V.A. MED. CTR. DIALYSIS CTR.
MEMPHIS,   TN   38104

V.A. MED. CTR./ SALEM, VA
SALEM   VA   24153

V.A. MED. CTR./CINCINNATI, OH
CINCINNATI   OH   45220

V.A. MED. CTR./DALLAS, TX
DALLAS   TX   75216

V.A. MED. CTR./DAYTON, OH
DAYTON   OH   45428

V.A. MED. CTR./DECATUR, GA
DECATUR   GA   30033

V.A. MED. CTR./IOWA CTY., IA
IOWA CITY   IA   52240

V.A. MED. CTR./LONG BEACH, CA
LONG BEACH   CA   90822

V.A. MED. CTR./MIAMI, FL
MIAMI   FL   33125

V.A. MED. CTR./NASHVILLE, TN
NASHVILLE   TN   37203

V.A. MED. CTR./NEW ORLEANS, LA
NEW ORLEANS   LA   70146

V.A. MED. CTR./PALO ALTO, CA
PALO ALTO   CA   94304

V.A. MED. CTR./PITTSBURGH, PA
PITTSBURGH   PA   15261

V.A. MED. CTR./SAN DIEGO, CA
SANDIEGO,   CA   92161

V.A. MED. CTR./SLT. LK. CITY UT
SALT LAKE CITY   UT   84148

V.A. MED. CTR./ST. LOUIS, MO
ST. LOUIS   MO   63106

V.A. MED. CTR./TUCSON, AZ
TUCSON   AZ 85723

V.A. MED. CTR./WOOD, WI
WOOD   WI 53193

V.A. MED. CTR/OKLAHOMA CITY, OK
OKLAHOMA CITY   OK 73104

VA MEDICAL CENTER - EAST ORANGE
EAST ORANGE   NJ 07019

VALLEY DIALYSIS ASSOCIATES, INC
BURBANK   CA 91506

VAMC NORTHPORT, NY
NORTHPORT,   NY 11768

W.W. WISE MEMORIAL DIALYSIS CTR
HARLINGEN   TX 78550

WADLEY HOSPITAL
TEXARKANA   TX 75501

WALTER REED ARMY MEDICAL CENTER
WASHINGTON   DC 20012

WALTER REED MEM. HOSP.
GLOUCHESTER   VA 23061

WARRENTON DIAL. FACILITY, INC.
WARRENTON   VA 22186

WASHINGTON HOSPITAL
FREMONT   CA 94538

WASHINGTON REGIONAL MED. CTR
FAYETTEVILLE   AR 72701

WASHOE MEDICAL CENTER
RENO   NV 89520

WATERBURY HOSPITAL HEALTH CTR
WATERBURY   CT 06708

WATSON CLINIC KIDNEY CTR
LAKELAND   FL 33805

WATSON W WISE DIALYSIS CENTER
DENISON   TX 75020

WATSON W WISE REG. DIAL. CTR
TYLER   TX 75701

WEISS RENAL CENTER
SUFFERN   NY 10901

WEST HAVEN V. A. MEDICAL CENTER
WEST HAVEN   CT 06516

WEST MANHATTAN KIDNEY CENTER
NEW YORK   NY 10024

WEST VA. HEALTH CARE COOP. INC.
MORGANTOWN   WV 26505

WESTCHESTER COUNTY MEDICAL CTR
VALHALLA   NY 10595

WESTERN DIALYSIS CENTER, P.C.
LAKEWOOD   CO 80214-1434

WESTERN MASSACHUSETTS KIDNEY CENTER
SPRINGFIELD   MA 01103

WHITTIER DIALYSIS CENTER
WHITTIER   CA 90603

WILLIAM BACKUS HOSPITAL
NORWICH   CT 06360

WILLIAM BEAUMONT HOSPITAL
TROY   MI 48098

WM. MIDDLETON MEM. VA HOSPITAL
MADISON,   WI 53705

WOODLAND DIALYSIS FACILITY
ELIZABETHTOWN,   KY 42701

WORCESTER MEMORIAL DIALYSIS
WORCESTER   MA 01605

YORK HOSPITAL DIALYSIS CENTER
YORK,   PA 17405

YOUNGSTOWN HOSPITAL ASSOCIATION
YOUNGSTOWN   OH 44501

Appendix III

Bibliography of the National CAPD Registry of the National Institutes of Health (1981–1988)

1988

Nolph KD, Lindblad AS, Novak JW. Current concepts: continuous ambulatory peritoneal dialysis. N Engl J Med 318: 1595–1600, 1988.

Nolph KD. Comparison of continuous ambulatory peritoneal dialysis and hemodialysis. Kidney Int 33(Supplement) 1988 Mar; 24: S123–131.

Nolph KD. The CAPD USA Registry. In: LaGreca, Chiaramonte, Fabris, Feriania, Ronco, eds. Peritoneal Dialysis. Milan: Wichtig Editorie, 1988: 203–205.

Lindblad AS, Novak JW, Nolph KD, Stablein DM, Cutler SJ. The 1987 USA National CAPD Registry Report. Trans Am Soc Artif Intern Organs 1988 Apr-Jun; 34(2): 150–156.

Lindblad AS, Novak JW, Nolph KD. The USA CAPD Registry characteristics of participants and selected outcome measures for the period of January 1, 1981 through August 31, 1987. In: Nolph KD ed. Peritoneal Dialysis. New York, Field and Rich (in press).

Lindblad AS, Nolph KD, Novak JW, Friedman EA. A survey of the NIH CAPD Registry with end-stage renal disease attributed to diabetic nephropathy. J Diabetic Complications (in press).

Lindblad AS, Hamilton RW, Nolph KD, Novak JW. A retrospective analysis of catheter configuration and cuff type. A National CAPD Registry Report. Peritoneal Dial Bull (accepted).

Stablein DM, Hamburger RJ, Lindblad AS, Nolph KD, Novak JW. The effect of CAPD on hypertension control. A Report of the National CAPD Registry. Peritoneal Dial Bull (accepted).

Lindblad AS, Novak JW, Nolph KD, Stablein DM, Cutler SJ. Highlights of the 1987 USA National CAPD Registry Report. ASAIO Trans (accepted).

Alexander S, Lindblad AS, Nolph KD, Novak JW. Pediatric CAPD/CCPD in the United States. A review of the experiences of the National CAPD Registry's pediatric population for the period January 1, 1981 through August 31, 1986. Submitted for publication.

1987

Nolph KD, Cutler SJ, Steinberg SM, Novak JW, Hirschman GH. Factors associated with morbidity and mortality among patients on CAPD. Trans Am Soc Artif Intern Organs 1987 Apr-Jun; 33(2): 57–65.

292

Report of the National CAPD Registry of the National Institutes of Health. Lindblad AS, Novak JW, Stablein DM, Cutler SJ, Nolph KD, eds. Potomac: EMMES, 1987.

Van Stone JC, Nolph KD. Dialysis. In: Gonick HC, ed. Current Nephrology. Vol. 10. Chicago: Year Book Medical Publications, Inc., 1987: 325–376.

Nolph KD. Continuous ambulatory peritoneal dialysis (CAPD) 1987: a therapy in evolution. Contemp Dial & Nephrol 1987 Sept; 8(9): 26–29.

1986

Cutler SJ, Steinberg SM, Nolph KD, Novak JW. Overview of three year experience of the National CAPD Registry of the National Institutes of Health. In: Maher JF, Winchester JF, eds. Frontiers in Peritoneal Dialysis. New York: Field and Rich, 1986: 291–292.

Nolph KD, Cutler SJ, Steinberg SM, Novak JW. Special studies from the NIH USA CAPD Registry. Peritoneal Dial Bull 1986 Jan-Mar; 6(1): 28–35.

Nolph KD. Peritoneal dialysis. In: Brenner BM, Rector FC, Jrs, eds. The Kidney. Philadelphia: W.B. Saunders Company, 1986: 1847–1906.

Nolph KD. Peritoneal dialysis. In: Gonick HC, ed. Current Nephrology. Vol. 9. Chicago: Year Book Medical Publishers, Inc., 1986: 1–65.

Steinberg SM, Cutler SJ, Novak JW, Nolph KD. Report of NIH National CAPD Registry. January, 1986.

1985

Steinberg SM, Cutler SJ, Novak JW, Nolph KD. The USA CAPD Registry. In: Nolph KD, ed. Peritoneal Dialysis. Second Edition. Boston: Martinus Nijhoff, 1985: 597–636.

Nolph KD, Cutler SJ, Steinberg SM, Novak JW. Continuous ambulatory peritoneal dialysis in the United States: a three year study. Kidney Int 1985 Aug; 28(2): 198–205.

Nolph KD, Steinberg SM, Cutler SJ, Novak JW. Diabetic nephropathy and the CAPD Registry. Diabetic Nephropathy 1985 Nov; 4(4): 161–162.

Steinberg SM, Cutler SJ, Novak JW, Nolph KD. Prognostic factors associated with the first episode of peritonitis in patients treated with continuous ambulatory peritoneal dialysis (CAPD). ASAIO J 1985; 4: 238–243.

Steinberg SM, Cutler SJ, Novak JW, Nolph KD. Prognostic factors associated with peritonitis among patients on continuous ambulatory peritoneal dialysis (CAPD). Trans Am Soc Artif Intern Organs 1985; 31: 565–567.

Nolph KD, Cutler SJ, Steinberg SM, Novak JW. Findings from the NIH National CAPD Registry, January 1985. Trans Am Soc Artif Intern Organs 1985; 31: 333–337.

Nolph KD. Peritoneal dialysis. In: Bayless TM, Brain MC, Cherniack RM, eds. Current Therapy in Internal Medicine. Toronto: BC Decker, Inc., 1984–1985: 1185–1191.

Steinberg SM, Cutler SJ, Novak JW, Nolph KD. Report of the National CAPD Registry. January, 1985.

Nolph KD. Peritoneal dialysis. In: Gonick HC, ed. Current Nephrology. Vol. 8. New York: John Wiley & Sons, Inc., 1985: 469–514.

1984

Steinberg SM, Cutler SJ, Nolph KD, Novak JW. A comprehensive report on the experience of patients on continuous ambulatory peritoneal dialysis for the treatment of end stage renal disease. Am J Kid Diseases 1984; 4(3): 233–241.

Nolph KD. Peritoneal dialysis. In: Gonick HC, ed. Current Nephrology. Vol. 7. New York: John Wiley & Sons, Inc., 1984: 1–56.

Steinberg SM, Cutler SJ, Novak JW, Nolph KD. Report of the National CAPD Registry. January, 1984.

Nolph KD, Popovich RP. A comparison of ambulatory peritoneal dialysis (CAPD) and continuous cyclic peritoneal dialysis (CCPD). In: Controversies in Nephrology. Washington, DC: Georgetown University, 1984; 4: 217–224.

Nolph KD. Peritoneal dialysis. In: Glassock RJ, ed. Current Therapy in Nephrology and Hypertension 1984–1985. Toronto: BC Decker, Inc., The C.V. Mosby Company, 1984: 269–274.

Khanna R, Nolph KD. Advances in peritoneal dialysis. Dial & Transplant 1984 Aug; 13(8): 526–531.

Nolph KD. Summary of a Working Party on Advanced Peritoneal Studies in Kings Fund Center, London, May 24–25, 1984. Peritoneal Dial Bull 1984 Jul-Sept; 4(3): 170–173.

Khanna R, Nolph KD, Prowant BF, Twardowski ZJ. Choosing a dialysis therapy: Introduction to mini-symposium. Am J Kid Diseases 1984; 4(3): 217.

Steinberg SM, Cutler SJ, Novak JW, Nolph KD. Report of the National CAPD Registry. July, 1984.

Nolph KD, Pyle WK, Hyatt M. Present status of continuous ambulatory peritoneal dialysis in the United States. In: Maekawa M, Nolph KD, Kishimoto T, Moncrief JW, eds. Machine-Free Dialysis for Patient Convenience. Cleveland: ISAO Press, 1984: 17–19.

Nolph KD. Present problems and future prospects of continuous ambulatory peritoneal dialysis. In: Maekawa M, Nolph KD, Kishimoto T, Moncrief JW, eds. Machine-Free Dialysis for Patient Convenience. Cleveland: ISAO Press, 1984: 145–146.

Twardowski ZJ, Nolph KD. USA CAPD Registry with special emphasis on diabetes mellitus. Continuous Ambulatory Peritoneal Dialysis, Proceedings of the Fourth Benelux Symposium, Rotterdam, The Netherlands, 1984: 41–57.

1983

Nolph KD, Boen ST, Farrell P, Pyle K. Continuous ambulatory peritoneal dialysis in Australia, Europe, and the U.S. 1981. Kidney Int 1983 Jan; 23(1): 3–9

Nolph KD, Van Stone JC. Peritoneal dialysis. In: Gonick HC, ed. Current Nephrology. New York: John Wiley & Sons, 1983; 6: 75–113.

Nolph KD. Dialysis and transplantation in the U.S. and the impact of continuous ambulatory peritoneal dialysis (CAPD). In: Parsons FM, Ogg CS, eds. Renal Failure Who Cares? Lancaster, England: MTP Press Limited, 1983: 75–88.

Nolph KD. CAPD Results An International Compilation. In: Edited Proceedings of Canada's First International Symposium on Peritoneal Dialysis, May 1982. Peritoneal Dialysis The State of the Art. New Jersey: Communications Media for Education, Inc., 1983: 27.

Nolph KD. The adequacy of dialysis in patients on CAPD. Peritoneal Dial Bull 1983 Jan-Mar; 3(1): 3–4.

Nolph KD. Foreword for Supplement of the Peritoneal Dialysis Bulletin, Endocrine and Metabolic Implications of CAPD 1983; 3: S1.

Nolph KD, Pyle WK. NIH CAPD Patient Registry Report: Population demographics and outcomes for the period 1/1/82–12/31/82. April, 1983.

Nolph KD, Sorkin MI. Peritoneal dialysis limitations and continuous ambulatory peritoneal dialysis. In: Marti M, Locatelli A, eds. Dialysis Peritoneal Cronica. Buenos Aires, 1983: 29–41.

Gloor HJ, Nolph KD. Care of the patient on acute and chronic peritoneal dialysis. In: Martinez-Maldonado M, ed. Handbook of Renal Therapeutics. New York: Plenum Publishing Corporation, 1983:487.

Nolph KD, Pyle WK, Hiatt M. Mortality and morbidity in continuous ambulatory peritoneal dialysis: Full and selected registry populations. ASAIO J 1983 Oct-Dec; 6(4):220–226.

Nolph KD. Results of the USA CAPD Registry. Abstracts of the 4th ISAO Official Satellite Symposium on CAPD. November, 1983.

1982

Nolph KD. United States National Registry of continuous ambulatory peritoneal dialysis (CAPD). Nefrologia 1982; 2:9–11.

Nolph KD. Second Annual National Conference on Pediatric and Adult CAPD; Kansas City, Missouri, February 15–17. Peritoneal Dial Bull 1982 Apr-Jun; 2(2):87–89.

Prowant B, Nolph KD. Five year's experience with peritonitis in a CAPD program. Peritoneal Dial Bull 1982 Oct-Dec; 2(4):169–171.

Nolph KD. What are the contraindications of CAPD, if any? Peritoneal Dial Bull 1982 Oct-Dec; 2(4):182–183.

Nolph KD, Pyle WK. NIH CAPD Patient Registry Report: Registered population demographics for the period 1/1/81–12/31/81. January, 1982.

Nolph KD, Pyle WK. NIH CAPD Patient Registry Report: The Registry pilot project for the period 1/1/81–12/31/81. April, 1982.

Nolph KD, Pyle WK. NIH CAPD Patient Registry Report: Population demographics and outcomes for the period 1/1/81–3/31/82. July, 1982.

1981

Nolph KD. Overview of chronic dialysis in the United States. In: End-Stage Renal Disease: Pathophysiology, Dialysis, and Transplantation. Monograph Series, U.S. Department of Health and Human Services, May 1981.

Nolph KD. The National Registry Pilot Study Group: The National Registry of CAPD patients. Dial & Transplant 1981 Sept; 10(9):744–750.

Nolph KD. Continuous ambulatory peritoneal dialysis (CAPD). Am J Neph 1981 Apr; 1:1–10.

Abstracts and presentations

1988

Nolph KD. Keynote Address: State of the Art, Peritoneal Dialysis 1988. Presented at the Seminar for Nephrologists, Laguna-Niguel, California, June 1988.

Nolph KD. The USA NIH CAPD Registry. Presented at the 3rd International Course on Peritoneal Dialysis, Vicenza, Italy, May 1988.

Nolph KD. Update of CAPD in the USA. Presented at the Symposium of the Scottish Renal Association on CAPD in the United Kingdom after the first ten years, Western General Hospital, Edinburgh, Scotland, May 1988.

Nolph KD. The NIH Registry and CAPD. Presented at the scientific session on issues in new solutions for peritoneal dialysis, Symposium: Ten Years of CAPD in Germany, University of Dusseldorf and University of Freiburg, Grainu, Germany, May, 1988.

Nolph KD. CAPD, CCPD Overview: NIH National Registry. Presented at the 8th National CAPD Conference, Kansas City, Missouri, February 1988.

Nolph KD. Special Diabetes Study from the NIH Registry. Presented at the 8th National CAPD Conference, Kansas City, Missouri, February 1988.

Nolph KD. Special Catheter Study from the NIH CAPD Registry. Presented at the 8th National CAPD Conference, Kansas City, Missouri, February 1988.

Nolph KD. Comprehensive Update in Nephrology and Hypertension. Presented at the Regional National Kidney Foundation Meeting, Fort Lauderdale, Florida, March 1988.

Nolph KD. Analysis of the CAPD Registry. Presented at the Comprehensive Update in Nephrology and Hypertension Regional National Kidney Foundation Meeting, Fort Lauderdale, Florida, March 1988.

Nolph KD. Advances in Techniques of Peritoneal Dialysis. Presented at the Update in Nephrology and Hypertension Regional National Kidney Foundation Meeting, Fort Lauderdale, Florida, March 1988.

Nolph KD. Treatment of Peritonitis. Presented at the Update in Nephrology and Hypertension -Regional National Kidney Foundation Meeting, Fort Lauderdale, Florida, March 1988.

Nolph KD. New findings from the NIH USA CAPD Registry. Presented at the American Society for Artificial Internal Organs, National Meeting, Reno, Nevada, May 1988.

Nolph KD. Renal replacement therapy: the role of and advances in peritoneal dialysis. Presented at the University of Missouri-Rolla, Rolla, Missouri, April 1988.

1987

Nolph K, Lindblad A, Novak J, Cutler S. USA CAPD Registry-1987 Report. Abstracts of the Fourth International Symposium on Peritoneal Dialysis. Peritoneal Dial Bull 1987; 7(Supplement):S57.

Nolph KD. Recent findings from the NIH CAPD Registry. Presented at the Travenol CAPD Consultant Meeting, Naples, Florida, January 1987.

Nolph KD. Advances in peritoneal dialysis and recent data from the USA CAPD Registry. Presented at the University of Colorado, School of Medicine, Denver, Colorado, February 1987.

Nolph KD. Recent data from the USA CAPD Registry. Presented at the Fitzsimmons Army Medical Center, Denver, Colorado, February 1987.

Nolph KD. CAPD/CCPD Overview, NIH National Registry. Presented at the 7th National Conference on CAPD, Kansas City, Missouri, February 1987.

Nolph KD. Dropout information from the NIH USA CAPD Registry. Presented at the 7th National Conference on CAPD, Kansas City, Missouri, February 1987.

Nolph KD. An update on the CAPD Registry. Presented at St. Luke's Hospital, Bethlehem, Pennsylvania, April 1987.

Nolph KD. Highlights of the upcoming CAPD Registry Report. Presented at the Allentown Hospital, Allentown, Pennsylvania, April 1987.

Nolph KD. The development and growth of CAPD. Presented at the Seminar on patient development and biotechnology transfer programs, St. Louis, Missouri, June 1987.

Nolph KD. An overview of CAPD from the NIH CAPD Registry. Presented at the Swiss CAPD meeting, Bern, Switzerland, June 1987.

Nolph KD, Lindblad A, Novak J, Cutler S. USA CAPD registry 1987 report. Presented at the Fourth Congress of the International Society for Peritoneal Dialysis, Venice, Italy, July 1987.

Nolph KD. NIH Registry. Presented at the Fourth Congress of the Inter-national Society for Peritoneal Dialysis, Venice, Italy, July 1987.

Nolph KD. State of the Art in Peritoneal Dialysis 1987. Presented at the Symposium for Nephrologists; Perspectives on Peritoneal Dialysis, Laguna- Niguel, California, October 1987.

Nolph KD. Peritoneal Dialysis. Presented at the Nephrology Update, ANNA and the University of Alabama, Birmingham, Alabama, November 1987.

Nolph KD. A survey of the NIH CAPD Registry population with end-stage renal disease attributed to diabetic nephropathy. Presented at the NIH CAPD Registry Executive Advisory Committee Meeting, Washington D.C., November 1987.

Nolph KD. A survey of the NIH CAPD Registry population with end-stage renal disease attributed to diabetic nephropathy. Presented at the seminar on the diabetic renal-retinal syndrome, State University of New York, New York City, November 1987.

Nolph KD. Data from the USA NIH CAPD Registry. Presented at the Michigan Kidney Foundation, Ann Arbor, Michigan, December 1987.

1986

Nolph KD. NIH Registry Results. Presented at the Meeting of Travenol North American Consulting Nephrologists, Phoenix, Arizona, January 1986.

Nolph KD. CAPD, CCPD overview from the NIH National Registry. Presented at the Sixth National Conference on CAPD, Kansas City, Missouri, February 1986.

Nolph KD. Peritonitis risk factors in the CAPD Registry. Presented at the Sixth National Conference on CAPD, Kansas City, Missouri, February 1986.

Nolph KD. Is CAPD a preferred therapy? Presented at the Dialysis and Transplantation Workshop of the Australasian Society of Nephrology, Perth, Australia, February 1986.

Nolph KD. CAPD, State of the Art. Presented at the 22nd Annual Meeting of the Australasian Society of Nephrology, Perth, Australia, February 1986.

Nolph KD. Anatomical, physiological, and practical aspects of peritoneal dialysis. Presented at the University of Wisconsin Medical School, Madison, Wisconsin, April 1986.

Nolph KD. Data from the USA NIH CAPD Registry. Presented at the UCLA Harbor Medical Center, Los Angeles California, May 1986.

Nolph KD. Lessons from the CAPD Registry. Presented at the American Society for Artificial Internal Organs, Los Angeles, California, May 1986.

Nolph KD. Experiences with peritoneal dialysis problem patients. Presented at the Peritoneal Dialysis Seminar on Advances in Therapy, Philadelphia, Pennsylvania, June 1986.

Nolph KD. Significant trends in the Peritoneal Dialysis Registry. Presented at the Symposium on Recent Advances in Dialysis, The National Kidney Foundation of Florida and the Watson Clinic Foundation of Lakeland, Florida, Daytona Beach, Florida, August 1986.

Nolph KD. CAPD Case Studies. Presented at the Peritoneal Dialysis Seminar 'Advances in Therapy', Atlanta, Georgia, August 1986.

Nolph KD. Clinical Case Studies of CAPD Problem Patients. Presented at the Peritoneal Dialysis Seminar 'Advances in Therapy', Chicago, Illinois, September 1986.

Nolph KD. Recent advances in peritoneal dialysis. Presented at the Eleventh renal symposium of the Kidney Foundation of Ohio, Cleveland, Ohio, September 1986.

Nolph KD. CAPD Registry Report. Presented at the Symposium on Clinical Concerns in Nephrology, 1986, American Nephrology Nurses Association, Chicago, Illinois, October 1986.

1985

Piraino B, Bernardini J, Steinberg SM, Sorkin M. The relationship of exit site infection to peritonitis in CAPD patients. Abstr Am Soc Artif Intern Organs 1985; 14:50.

Steinberg SM, Cutler SJ, Novak JW, Nolph KD. Risk factors for development of peritonitis in patients treated for ESRD by means of CAPD findings in 5,984 patients. Abstr Am Soc Artif Intern Organs 1985; 14:41.

Steinberg SM, Cutler SJ, Novak JW, Nolph KD. Findings from the NIH National CAPD Registry: January 1985. Abstr Am Soc Artif Intern Organs 1985; 14:41.

Nolph KD. Update on NIH/CAPD Registry results. Presented at the Travenol Laboratories Consultants Meeting, Key Biscayne, Florida, January 1985.

Nolph KD. Results with long-term patients in the NIH-CAPD Registry. Presented at the Travenol Laboratories Consultants Meeting, Key Biscayne, Florida, January 1985.

Nolph KD. The Impact of the Multi-Center Ultraviolet Study, the CAPD National Registry analysis of Risk Factors and the International Ultra-filtration Survey on the Designs of Future Clinical Trials in CAPD Patients. Presented at the Meeting of Canadian Nephrologist Consultants to Travenol, Acapulco, Mexico, January 1985.

Nolph KD. Major problems with CAPD in the USA. Presented at the 5th National CAPD Conference, Kansas City, Missouri, February 1985.

Nolph KD. Sclerosing peritonitis. Presented at the Symposium for Texans Active in Renal Therapy, Austin, Texas, March 1985.

Nolph KD. Continuous ambulatory peritoneal dialysis. State of the art. Presented at Medical Grand Rounds, Brooke Army Medical Center, Fort Sam Houston, San Antonio, Texas, March 1985.

Nolph KD. Peritoneal dialysis 1985. Presented at Medical Grand Rounds, Middlesex General-Rutgers University Hospital, New Brunswick, New Jersey. April 1985.

Nolph KD. Highlights of the 5th National CAPD Conference. Presented at the Quarterly Meeting CAPD Nurses of Connecticut, Hartford, Connecticut. April 1985.

Nolph KD, Steinburg S, Cutler S, Novak J. Findings from the NIH National CAPD Registry: January 1985. Presented at the National Meeting of the American Society for Artificial Internal Organs. Atlanta, Georgia. May 1985.

Nolph K, Steinberg S, Cutler S, Novak J. Risk factors for development of peritonitis in patients treated for ESRD by means of CAPD. Findings in 5,984 patients. Presented at the National Meeting of the American Society for Artificial Internal Organs, Atlanta, Georgia, May 1985.

Nolph KD. Symposium on Advances in CAPD. Presented at the Cedars-Sinai Medical Center, Los Angeles, California, June 1985.

Nolph KD. The Future of CAPD. Presented at the Symposium on 'Today's Therapy in Nephrology', Nephrology Society of New Jersey and the American Kidney Fund, Atlantic City, New Jersey, June 1985.

Nolph KD. An Update on CAPD. Presented at the CAPD Seminars. Tokyo, Japan; Kanazawa, Japan; Osaka, Japan; Hirosaki, Japan; Sapporo, Japan; Fukuoka, Japan, August 1985.

Nolph KD. The USA CAPD Registry. Presented at the Annual Meeting of the United Kingdom CAPD Hemodialysis Multistudy Group, London, United Kingdom, September 1985.

Nolph KD. Anatomical physiological and practical aspects of CAPD. Presented at the 3rd National Convention on Peritoneal Dialysis, S. Margherita, Ligure, Italy, September 1985.

Nolph KD. Continuous ambulatory peritoneal dialysis. Presented at Medical Grand Rounds, University of Iowa School of Medicine, Iowa City, Iowa, October 1985.

Nolph KD. Hemodialysis vs. CAPD. Presented at the International Forum on Contemporary Management of Renal Failure, Marrakech, Morocco, November 1985.

Nolph KD. The CAPD Registry. Presented at the National Meeting of the American Society of Nephrology, New Orleans, Louisiana, December 1985.

1984

Nolph K, Steinberg SM, Cutler SJ, Novak JW. USA CAPD Registry of the National Institutes of Health. Peritoneal Dial Bull 1984; 4:S46.

Nolph KD. CAPD in the USA. Presented at the CAPD Symposium, Murnau, Germany, January 1984.

Nolph KD. CAPD Update: University of Missouri, USA and European Results. Presented at the CAPD Symposium, University of Brescia, Brescia, Italy, January 1984.

Nolph KD. CAPD Update: University of Missouri, USA and European Results. Presented at the Interregional Meeting of the Tuscany-Ligure Societies of Nephrology, Santa Margherita, Ligure, February 1984.

Nolph KD. CAPD Update: University of Missouri, USA and European Results. Presented at the CAPD Symposium, University of Torino, Torino, Italy, February 1984.

Nolph KD. Morbidity and mortality with CAPD in the USA. Presented at the Fourth National CAPD Conference, Kansas City, Missouri, February 1984.

Nolph KD. Clinical experiences with peritoneal dialysis at the University of Missouri and in the USA. Presented at the Royal Victoria Hospital, McGill University, Montreal, Canada, March 1984.

Nolph KD. Adequacy of peritoneal dialysis in acute renal failure. Presented at the Symposium on nutrition and adequacy of dialysis in acute and chronic renal failure, University of Oklahoma and the Network 10 ESRD Coordinating Council, Tulsa, Oklahoma, March 1984.

Nolph KD. CAPD Today. Presented at the Symposium, F. Florida, Kidney Foundation and NAPHT, Tampa, FL., April 1984.

Nolph KD. CAPD patient demographics. Presented at the Annual Meeting of the Coordinating Counsel of the Indiana End-Stage Renal Disease Network Inc., Bloomington, Indiana, April 1984.

Nolph KD. The CAPD Registry 1983. Presented at the Kidney Disease Symposium of the National Kidney Foundation of Michigan, Grand Rapids, Michigan, May 1984.

Nolph KD. Epidemiology of the problem of ultrafiltration loss in CAPD. Working Party on Advance Peritoneal Studies. Presented at the University Department of Medicine, Royal Infirmary, Glasgow University and Travenol Laboratories, London, England, May 1984.

Nolph KD. USA Registry of the National Institutes of Health. Poster presentation. Presented at the Third International Symposium on Peritoneal Dialysis, Washington, D.C., June 1984.

Nolph KD. Results of the USA CAPD Registry. Panel participant. Presented at the Third International Symposium on Peritoneal Dialysis, Washington, D.C., June 1984.

Nolph KD. Three year results of the USA CAPD Registry. Presented at the Latin American Nephrologists meeting, Miami, Florida, June 1984.

Nolph KD. Loss of ultrafiltration during peritoneal dialysis. Presented at the Meeting of Latin American Nephrologists, Miami, Florida, June 1984.

Nolph KD. Peritoneal dialysis concepts. Presented at the 3rd North American Symposium on Dialysis and Transplantation, Maui, Hawaii, July 1984.

Nolph KD. CAPD is a promise fulfilled. Presented at the 24th Annual Scientific Symposium on Kidney Disease, National Kidney Foundation of Southern California, Los Angeles, California, September 1984.

Nolph KD. Rehabilitation and quality of life with CAPD. Panel Presentation, Presented at the 24th Annual Scientific Symposium on Kidney Disease, National Kidney Foundation of Southern California, Los Angeles, California, September 1984.

Nolph KD. CAPD as an alternative dialysis treatment. Presented at the Third Annual National Kidney Foundation lecturer, Singapore, September 1984.

Nolph KD. The future of CAPD. Presented at the Melbourne CAPD Seminar, Melbourne, Australia, September 1984.

Nolph KD. Ambulatory peritoneal dialysis. Presented at the 27th Annual Physicians Alumni Weekend School of Medicine, University of Missouri, Columbia, Missouri, October 1984.

Nolph KD. Continuous ambulatory peritoneal dialysis. Presented at the Faculty Forum (Medical School Wide Lecture), Columbia, Missouri, November 1984.

Nielsen LH, Nolph KD, Khanna R, Moore H. Sclerosing peritonitis on CAPD: The acetatelactate controversy. Presented at the 17th Annual Meeting of the American Society of Nephrology, Washington, D.C., December 1984.

Nolph KD. The National CAPD Registry Model. Presented at the Executive Committee Meeting of the North American Pediatric Dialysis Registry, Washington, D.C., December 1984.

1983

Nolph KD. CAPD Registry report long time survival. Advanced Nephrology for the Consultant. Presented at the University of California, San Diego School of Medicine, San Diego, California, January 1983.

Nolph KD. Current clinical problems in the CAPD patient. Advanced Nephrology for the Consultant. Presented at the University of California, San Diego School of Medicine, San Diego, California, January 1983.

Nolph KD. The National CAPD Registry. Presented at the Third National Conference on Continuous Ambulatory Peritoneal Dialysis, Kansas City, Missouri, February 1983.

Nolph KD. Nutrition in CAPD. Presented at the Third National Conference on Continuous Ambulatory Peritoneal Dialysis, Kansas City, Missouri, February 1983.

Nolph KD. CAPD in the United States. Presented at the CAPD meeting of French nephrologists, Paris, France, March 1983.

Nolph KD. The CAPD National Registry. Presented at the CAPD Seminar, University of Maryland, Baltimore, Maryland, April 1983.

Nolph KD. Mortality and morbidity. CAPD, hemodialysis and hemofiltration. Panel presentation. Presented at the National Meeting of the American Society for Artificial Internal Organs, Toronto, Ontario, Canada, April 1983.

Nolph KD. Current status of peritoneal dialysis. Presented at Medical Grand Rounds (Murray Memorial Lecture), University of Pennsylvania, School of Medicine, Philadelphia, Pennsylvania, May 1983.

Nolph KD. National Registry of CAPD patients an update. Presented at the CAPD Seminar for Travenol consultants, Asheville, North Carolina, June 1983.

Nolph KD. CAPD, a critical appraisal. Presented at the symposium on dialysis and transplantation, the Illinois experience, ESRD Network 5, the National Kidney Foundation of Illinois, the Illinois Transplant Society, and the University of Illinois, Chicago, Illinois, October 1983.

Nolph KD. Chronic peritoneal dialysis therapy in chronic renal failure. Presented at the American Kidney Fund Nephrology Conference, Boston University Medical Center, Brigham and Women's Hospital, Massachusetts General Hospital and The New England Medical Center, Boston, Massachusetts, October 1983.

Nolph KD. Present status of CAPD in the USA. Presented at the Fourth ASAIO Official Satellite Symposium on CAPD, Kyoto, Japan, November 1983.

Nolph KD. Lectures on peritoneal dialysis. Presented at the CAPD seminars, Ngoya, Japan; Tokyo, Japan; Osaka, Japan, November 1983.

1982

Nolph KD. Peritonitis detection and treatment. Presented at the Symposium on CAPD, St. Thomas Medical Center, Akron, Ohio, January 1982.

Nolph KD. CAPD, complications, and considerations. Presented at the Symposium on CAPD, St. Thomas Hospital Medical Center, Akron, Ohio, January 1982.

Nolph KD. CAPD or CCPD Which is better? Presented at the Symposium, 'Controversies in Nephrology 1982', Georgetown University Medical Center, Washington, D.C., January 1982.

Nolph KD. Selection of patients for CAPD and future trend. Presented at the Symposium on CAPD, Manchester Royal Infirmary, Manchester, England, January 1982.

Nolph KD. CAPD National Registry Data. Presented at the Second Annual National Conference on Pediatric and Adult Continuous Ambulatory Peritoneal Dialysis, Kansas City, Missouri, February 1982.

Nolph KD. Clinical management and complications of the CAPD patient. Presented at the Second Annual National Conference on Pediatric and Adult Continuous Ambulatory Peritoneal Dialysis, Kansas City, Missouri, February 1982.

Nolph KD. Current status of CAPD as a treatment modality for ESRD. Data from the National Registry. Presented at the Symposium on Critical Aspects of Longterm CAPD Management, Yale University School of Medicine, New Haven, Connecticut, March 1982.

Nolph KD. Report on the National Registry of CAPD in the USA. Presented at the 2nd Symposium on Peritoneal Dialysis, Toledo, Spain, March 1982.

Nolph KD. Criteria for the diagnosis of peritonitis, University of Missouri. Presented at the 2nd Symposium on Peritoneal Dialysis, Toledo, Spain, March 1982.

Nolph KD. Peritonitis in CAPD, incidence, prevention, and treatment in the USA. Presented at the 2nd Symposium on Peritoneal Dialysis, Toledo, Spain, March 1982.

Nolph KD. CAPD physiology and kinetics. Presented at the CAPD Update, University of Miami School of Medicine, Miami, Florida, April 1982.

Nolph KD. Clinical results of CAPD. Presented at the continuous ambulatory peritoneal dialysis update, University of Miami School of Medicine, Miami, Florida, April 1982.

Nolph KD. Peritonitis, diagnosis and treatment. Presented at the CAPD Update, University of Miami School of Medicine, Miami, Florida, April 1982.

Nolph KD. The North American experience in treating end-stage renal failure. Presented at the Symposium on renal failure, University of East Anglia, Norwich, England, April 1982.

Nolph KD. Presentation on status of continuous ambulatory peritoneal dialysis, to the Subcommittee on Oversight Committee on Ways and Means, U.S. House of Representatives. Presented at the Dialysis Reimbursement Hearing, Washington, D.C., April 1982.

Nolph KD. CAPD, 1982. Presented at the Nephrology Update 1982, University of Alabama School of Medicine, Birmingham, Alabama, May 1982.

Nolph KD. Peritonitis diagnosis and treatment. Presented at Canada's First International Symposium on Peritoneal Dialysis, University of British Columbia Faculty of Medicine, Vancouver, B.C., May 1982.

Nolph KD. CAPD concepts and experiences. Presented at the 21st Annual Kidney Disease Symposium, National Kidney Foundation of Michigan in conjunction with Hurley Medical Center, Flint, Michigan, May 1982.

Nolph KD. Continuous ambulatory peritoneal dialysis. Presented at the 9th Annual Kidney Symposium, Midwest Organ Bank and The National Kidney Foundation, Kansas City, Missouri, May 1982.

Nolph KD. Diagnosis and treatment of peritonitis. Presented at the Symposium on CAPD, Pugnochiuso, Italy, May 1982.

Nolph KD. Results of the USA CAPD Registry. Presented at the CAPD Symposium, Pugnochiuso, Italy, May 1982.

Nolph KD. The impact of peritonitis on CAPD outcome. Presented at the Meeting of Travenol Consultants, Hilton Head Island, South Carolina, June 1982.

Nolph KD. CAPD A National Perspective. Presented at the Symposium, University of North Carolina at Chapel Hill School of Medicine, Chapel Hill, North Carolina, June 1982.

Nolph KD. Peritoneal Dialysis, 5th Comprehensive Nephrology Review Course. Presented at the UCLA School of Medicine and the Cedar Sinai Medical Center, Los Angeles, California, September 1982.

Nolph KD. Historical perspective of CAPD. Presented at the Symposium on Peritoneal Dialysis, University of Pittsburgh, Pittsburgh, Pennsylvania, September 1982.

Nolph KD. Trends in Peritoneal Dialysis Research. Presented at the Research Presentation, University of Pittsburgh, Pittsburgh, Pennsylvania, September 1982.

Nolph KD. Peritoneal Transport and CAPD experiences (two lectures). Presented at the Symposium on CAPD, Helsinki, Finland, September 1982.

Nolph KD. Peritoneal transport physiology and clinical status of CAPD (two lectures). Presented at the Symposium on CAPD for the nephrologists of Denmark, Copenhagan, Denmark, September 1982.

Nolph KD. CAPD concepts and experiences. Presented at the CAPD Seminar for Norwegian nephrologists, Oslo, Norway, September 1982.

Nolph KD. CAPD concepts and experiences. Presented at the CAPD Seminar for Swedish nephrologists, Stockholm, Sweden, September 1982.

Nolph KD. CAPD experiences. Presented at the CAPD Seminar for nephrologists of Southern Sweden, Grenna, Sweden, September 1982.

Nolph KD. Continuous ambulatory peritoneal dialysis. Presented at the Seminar on CAPD for nephrologists of Austria, Vienna, Austria, September 1982.

Nolph KD. Current status of CAPD in the United States. Presented at the Seminar on CAPD for nephrologists of The Netherlands, University of Amsterdam Medical Center, Amsterdam, Netherlands, September 1982.

Nolph KD. Current status of CAPD in the United States. Presented at the Seminar for British Press, The Royal Society of Medicine, London, England, October 1982.

Nolph KD. The past, present, and future of peritoneal dialysis. Presented at the Meeting of the End-Stage Renal Disease Network of Virginia and West Virginia, Virginia Beach, Virginia, October 1982.

Nolph KD. National CAPD Registry. Presented at the Seminar on Perspectives in Continuous Ambulatory Peritoneal Dialysis, Medical College of Virginia, Virginia Beach, Virginia, October 1982.

1981

Nolph KD. Multi-Center Study and National Registry plans for CAPD. Presented at the National Conference on CAPD, Kansas City, Missouri, February 1981.

Nolph KD. Patient selection for CAPD. Presented at the First National Symposium on CAPD, Siena, Italy, March 1981.

Nolph KD. Infection and nutrition in CAPD. Presented in Toulose, France, March 1981.

Nolph KD. CAPD: State of the art. Presented at the Department of Medicine Grand Rounds, Duke University Medical Center, Durham, North Carolina, March 1981.

Nolph KD. Advances in CAPD. Presented at Grand Rounds at Good Samaritan Hospital, Phoenix, Arizona, April 1981.

Nolph KD. Four lectures. Presented at the Seminar on CAPD, Loma Linda University, Newport Beach, California, May 1981.

Nolph KD. New developments in CAPD. Presented at the CAPD Symposium, Munich, Germany, June 1981.

Nolph KD. Panel presentation Preliminary results of the National CAPD Registry. Presented at the 2nd International Symposium on Peritoneal Dialysis, Berlin, West Germany, June 1981.

Nolph KD. Advances in peritoneal dialysis. Presented at the University of Amsterdam, School of Medicine, Amsterdam, The Netherlands, June 1981.

Nolph KD. Understanding peritoneal dialysis and CAPD. Presented at the CAPD Symposium, Zurich, Switzerland, June 1981.

Nolph KD. The National CAPD Registry. Presented at the CAPD Consultants Meeting, Travenol Corporate Headquarters, Deerfield, Illinois, July 1981.

Nolph KD. CAPD National Institutes of Health Studies. Presented at the Symposium on Infection Control in Continuous Ambulatory Peritoneal Dialysis, Atlanta, Georgia, August 1981.

Nolph KD. Experiences with CAPD. Presented at the Symposium on CAPD, University of Indiana School of Medicine, Indianapolis, Indiana, September 1981.

Nolph KD. Peritoneal Dialysis State of the Art. Presented at the 12th Annual Meeting of the Western Dialysis and Transplant Society, Honolulu, Hawaii, October 1981.

Nolph KD. Rehabilitation in continuous ambulatory peritoneal dialysis. Presented at the Social Worker's Meeting at the 12th Annual Meeting of the Western Dialysis and Transplant Society, Honolulu, Hawaii, October 1981.

Nolph KD. Experiences with peritonitis in CAPD: The state of the art. Presented at the Symposium on Peritonitis and CAPD, University of Pennsylvania, Philadelphia, Pennsylvania, October 1981.

Nolph KD. Advances in peritoneal dialysis. Presented at the Advances in Dialytic Therapy Seminar, American Association of Nephrology Nurses and Technicians, New York City, New York, November 1981.

Nolph KD. Chairman's Address, Advances in Peritoneal Dialysis. Presented at the National Meeting of the American Society of Nephrology, Washington, D.C., November 1981.

Developments in Nephrology

1. Cheigh, J.S., Stenzel, K.H. and Rubin, A.L. (eds.): Manual of Clinical Nephrology of the Rogosin Kidney Center. 1981   ISBN 90-247-2397-3
2. Nolph, K.D. (ed.): Peritoneal Dialysis. 1981 ed.: out of print
   3rd revised and enlarged ed. 1988 (not in this series) ISBN 0-89838-406-0
3. Gruskin, A.B. and Norman, M.E. (eds.): Pediatric Nephrology. 1981
   ISBN 90-247-2514-3
4. Schück, O.: Examination of the Kidney Function. 1981
   ISBN 0-89838-565-2
5. Strauss, J. (ed.): Hypertension, Fluid-electrolytes and Tubulopathies in Pediatric Nephrology. 1982   ISBN 90-247-2633-6
6. Strauss, J. (ed.): Neonatal Kidney and Fluid-electrolytes. 1983
   ISBN 0-89838-575-X
7. Strauss, J. (ed.): Acute Renal Disorders and Renal Emergencies. 1984
   ISBN 0-89838-663-2
8. Didio, L.J.A. and Motta, P.M. (eds.): Basic, Clinical, and Surgical Nephrology. 1985   ISBN 0-89838-698-5
9. Friedman, E.A. and Peterson, C.M. (eds.): Diabetic Nephropathy: Strategy for Therapy. 1985   ISBN 0-89838-735-3
10. Dzúrik, R., Lichardus, B. and Guder, W. (eds.): Kidney Metabolism and Function. 1985   ISBN 0-89838-749-3
11. Strauss, J. (ed.): Homeostasis, Nephrotoxicity, and Renal Anomalies in the Newborn. 1986   ISBN 0-89838-766-3
12. Oreopoulos, D.G. (ed.): Geriatric Nephrology. 1986
   ISBN 0-89838-781-7
13. Paganini, E.P. (ed.): Acute Continuous Renal Replacement Therapy. 1986   ISBN 0-89838-793-0
14. Cheigh, J.S., Stenzel, K.H. and Rubin, A.L. (eds.): Hypertension in Kidney Disease. 1986   ISBN 0-89838-797-3
15. Deane, N., Wineman, R.J. and Benis, G.A. (eds.): Guide to Reprocessing of Hemodialyzers. 1986   ISBN 0-89838-798-1
16. Ponticelli, C., Minetti, L. and D'Amico, G. (eds.): Antiglobulins, Cryoglobulins and Glomerulonephritis. 1986   ISBN 0-89838-810-4
17. Strauss, J. (ed.), with the assistance of L. Strauss: Persistent Renalgenitourinary Disorders. 1987   ISBN 0-89838-845-7
18. Andreucci, V.E. and Dal Canton, A. (eds.): Diuretics: Basic, Pharmacological, and Clinical Aspects. 1987   ISBN 0-89838-885-6
19. Bach, P.H. and Lock, E.H. (eds.): Nephrotoxicity in the Experimental and Clinical Situation, Part 1. 1987   ISBN 0-89838-977-1

20. Bach, P.H. and Lock, E.H. (eds.): Nephrotoxicity in the Experimental and Clinical Situation, Part 2. 1987   ISBN 0-89838-980-2
21. Gore, S.M. and Bradley, B.A. (eds.): Renal Transplantation: Sense and Sensitization. 1988   ISBN 0-89838-370-6
22. Minetti, L., D'Amico, G. and Ponticelli, C. (eds.): The Kidney in Plasma Cell Dyscrasias. 1988   ISBN 0-89838-385-4
23. Lindblad, A.S., Novak, J.W. and Nolph, K.D. (eds.): Continuous Ambulatory Peritoneal Dialysis in the USA. 1989   ISBN 0-7923-0179-X
24. Andreucci, V.E. and Dal Canton, A. (eds.): Current Therapy in Nephrology. 1989   ISBN 0-7923-0206-0
25. Kovács, L. and Lichardus, B.: Vasopressin – Disturbed secretion and its effects. 1989   ISBN 0-7923-0249-4
26. De Broe, M.E. and Coburn, J.W. (eds.): Aluminium and Renal Failure. 1989   ISBN 0-7923-0347-4
27. Gardner, Jr., K.D. and Willebrand, J. (eds.): Oceanic Circulation Models: Combining Data and Dynamics. 1989   ISBN 0-7923-0392-X

Kluwer Academic Publishers
DORDRECHT / BOSTON / LONDON